CAPOZIDE® 25/15
CAPOZIDE® 25/25
CAPOZIDE® 50/15
CAPOZIDE® 50/25
Captopril-Hydrochlorothiazide Tablets

DESCRIPTION
CAPOZIDE (Captopril-Hydrochlorothiazide Tablets) for oral administration combines two antihypertensive agents: CAPOTEN® (captopril) and hydrochlorothiazide. Captopril, the first of a new class of antihypertensive agents, is a specific competitive inhibitor of angiotensin I-converting enzyme (ACE), the enzyme responsible for the conversion of angiotensin I to angiotensin II. Hydrochlorothiazide is a benzothiadiazide (thiazide) diuretic-antihypertensive. CAPOZIDE tablets are available in four combinations of captopril with hydrochlorothiazide: 25 mg with 15 mg, 25 mg with 25 mg, 50 mg with 15 mg, and 50 mg with 25 mg. Inactive ingredients: cellulose, colorant (FD&C Yellow No. 6), lactose, magnesium stearate, pregelatinized starch, and stearic acid.

Captopril is designated chemically as 1-[(2S)-3-mercapto-2-methylpropionyl]-L-proline; hydrochlorothiazide is 6-Chloro-3,4-dihydro-2H-1,2,4-benzothiadiazine-7-sulfonamide 1,1-dioxide.

Captopril is a white to off-white crystalline powder that may have a slight sulfurous odor; it is soluble in water (approx. 160 mg/mL), methanol, and ethanol and sparingly soluble in chloroform and ethyl acetate.

Hydrochlorothiazide is a white crystalline powder slightly soluble in water but freely soluble in sodium hydroxide solution.

CLINICAL PHARMACOLOGY
Captopril
Mechanism of Action
The mechanism of action of captopril has not yet been fully elucidated. Its beneficial effects in hypertension and heart failure appear to result primarily from suppression of the renin-angiotensin-aldosterone system. However, there is no consistent correlation between renin levels and response to the drug. Renin, an enzyme synthesized by the kidneys, is released into the circulation where it acts on a plasma globulin substrate to produce angiotensin I, a relatively inactive decapeptide. Angiotensin I is then converted by angiotensin converting enzyme (ACE) to angiotensin II, a potent endogenous vasoconstrictor substance. Angiotensin II also stimulates aldosterone secretion from the adrenal cortex, thereby contributing to sodium and fluid retention.

Captopril prevents the conversion of angiotensin I to angiotensin II by inhibition of ACE, a peptidyldipeptide carboxy hydrolase. This inhibition has been demonstrated in both healthy human subjects and in animals by showing that the elevation of blood pressure caused by exogenously administered angiotensin I was attenuated or abolished by captopril. In animal studies, captopril did not alter the pressor responses to a number of other agents, including angiotensin II and norepinephrine, indicating specificity of action.

ACE is identical to "bradykininase," and captopril may also interfere with the degradation of the vasodepressor peptide, bradykinin. Increased concentrations of bradykinin or prostaglandin E_2 may also have a role in the therapeutic effect of captopril.

Inhibition of ACE results in decreased plasma angiotensin II and increased plasma renin activity (PRA), the latter resulting from loss of negative feedback on renin release caused by reduction in angiotensin II. The reduction of angiotensin II leads to decreased aldosterone secretion, and, as a result, small increases in serum potassium may occur along with sodium and fluid loss.

The antihypertensive effects persist for a longer period of time than does demonstrable inhibition of circulating ACE. It is not known whether the ACE present in vascular endothelium is inhibited longer than the ACE in circulating blood.

Pharmacokinetics
After oral administration of therapeutic doses of captopril, rapid absorption occurs with peak blood levels at about one hour. The presence of food in the gastrointestinal tract reduces absorption by about 30 to 40 percent; captopril therefore should be given one hour before meals. Based on carbon-14 labeling, average minimal absorption is approximately 75 percent. In a 24-hour period, over 95 percent of the absorbed dose is eliminated in the urine; 40 to 50 percent is unchanged drug; most of the remainder is the disulfide dimer of captopril and captopril-cysteine disulfide.

Approximately 25 to 30 percent of the circulating drug is bound to plasma proteins. The apparent elimination half-life for total radioactivity in blood is probably less than three hours. An accurate determination of half-life of unchanged captopril is not, at present, possible, but it is probably less than two hours. In patients with renal impairment, however, retention of captopril occurs (see DOSAGE AND ADMINISTRATION).

Pharmacodynamics
Administration of captopril results in a reduction of peripheral arterial resistance in hypertensive patients with either no change, or an increase, in cardiac output. There is an increase in renal blood flow following administration of captopril and glomerular filtration rate is usually unchanged. In patients with heart failure, significantly decreased peripheral (systemic vascular) resistance and blood pressure (afterload), reduced pulmonary capillary wedge pressure (preload) and pulmonary vascular resistance, increased cardiac output, and increased exercise tolerance time (ETT) have been demonstrated.

Reductions of blood pressure are usually maximal 60 to 90 minutes after oral administration of an individual dose of captopril. The duration of effect is dose related. The reduction in blood pressure may be progressive, so to achieve maximal therapeutic effects, several weeks of therapy may be required. The blood pressure lowering effects of captopril and thiazide-type diuretics are additive. In contrast, captopril and beta-blockers have a less than additive effect.

Blood pressure is lowered to about the same extent in both standing and supine positions. Orthostatic effects and tachycardia are infrequent but may occur in volume-depleted patients. Abrupt withdrawal of captopril has not been associated with a rapid increase in blood pressure.

Studies in rats and cats indicate that captopril does not cross the blood-brain barrier to any significant extent.

Hydrochlorothiazide
Thiazides affect the renal tubular mechanism of electrolyte reabsorption. At maximal therapeutic dosage all thiazides are approximately equal in their diuretic potency.

Thiazides increase excretion of sodium and chloride in approximately equivalent amounts. Natriuresis causes a secondary loss of potassium and bicarbonate.

The mechanism of the antihypertensive effect of thiazides is unknown. Thiazides do not affect normal blood pressure.

The mean plasma half-life of hydrochlorothiazide in fasted individuals has been reported to be approximately 2.5 hours.

Onset of diuresis occurs in two hours and the peak effect at about four hours. Its action persists for approximately six to twelve hours. Hydrochlorothiazide is eliminated rapidly by the kidney.

INDICATIONS AND USAGE
CAPOZIDE (Captopril-Hydrochlorothiazide Tablets) is indicated for the treatment of hypertension. The blood pressure lowering effects of captopril and thiazides are approximately additive.

This fixed combination drug is not indicated for initial therapy of hypertension. If the fixed combination represents the dose titrated to the individual patient's needs, it may be more convenient than the separate components.

In using CAPOZIDE, consideration should be given to the risk of neutropenia/agranulocytosis (see WARNINGS).

CAPOZIDE may be used for patients with normal renal function, in whom the risk is relatively low. In patients with impaired renal function, particularly those with collagen vascular disease, CAPOZIDE should be reserved for hypertensives who have either developed unacceptable side effects on other drugs, or have failed to respond satisfactorily to other drug combinations.

CONTRAINDICATIONS
Hydrochlorothiazide
Hydrochlorothiazide is contraindicated in anuria. It is also contraindicated in patients who have previously demonstrated hypersensitivity to hydrochlorothiazide or other sulfonamide-derived drugs.

WARNINGS
Captopril
Neutropenia/Agranulocytosis
Neutropenia ($<1000/mm^3$) with myeloid hypoplasia has resulted from use of captopril. About half of the neutropenic patients developed systemic or oral cavity infections or other features of the syndrome of agranulocytosis.

The risk of neutropenia is dependent on the clinical status of the patient:

In clinical trials in patients with hypertension who have normal renal function (serum creatinine less than 1.6 mg/dL and no collagen vascular disease), neutropenia has been seen in one patient out of over 8,600 exposed.

In patients with some degree of renal failure (serum creatinine at least 1.6 mg/dL) but no collagen vascular disease, the risk of neutropenia in clinical trials was about 1 per 500, a frequency over 15 times that for uncomplicated hypertension. Daily doses of captopril were relatively high in these patients, particularly in view of their diminished renal function. In foreign marketing experience in patients with renal failure, use of allopurinol concomitantly with captopril has been associated with neutropenia but this association has not appeared in U.S. reports.

In patients with collagen vascular diseases (e.g., systemic lupus erythematosus, scleroderma) and impaired renal function, neutropenia occurred in 3.7 percent of patients in clinical trials.

While none of the over 750 patients in formal clinical trials of heart failure developed neutropenia, it has occurred during the subsequent clinical experience. About half of the reported cases had serum creatinine ≥1.6 mg/dL and more than 75 percent were in patients also receiving procainamide. In heart failure, it appears that the same risk factors for neutropenia are present.

The neutropenia has usually been detected within three months after captopril was started. Bone marrow examinations in patients with neutropenia consistently showed myeloid hypoplasia, frequently accompanied by erythroid hypoplasia and decreased numbers of megakaryocytes (e.g., hypoplastic bone marrow and pancytopenia); anemia and thrombocytopenia were sometimes seen.

In general, neutrophils returned to normal in about two weeks after captopril was discontinued, and serious infections were limited to clinically complex patients. About 13 percent of the cases of neutropenia have ended fatally, but almost all fatalities were in patients with serious illness, having collagen vascular disease, renal failure, heart failure or immunosuppressant therapy, or a combination of these complicating factors.

Evaluation of the hypertensive or heart failure patient should always include assessment of renal function.

If captopril is used in patients with impaired renal function, white blood cell and differential counts should be evaluated prior to starting treatment and at approximately two-week intervals for about three months, then periodically.

In patients with collagen vascular disease or who are exposed to other drugs known to affect the white cells or immune response, particularly when there is impaired renal function, captopril should be used only after an assessment of benefit and risk, and then with caution.

All patients treated with captopril should be told to report any signs of infection (e.g., sore throat, fever). If infection is suspected, white cell counts should be performed without delay.

Since discontinuation of captopril and other drugs has generally led to prompt return of the white count to normal, upon confirmation of neutropenia (neutrophil count $<1000/mm^3$) the physician should withdraw captopril and closely follow the patient's course.

Proteinuria—Total urinary proteins greater than 1 g per day were seen in about 0.7 percent of patients receiving captopril. About 90 percent of affected patients had evidence of prior renal disease or received relatively high doses of captopril (in excess of 150 mg/day), or both. The nephrotic syndrome occurred in about one-fifth of proteinuric patients. In most cases, proteinuria subsided or cleared within six months whether or not captopril was continued. Parameters of renal function, such as BUN and creatinine, were seldom altered in the patients with proteinuria.

Since most cases of proteinuria occurred by the eighth month of therapy with captopril, patients with prior renal disease or those receiving captopril at doses greater than 150 mg per day, should have urinary protein estimations (dip-stick on first morning urine) prior to treatment, and periodically thereafter.

Hypotension—Excessive hypotension was rarely seen in hypertensive patients but is a possible consequence of captopril use in severely salt/volume depleted persons such as those treated vigorously with diuretics, for example, patients with severe congestive heart failure (see PRECAUTIONS [Drug Interactions]).

Hydrochlorothiazide

Thiazides should be used with caution in severe renal disease. In patients with renal disease, thiazides may precipitate azotemia. Cumulative effects of the drug may develop in patients with impaired renal function.

Thiazides should be used with caution in patients with impaired hepatic function or progressive liver disease, since minor alterations of fluid and electrolyte balance may precipitate hepatic coma.

Sensitivity reactions may occur in patients with or without a history of allergy or bronchial asthma.

The possibility of exacerbation or activation of systemic lupus erythematosus has been reported.

PRECAUTIONS
General
Captopril

Impaired Renal Function—Some patients with renal disease, particularly those with severe renal artery stenosis, have developed increases in BUN and serum creatinine after reduction of blood pressure with captopril. Captopril dosage reduction and/or discontinuation of diuretic may be required. For some of these patients, it may not be possible to normalize blood pressure and maintain adequate renal perfusion (see CLINICAL PHARMACOLOGY, DOSAGE AND ADMINISTRATION, ADVERSE REACTIONS [Altered Laboratory Findings]).

Surgery/Anesthesia—In patients undergoing major surgery or during anesthesia with agents that produce hypotension, captopril will block angiotensin II formation secondary to compensatory renin release. If hypotension occurs and is considered to be due to this mechanism, it can be corrected by volume expansion.

Hydrochlorothiazide

All patients receiving thiazide therapy should be observed for clinical signs of fluid or electrolyte imbalance; namely hyponatremia, hypochloremic alkalosis, and hypokalemia. Serum and urine electrolyte determinations are particularly important when the patient is vomiting excessively or receiving parenteral fluids. Warning signs, irrespective of cause include dryness of mouth, thirst, weakness, lethargy, drowsiness, restlessness, muscle pains or cramps, muscular fatigue, hypotension, oliguria, tachycardia, and gastrointestinal disturbances such as nausea and vomiting.

Hypokalemia may develop, especially with brisk diuresis, when severe cirrhosis is present. Interference with adequate oral electrolyte intake will also contribute to hypokalemia. Hypokalemia can sensitize or exaggerate the response of the heart to the toxic effects of digitalis (e.g., increased ventricular irritability). Because captopril reduces the production of aldosterone, concomitant therapy with captopril reduces the diuretic-induced hypokalemia. Fewer patients may require potassium supplements and/or foods with a high potassium content (see Drug Interactions, Agents Increasing Serum Potassium).

Any chloride deficit is generally mild and usually does not require specific treatment except under extraordinary circumstances (as in liver disease or renal disease). Dilutional hyponatremia may occur in edematous patients in hot weather; appropriate therapy is water restriction, rather than administration of salt except in rare instances when the hyponatremia is life-threatening. In actual salt depletion, appropriate replacement is the therapy of choice.

Hyperuricemia may occur or frank gout may be precipitated in certain patients receiving thiazide therapy.

Diabetes mellitus which has been latent may become manifest during thiazide administration.

The antihypertensive effects of the drug may be enhanced in the postsympathectomy patient.

If progressive renal impairment becomes evident, as indicated by rising nonprotein nitrogen or blood urea nitrogen, a careful reappraisal of therapy is necessary with consideration given to withholding or discontinuing diuretic therapy.

Thiazides may decrease serum PBI levels without signs of thyroid disturbance.

Calcium excretion is decreased by thiazides. Pathologic changes in the parathyroid gland with hypercalcemia and hypophosphatemia have been observed in a few patients on prolonged thiazide therapy. The common complications of hyperparathyroidism have not been seen.

Information for Patients

Patients should be told to report promptly any indication of infection (e.g., sore throat, fever), which may be a sign of neutropenia, or of progressive edema which might be related to proteinuria and nephrotic syndrome.

All patients should be cautioned that excessive perspiration and dehydration may lead to an excessive fall in blood pressure because of reduction in fluid volume. Other causes of volume depletion such as vomiting or diarrhea may also lead to a fall in blood pressure; patients should be advised to consult with the physician.

Patients should be warned against interruption or discontinuation of medication unless instructed by the physician.

Heart failure patients on captopril therapy should be cautioned against rapid increases in physical activity.

Patients should be informed that CAPOZIDE (Captopril-Hydrochlorothiazide Tablets) should be taken one hour before meals (see DOSAGE AND ADMINISTRATION).

Laboratory Tests

Serum and urine electrolyte levels should be regularly monitored (see WARNINGS, [Captopril and Hydrochlorothiazide], also PRECAUTIONS [General, Hydrochlorothiazide]).

Drug Interactions
Captopril

Hypotension—Patients on Diuretic Therapy: Patients on diuretics and especially those in whom diuretic therapy was recently instituted, as well as those on severe dietary salt restriction or dialysis, may occasionally experience a precipitous reduction of blood pressure usually within the first hour after receiving the initial dose of captopril.

The possibility of hypotensive effects with captopril can be minimized by either discontinuing the diuretic or increasing the salt intake approximately one week prior to initiation of treatment with captopril or initiating therapy with small doses (6.25 or 12.5 mg). Alternatively, provide medical supervision for at least one hour after the initial dose. If hypotension occurs, the patient should be placed in a supine position and, if necessary, receive an intravenous infusion of normal saline. This transient hypotensive response is not a contraindication to further doses which can be given without difficulty once the blood pressure has increased after volume expansion.

Agents Having Vasodilator Activity: Data on the effect of concomitant use of other vasodilators in patients receiving captopril for heart failure are not available; therefore, nitroglycerin or other nitrates (as used for management of angina) or other drugs having vasodilator activity should, if possible, be discontinued before starting captopril. If resumed during captopril therapy, such agents should be administered cautiously, and perhaps at lower dosage.

Agents Causing Renin Release: Captopril's effect will be augmented by antihypertensive agents that cause renin release. For example, diuretics (e.g., thiazides) may activate the renin-angiotensin-aldosterone system.

Agents Affecting Sympathetic Activity: The sympathetic nervous system may be especially important in supporting blood pressure in patients receiving captopril alone or with diuretics. Therefore, agents affecting sympathetic activity (e.g., ganglionic blocking agents or adrenergic neuron blocking agents) should be used with caution. Beta-adrenergic blocking drugs add some further antihypertensive effect to captopril, but the overall response is less than additive.

Agents Increasing Serum Potassium: Since captopril decreases aldosterone production, elevation of serum potassium may occur. Potassium-sparing diuretics such as spironolactone, triamterene, or amiloride, or potassium supplements, should be given only for documented hypokalemia, and then with caution, since they may lead to a significant increase of serum potassium. Salt substitutes containing potassium should also be used with caution.

Inhibitors Of Endogenous Prostaglandin Synthesis: It has been reported that indomethacin may reduce the antihypertensive effect of captopril, especially in cases of low renin hypertension. Other nonsteroidal anti-inflammatory agents (e.g., aspirin) may also have this effect.

Hydrochlorothiazide

When administered concurrently the following drugs may interact with thiazide diuretics:

Alcohol, barbiturates, or narcotics—potentiation of orthostatic hypotension may occur.

Antidiabetic drugs (oral agents and insulin)—hyperglycemia induced by thiazides may require dosage adjustment of the antidiabetic drug.

Other antihypertensive drugs—additive effect or potentiation. Potentiation occurs with ganglionic or peripheral adrenergic blocking drugs.

Corticosteroids, ACTH—intensified electrolyte depletion, particularly hypokalemia.

Preanesthetic and anesthetic agents—effects of preanesthetic and anesthetic agents may be potentiated; adjust dosage of these agents accordingly.

Pressor amines (e.g., norepinephrine)—possible decreased response to pressor amines but not sufficient to preclude their use.

Skeletal muscle relaxants, nondepolarizing (e.g., tubocurarine)—possible increased responsiveness to the muscle relaxant.

Lithium—should not generally be given with diuretics; diuretic agents reduce the renal clearance of lithium and add a high risk of lithium toxicity. Refer to the package insert for lithium preparations before use of such preparations with CAPOZIDE (Captopril-Hydrochlorothiazide Tablets).

Drug/Laboratory Test Interactions
Captopril

Captopril may cause a false-positive urine test for acetone.

Hydrochlorothiazide

Thiazides should be discontinued before carrying out tests for parathyroid function (see PRECAUTIONS [General, Hydrochlorothiazide]).

Carcinogenesis, Mutagenesis, Impairment of Fertility
Captopril

Two-year studies with doses of 50 to 1350 mg/kg/day in mice and rats failed to show any evidence of carcinogenic potential.

Studies in rats have revealed no impairment of fertility.

Animal Toxicology

Chronic oral toxicity studies were conducted in rats (2 years), dogs (47 weeks; 1 year), mice (2 years), and monkeys (1 year). Significant drug-related toxicity included effects on hematopoiesis, renal toxicity, erosion/ulceration of the stomach, and variation of retinal blood vessels.

Reductions in hemoglobin and/or hematocrit values were seen in mice, rats, and monkeys at doses 50 to 150 times the maximum recommended human dose (MRHD). Anemia, leukopenia, thrombocytopenia, and bone marrow suppression occurred in dogs at doses 8 to 30 times MRHD. The reductions in hemoglobin and hematocrit values in rats and mice were only significant at 1 year and returned to normal with continued dosing by the end of the study. Marked anemia was seen at all dose levels (8 to 30 times MRHD) in dogs, whereas moderate to marked leukopenia was noted only at 15 and 30 times MRHD and thrombocytopenia at 30 times MRHD. The anemia could be reversed upon discontinuation of dosing. Bone marrow suppression occurred to a varying degree, being associated only with dogs that died or were sacrificed in a moribund condition in the 1-year study. However, in the 47-week study at a dose 30 times MRHD, bone marrow suppression was found to be reversible upon continued drug administration.

Captopril caused hyperplasia of the juxtaglomerular apparatus of the kidneys at doses 7 to 200 times the MRHD in rats and mice, at 20 to 60 times MRHD in monkeys, and at 30 times the MRHD in dogs.

Gastric erosions/ulcerations were increased in incidence at 20 and 200 times MRHD in male rats and at 30 and 65 times MRHD in dogs and monkeys, respectively. Rabbits developed gastric and intestinal ulcers when given oral doses approximately 30 times MRHD for only five to seven days.

In the two-year rat study, irreversible and progressive variations in the caliber of retinal vessels (focal sacculations and constrictions) occurred at all dose levels (7 to 200 times MRHD) in a dose-related fashion. The effect was first observed in the 88th week of dosing, with a progressively increased incidence thereafter, even after cessation of dosing.

Hydrochlorothiazide

Long-term studies in animals have not been performed to evaluate carcinogenic potential, mutagenesis, or whether this drug affects fertility in males or females.

Pregnancy—Category C
Captopril
Captopril was embryocidal in rabbits when given in doses about 2 to 70 times (on a mg/kg basis) the maximum recommended human dose, and low incidences of craniofacial malformations were seen. These effects in rabbits were most probably due to the particularly marked decrease in blood pressure caused by the drug in this species.

Captopril given to pregnant rats at 400 times the recommended human dose continuously during gestation and lactation caused a reduction in neonatal survival.

No teratogenic effects (malformations) have been observed after large doses of captopril in hamsters and rats.

Captopril crosses the human placenta.

Hydrochlorothiazide
Teratology studies have been performed in pregnant rats using captopril and hydrochlorothiazide individually and in combination; each agent was administered in doses up to 1350 mg/kg (400 times the maximum recommended human dose for hydrochlorothiazide). No evidence of embryotoxicity, fetotoxicity, or teratogenicity was found in any group.

There are no adequate and well-controlled studies with captopril and hydrochlorothiazide in pregnant women. Because animal reproduction studies are not always predictive of human response, CAPOZIDE should be used during pregnancy, or for patients likely to become pregnant, only if the potential benefit justifies a potential risk to the fetus.

Pregnancy—Nonteratogenic Effects
Hydrochlorothiazide
Thiazides cross the placental barrier and appear in cord blood. The use of thiazides in pregnant women requires that the anticipated benefit be weighed against possible hazards to the fetus. These hazards include fetal or neonatal jaundice, thrombocytopenia, and possibly other adverse reactions which have occurred in the adult.

Nursing Mothers
Both captopril and hydrochlorothiazide are excreted in human milk. Because of the potential for serious adverse reactions in nursing infants from both drugs, a decision should be made whether to discontinue nursing or to discontinue therapy taking into account the importance of CAPOZIDE (Captopril-Hydrochlorothiazide Tablets) to the mother.

Pediatric Use
Safety and effectiveness in children have not been established although there is limited experience with the use of captopril in children from 2 months to 15 years of age with secondary hypertension and varying degrees of renal insufficiency. Dosage, on a weight basis, was comparable to that used in adults. CAPOZIDE (Captopril-Hydrochlorothiazide Tablets) should be used in children only if other measures for controlling blood pressure have not been effective.

ADVERSE REACTIONS
Captopril
Reported incidences are based on clinical trials involving approximately 7000 patients.

Renal—About one of 100 patients developed proteinuria (see WARNINGS).

Each of the following has been reported in approximately 1 to 2 of 1000 patients and is of uncertain relationship to drug use: renal insufficiency, renal failure, polyuria, oliguria, and urinary frequency.

Hematologic—Neutropenia/agranulocytosis has occurred (see WARNINGS). Cases of anemia, thrombocytopenia, and pancytopenia have been reported.

Dermatologic—Rash, often with pruritus, and sometimes with fever, arthralgia, and eosinophilia, occurred in about 4 to 7 (depending on renal status and dose) of 100 patients, usually during the first four weeks of therapy. It is usually maculopapular, and rarely urticarial. The rash is usually mild and disappears within a few days of dosage reduction, short-term treatment with an antihistaminic agent, and/or discontinuing therapy; remission may occur even if captopril is continued. Pruritus, without rash, occurs in about 2 of 100 patients. Between 7 and 10 percent of patients with skin rash have shown an eosinophilia and/or positive ANA titers. A reversible associated pemphigoid-like lesion, and photosensitivity, have also been reported.

Angioedema of the face, mucous membranes of the mouth, or of the extremities has been observed in approximately 1 of 1000 patients and is reversible on discontinuance of captopril therapy. One case of laryngeal edema has been reported.

Flushing or pallor has been reported in 2 to 5 of 1000 patients.

Cardiovascular—Hypotension may occur; see WARNINGS and PRECAUTIONS (Drug Interactions) for discussion of hypotension on initiation of captopril therapy.

Tachycardia, chest pain, and palpitations have each been observed in approximately 1 of 100 patients.

Angina pectoris, myocardial infarction, Raynaud's syndrome, and congestive heart failure have each occurred in 2 to 3 of 1000 patients.

Dysgeusia—Approximately 2 to 4 (depending on renal status and dose) of 100 patients developed a diminution or loss of taste perception. Taste impairment is reversible and usually self-limited (2 to 3 months) even with continued drug administration. Weight loss may be associated with the loss of taste.

The following have been reported in about 0.5 to 2 percent of patients but did not appear at increased frequency compared to placebo or other treatments used in controlled trials: gastric irritation, abdominal pain, nausea, vomiting, diarrhea, anorexia, constipation, aphthous ulcers, peptic ulcer, dizziness, headache, malaise, fatigue, insomnia, dry mouth, dyspnea, cough, alopecia, paresthesias.

Hydrochlorothiazide
Gastrointestinal System—anorexia, gastric irritation, nausea, vomiting, cramping, diarrhea, constipation, jaundice (intrahepatic cholestatic jaundice), pancreatitis, and sialadenitis.

Central Nervous System—dizziness, vertigo, paresthesias, headache, and xanthopsia.

Hematologic—leukopenia, agranulocytosis, thrombocytopenia, aplastic anemia, and hemolytic anemia.

Cardiovascular—orthostatic hypotension.

Hypersensitivity—purpura, photosensitivity, rash, urticaria, necrotizing angiitis (vasculitis; cutaneous vasculitis), fever, respiratory distress including pneumonitis, and anaphylactic reactions.

Other—hyperglycemia, glycosuria, hyperuricemia, muscle spasm, weakness, restlessness, and transient blurred vision.

Whenever adverse reactions are moderate or severe, thiazide dosage should be reduced or therapy withdrawn.

Altered Laboratory Findings
Elevations of liver enzymes have been noted in a few patients but no causal relationship to captopril use has been established. Rare cases of cholestatic jaundice and of hepatocellular injury with or without secondary cholestasis have been reported in association with captopril administration.

A transient elevation of BUN and serum creatinine may occur, especially in patients who are volume-depleted or who have renovascular hypertension. In instances of rapid reduction of longstanding or severely elevated blood pressure, the glomerular filtration rate may decrease transiently, also resulting in transient rises in serum creatinine and BUN.

Small increases in the serum potassium concentration frequently occur, especially in patients with renal impairment (see PRECAUTIONS).

OVERDOSAGE
Captopril
Correction of hypotension would be of primary concern. Volume expansion with an intravenous infusion of normal saline is the treatment of choice for restoration of blood pressure.

Captopril may be removed from the general circulation by hemodialysis.

Hydrochlorothiazide
In addition to the expected diuresis, overdosage of thiazides may produce varying degrees of lethargy which may progress to coma within a few hours, with minimal depression of respiration and cardiovascular function and without evidence of serum electrolyte changes or dehydration. The mechanism of thiazide-induced CNS depression is unknown. Gastrointestinal irritation and hypermotility may occur. Transitory increase in BUN has been reported, and serum electrolyte changes may occur, especially in patients with impaired renal function.

In addition to gastric lavage and supportive therapy for stupor or coma, symptomatic treatment of gastrointestinal effects may be needed. The degree to which hydrochlorothiazide is removed by hemodialysis has not been clearly established. Measures as required to maintain hydration, electrolyte balance, respiration, and cardiovascular and renal function should be instituted.

DOSAGE AND ADMINISTRATION
DOSAGE MUST BE INDIVIDUALIZED (SEE INDICATIONS AND USAGE).

CAPOZIDE (Captopril-Hydrochlorothiazide Tablets) should be taken one hour before meals.

The usual initial dose of captopril is 25 mg bid or tid. Hydrochlorothiazide is usually given at a total daily dose of 25 to 100 mg.

The approximate daily dose of captopril and hydrochlorothiazide, as determined by titration of the individual components (see INDICATIONS AND USAGE), may be administered by utilizing an appropriate potency of CAPOZIDE bid.

For example, CAPOZIDE may be administered beginning with the 25 mg/15 mg combination tablet bid. Increased captopril dosage may be obtained by utilizing the 50 mg/15 mg combination tablet bid or increased hydrochlorothiazide dosage may be obtained by utilizing the 25 mg/25 mg combination tablet bid. CAPOZIDE 25 mg/15 mg and 50 mg/15 mg tablets may also be utilized in tid dosage regimens to provide higher daily dosages.

If additional control beyond that provided by the 50 mg/15 mg tid CAPOZIDE dose is indicated, it is recommended that other antihypertensive agents be added to the regimen.

A maximum daily dose of 450 mg captopril should not be exceeded.

Beta-blockers may be used in conjunction with CAPOZIDE therapy (see PRECAUTIONS [Drug Interactions]), but the effects are less than additive. Other agents may be added gradually beginning with 50 percent of the usual recommended starting dose to avoid an excessive fall in blood pressure.

For patients with severe hypertension (e.g., accelerated or malignant hypertension), the dosage increments may be made more frequently than every two weeks with the patient under continuous medical supervision until a satisfactory blood pressure response is obtained or the maximal dose of captopril is reached.

Dosage Adjustment in Renal Impairment—Because captopril and hydrochlorothiazide are excreted primarily by the kidneys, excretion rates are reduced in patients with impaired renal function. These patients will take longer to reach steady-state captopril levels and will reach higher steady-state levels for a given daily dose than patients with normal renal function. Therefore, these patients may respond to smaller or less frequent doses of CAPOZIDE.

After the desired therapeutic effect has been achieved, the dose intervals should be increased or the total daily dose reduced until the minimal effective dose is achieved. When concomitant diuretic therapy is required in patients with severe renal impairment, a loop diuretic (e.g., furosemide), rather than a thiazide diuretic is preferred for use with captopril; therefore, for patients with severe renal dysfunction the captopril-hydrochlorothiazide combination tablet is not usually recommended.

HOW SUPPLIED
CAPOZIDE (Captopril-Hydrochlorothiazide Tablets)

25 mg captopril combined with 15 mg hydrochlorothiazide
in bottles of 100. Tablets are white with distinct orange mottling; they are biconvex rounded squares with quadrisect bars. Tablet identification no. **338**.

25 mg captopril combined with 25 mg hydrochlorothiazide
in bottles of 100. Tablets are peach-colored and may show slight mottling; they are biconvex rounded squares with quadrisect bars. Tablet identification no. **349**.

50 mg captopril combined with 15 mg hydrochlorothiazide
in bottles of 100. Tablets are white with distinct orange mottling; they are biconvex ovals with a bisect bar. Tablet identification no. **384**.

50 mg captopril combined with 25 mg hydrochlorothiazide
in bottles of 100. Tablets are peach-colored and may show slight mottling; they are biconvex ovals with a bisect bar. Tablet identification no. **390**.

STORAGE
Keep bottles tightly closed (protect from moisture); do not store above 86° F.

(J4-005C)

SPECIALTY BOARD REVIEW
FAMILY PRACTICE

THIRD EDITION

ARCO MEDICAL REVIEW SERIES

SPECIALTY BOARD REVIEW
FAMILY PRACTICE

THIRD EDITION

ERNEST YUH-TING YEN, M.D., M.P.H., Dr. P.H.

Cerritos, California

V. BUSHAN BHARDWAJ, M.D., B.S. (Lond.)

Gietzville, New York

APPLETON-CENTURY-CROFTS/Norwalk, Connecticut

86 87 88 89 / 10 9 8 7 6 5 4 3 2 1

Prentice-Hall of Australia, Pty. Ltd., Sydney
Prentice-Hall Canada, Inc.
Prentice-Hall Hispanoamericana, S.A., Mexico
Prentice-Hall of India Private Limited, New Delhi
Prentice-Hall International (UK) Limited, London
Prentice-Hall of Japan, Inc., Tokyo
Prentice-Hall of Southeast Asia (Pte.) Ltd., Singapore
Whitehall Books Ltd., Wellington, New Zealand
Editora Prentice-Hall do Brasil Ltda., Rio de Janeiro

ISBN: 0-8385-8628-8
ISBN: 0-8385-8627-9 (Squibb)
LC: 86-070436

PRINTED IN THE UNITED STATES OF AMERICA

To all our personal and professional friends
whose inspiration and support
have nurtured our continuous growth.

Contents

Preface

In recent years the American Board of Family Practice utilized modified multiple true-false questions and clinical set problems in the examinations. In this edition, these examination formats are explained and the examples provided for readers' review. There are many readers who prepare examinations which continue to utilize the standard multiple true-false questions and this type of question is preserved for readers' use.

Dr. Ludlow B. Creary, Chairman of the Department of Family Medicine, Charles R. Drew Postgraduate Medical School supported the work; Drs. Isaac English, Calvin Hicks, Russell Boxley, Eleanor Kong, Ron Edelstein, Karen Knighton, and Rabia Ahmed, all of the King-Drew Family Practice Residency contributed the questions included in this edition; Dr. T. Ouyang and Ms. L. Furman both of the University of North Dakota also provided the materials in this book; Ms. Louise T. Bryant and Ms. Ella Stokes edited and typed the manuscripts. Mr. Craig Percy of Appleton-Century-Crofts encouraged the completion of the project.

Introduction

HELPFUL TIPS FOR EXAMINATION

Applications for Taking Examinations

A petition to take the examination should be made early to allow for a possible delay in application procedures. Complete and accurate applications should be submitted along with all required documents and correct fees.

Preparation Plans

1. In drafting up a study schedule, it should be remembered that the date of the examination is the deadline date, by which all preparations are to be completed. It is important to stick to the study schedule and complete it.
2. Start early and allocate ample time for preparation.
3. Review all subject areas; start with those subjects which are less familiar and spend more time on those subjects that will probably constitute a large part of the examination.
4. Read familiar textbooks first; use question and answer books to assess the progress. Enhance weak areas through further readings of reference sources.
5. As the date of the examination approaches, the golden rule of Contentment is essential.
6. On the day before the examination, keep a clear head, calm mind, and confident outlook. A good night's sleep before the examination is beneficial. Do not take any sedatives which are unfamiliar.

On the Day of the Examination

1. Be sure to wake up in time—an alarm clock may be needed.
2. Do not get hypoglycemic. Eat a good, light breakfast and bring candies, soda, or gum with you.
3. Dress comfortably and casually; bring along a working watch, two pencils, and necessary identifications.
4. Arrive at the examination hall ahead of time, take into account a possible traffic jam.
5. If you must smoke, request special permission to leave the room for a break.
6. Ask permission for use of the toilet facilities.
7. Time yourself on the test. Reserve time for rechecking the answers. For multiple choice answers, plan to spend no more than 40 seconds per item.

8. Follow directions printed at the beginning of each section of the test. Follow the directions given for each special group of questions. Be aware of the changes in examination format (e.g., from the positive to the negative form of multiple choice questions).

9. Make sure that the answer corresponds correctly to the question and that the correct answer is given on the answer sheet.

10. Answer all multiple choice questions.

11. Try not to discuss the examination during the breaks; use the breaks to prepare for the next session.

COMMON TYPES OF MULTIPLE CHOICE EXAMINATION QUESTIONS

One Best Response Type

The question contains the stem followed by five suggested lettered answers (A, B, C, D, E). Only one answer is correct. The examinee is instructed to select only the best or most appropriate answer among five alternative answers given. There is a 20% (1 out of 5) chance of choosing the correct answer just by random guessing. Through the process of elimination (discussed later in this chapter), the examinee can guess intelligently to select the correct answer.

Excluded Term Type (Negative Term Type)

The stem of the question is followed by five suggested lettered answers (A, B, C, D, E) of which all but one (i.e., four answers) are applicable to the statement or situation described by the stem. The examinee is instructed to choose the one answer which is least applicable to the statement or situation of the stem. The commonly used negative words include *except, least,* and *not*. The examinee should remember that the "wrong" answer is the "correct" response.

Matching Type

A matching question consists of a list of lettered headings followed by a list of numbered words or phrases. The examinee is asked to select one or several headings most closely related to each of the numbered words or phrases. There are usually five lettered headings (A, B, C, D, E) and fewer than five numbered items (usually two or three). Only one lettered heading is matched with each numbered item, and each lettered heading can be used once, more than once, or not at all. To prepare for the matching questions, a familiarity with word association in medicine is useful.

Modified Matching Type

The list of numbered questions (often two or three) is followed by four lettered answers (A, B, C, D). The examinee is instructed to answer:

> **A,** if the numbered question is associated with A only.
> **B,** if the numbered question is associated with B only.
> **C,** if the numbered question is associated with both A and B.
> **D,** if the numbered question is associated with neither A nor B.

Each lettered answer (A, B, C, D) can be used once, more than once, or not at all. This type of question is used to make the examinee identify the similarity (association) of and difference between A and B, and the questions usually concern the differential diagnosis of A and B.

Standard Multiple True-False Type

This consists of a stem (a statement of a problem or a presentation of a question) followed by four true or false statements (statements 1, 2, 3, 4). The examinee is instructed to choose:

A, if only statements 1, 2, and 3 are correct.
B, if only statements 1 and 3 are correct.
C, if only statements 2 and 4 are correct.
D, if only statement 4 is correct.
E, if all statements (1, 2 3, 4) are correct.

This type of question will be further discussed later in this chapter.

Modified Multiple True-False Type

Each test item consists of an item followed by four or five lettered options (i.e., options A, B, C, D, or options A, B, C, D, E). The examinee is asked to evaluate all options, if the option is true (or correct), answer the option with "T"; if the option is false (or incorrect), answer the option with "F".

In this type of question, all options are listed randomly and do not denote priority or sequential relationships among options. All options may be correct or all may be incorrect, there is no specific pattern that can be identified. Although all options are somehow related to each other (e.g., describe the different aspects of the same illness) each option needs to be examined separately, independent of other options listed. This question type forms the basic unit of the clinical set problems.

Situation Type

Actual clinical conditions selected from medical practice are simulated to form situation questions. The examinee is usually given information in one or several of the following areas concerning a simulated patient: history, signs and symptoms, laboratory determinations, diagnosis and problems, treatment, and prognosis. Then the examinee is instructed to answer a series of questions on the appropriate actions to be taken and on the medical knowledge that is relevant to the situation presented. Examinees with diverse clinical experiences can expect that their experiences and the situations presented will be similar and should answer the questions logically, as they would in actual clinical situations. However, when examinees must analyze situations with which they have had little or no experience, they should not panic; rather they should apply basic principles and techniques of family medicine to answer the questions. More elaborate situation questions are called "Patient Management Problems" (PMP), which will be discussed further later in this chapter. Situation questions in the modified multiple true–false type is called "the clinical set problem."

Pictorial Quizzes

The pictorial quizzes may utilize all seven types of multiple choice questions (one best response type, excluded term type, matching type, modified matching type, standard and modified multiple true-false type, and situation type) in presenting the pictorial illustrations in the question either as numbered items or as lettered items. The pictorial illustration includes x-rays, EKGs, skin conditions, eye problems, eyegrounds, blood smears, bone marrow smears, urine sediments, audiograms, gross and microscopic specimens, experimental graphs, anatomical atlases, statistical charts, and summary tables. Pictures, graphs, tables, or x-rays that are used in the examination are usually typical cases, and the examinee should look for the central focus to select the correct responses. Whenever pictorial questions are accompanied by case histories, the examinee should review the case histories in detail *first*, then analyze the illustrations according to the characteristics expected from the case histories given in the question. The pictorial quizzes will be further discussed later in this chapter.

HELPFUL HINTS FOR GUESSING MULTIPLE CHOICE QUESTIONS WHEN THE ANSWERS ARE NOT KNOWN

1. Use the process of elimination. Cross out wrong responses, then eliminate the unlikely responses; then select the most probable response among the remaining ones.
2. Look for verbal cues. A statement with "may" is often correct; a statement containing "always," "never," or "100% of the patients" may be incorrect.
3. The content of one item may indicate the answer to another item. Similar questions are often repeated; often the same questions appear.
4. Look for the design of the alternatives. A statement that does not grammatically follow the stem of the question may be incorrect. The shortest or the longest alternative may be the correct one.
5. In the one best response type question, if two alternatives are similar, both may be incorrect. If they are contradictory, one may be correct.
6. A statement with unfamiliar technical terms may be an incorrect response.
7. "All of the above" or "None of the above" is usually the correct response.
8. In the situation type question, the answer is often related to the correct response for a previous question.
9. Generally, true-false tests have a greater number of true answers.
10. Occasionally, rely on your intuition.

THE ANSWERING STRATEGY FOR STANDARD MULTIPLE TRUE-FALSE QUESTIONS

Pictorial Summary of the Directions

In the multiple true-false question, the examinee is instructed to match statements 1, 2, 3, 4 to five lettered answers, A, B, C, D, and E according to the following keys:

A, if only 1, 2, and 3 are correct.
B, if only 1 and 3 are correct.
C, if only 2 and 4 are correct.
D, if only 4 is correct.
E, if 1, 2, 3, and 4 are all correct.

The above directions can be summarized with the following "5 × 4" table (Table 1).

Table 1. The Instruction Matrix.

Statement / Key	1	2	3	4
A	1	2	3	
B	1		3	
C		2		4
D				4
E	1	2	3	4

Letting " +" denote correct responses and "−" indicate incorrect responses, Table 1 can be transformed into Table 2, the response matrix.

Table 2. The Response Matrix.

Statement / Key	1	2	3	4
A	+	+	+	−
B	+	−	+	−
C	−	+	−	+
D	−	−	−	+
E	+	+	+	+

Useful Rules

From analysis of Table 2, the following rules can be obtained.

1. 1 and 3 are always together. When 1 is correct, 3 will be correct; when 3 is correct, 1 will be correct. When 1 is incorrect, 3 will be incorrect; when 3 is incorrect, 1 will be incorrect.
2. When 4 is incorrect, 1 and 3 will be correct; when 1 and 3 are incorrect, 4 will be correct. However, 1, 3 and 4 can all be correct; in this instance, 2 has to be correct, and the answer is E.

Decision Principle

Applying the above rules, Table 2 can be converted to Table 3, the decision matrix.

Table 3. The Decision Matrix.

Statement / Key	1	2	3	4
A		+		−
B	+	−		
C	−	+		
D	−	−		
E	+			+

As shown in Table 3, only two statements (instead of four) are required to make decisions on the lettered responses (A, B, C, D, E). This is due to the redundant information provided in the question according to the rules stated above. Table 3 can be transformed into Table 4, the simplified decision matrix.

Table 4. The Simplified Decision Matrix.

Key	+	−
A	2	4
B	1	2
C	2	1
D		1,2
E	1,4	

Table 4 enables the examinee to decide the correct lettered responses with partial knowledge of two statements instead of complete knowledge of four statements.

The Forward Approach

Tables 2, 3, and 4 can be summarized by means of the forward algorithm as shown in Flow Chart 1.

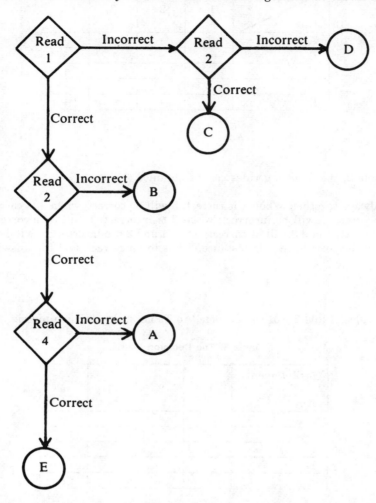

Figure 1. Flow Chart 1 (From Bhardwaj, V.B.; Yen, Y.-T. *Medical Examinations: A Preparation Guide.* New York: Arco, 1979).

The decision principle employed in Flow Chart 1 is shown in Table 5.

Table 5. The Forward Decision Strategy.

Statement / Key	1	2	3	4
A	+	+		−
B	+	−		
C	−	+		
D	−	−		
E	+	+		+

It is noteworthy that the forward decision strategy is less efficient than the decision principle described in Tables 3 and 4. Deciding on E and A requires information on three statements in Table 5 and only requires information on two statements in Tables 3 and 4. However, the forward decision strategy is easier to adopt in actual examination situations. Flow Chart 1 can further be simplified as shown in Table 6.

Table 6. The Forward Path.

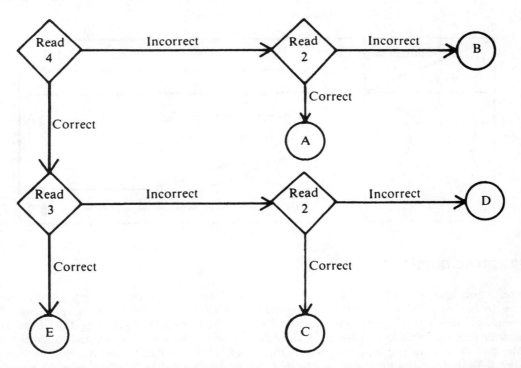

The Backward Approach

Alternatively, the examinee can also establish the backward approach, reading the statements from the bottom up (start from statement 4, proceed to statement 3, then to statement 2, and ignore statement 1 completely). The backward algorithm is shown in Flow Chart 2.

Figure 2. Flow Chart 2 (From Bhardwaj, V.B.; Yen, Y.-T. *Medical Examinations: A Preparation Guide*. New York: Arco, 1979).

Flow Chart 2 can be summarized in Table 7.

Table 7. The Backward Decision Strategy.

Key \ Statement	4	3	2	1
E	+	+		
D	+	−	−	
C	+	−	+	
B	−		−	
A	−		+	

The backward approach is as efficient as the forward approach but is less efficient than the decision principle described in Tables 3 and 4. However, it is a systematic way to approach the question; Table 8 (the backward path) illustrates this approach diagramatically.

Table 8. The Backward Path.

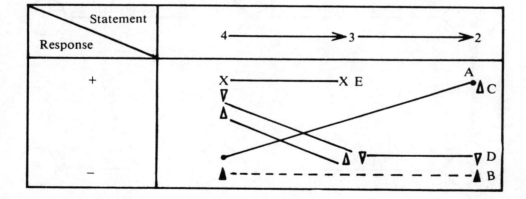

THE PICTORIAL QUIZZES

The pictorial quiz is a form of the multiple choice question. Each question concerning a pictorial illustration may have to be answered within 30 to 45 seconds, as with other multiple choice questions. Thus the examinee should concentrate on the recognition of specific patterns in the pictorial illustration related to the disease or problem situation presented in the question, so as to answer the question correctly within an allowable span of time, rather than spending a great deal of time analyzing and interpreting the pictorial illustrations. To do this, the examinee is expected to become thoroughly familiar with the popular topics listed on the following pages.

RADIOLOGY

Chest x-ray

1. Miliary tuberculosis
2. Interstitial pneumonitis
3. Pulmonary infarction
4. Diaphragmatic hernia
5. Staphylococcal pneumonia
6. Hiatus hernia
7. Mitral stenosis
8. Transposition of the vessels
9. Fallot's tetralogy
10. Retrosternal goiter
11. Posterior mediastinal tumor
12. Silicosis
13. Asbestosis
14. Hyaline membrane disease
15. Pneumothorax
16. Aspergilloma
17. Lobar pneumonia

Bones

1. Severe iron deficiency anemia—skull
2. Multiple myeloma
3. Paget's disease
4. Lead poisoning
5. Hyperparathyroidism
6. Rheumatoid arthritis
7. Gout
8. Psoriatic arthritis
9. Sarcoidosis
10. Osteoarthritis
11. Ankylosing spondylitis—spine
12. Osteoporosis
13. Osteomalacia
14. Congenital syphilis
15. Chronic osteomyelitis
16. Congenital dislocation of the hip
17. Tuberculosis of the spine
18. Femoral slipped epiphysis
19. Avascular necrosis of the femur head
20. Child abuse
21. Osteogenic sarcoma
22. Gaucher's disease
23. Osteogenesis imperfecta
24. Bursitis, muscle calcification
25. Fracture, radial styloid process
26. Fracture, femoral supracondyle

Gastrointestinal Tract

1. Carcinoma of the esophagus
2. Duodenal atresia
3. Chronic duodenal ulcer
4. Gastric carcinoma
5. Ulcerative colitis
6. Crohn's disease
7. Perforated bowel
8. Paralytic ileus
9. Volvulus
10. Intussusception
11. Intestinal mechanic obstruction
12. Diverticulosis
13. Polyposis coli
14. Chronic pancreatitis
15. Meconium ileus
16. Esophageal varices
17. Fecalith—appendix
18. Carcinoma of the cecum
19. Gallstones

Genitourinary Tract

1. Hydronephrosis
2. Wilm's tumor
3. Neuroblastoma
4. Vesicoureteric reflux
5. Renal stones

Skull and CT Scan

1. Subdural hematoma
2. Hydrocephalus
3. Brain tumor—astrocytoma
4. Meningioma
5. Intracranial calcification—toxoplasmosis, tuberous sclerosis, Sturge-Weber's syndrome, cytomegalovirus
6. Craniopharyngioma
7. Brain abscess

Bone Scan

1. Osteomyelitis
2. Bone cysts

Thyroid Scan: Cold and Hot Nodules

OPHTHALMOLOGY

1. Optic atrophy
2. Diabetic retinopathy
3. Hypertensive retinopathy
4. Central vein occlusion
5. Central artery occlusion
6. Choroiditis
7. Tay-Sachs' disease
8. Papilledema
9. Glaucoma
10. Kayser-Fleischer's ring
11. Subconjunctival hemorrhage
12. Chalazion
13. Pterygium
14. External hordeolum

AUDIOGRAM

1. Serous otitis media
2. Congenital deafness (rubella)
3. Meniere's disease
4. Otosclerosis
5. Noise exposure
6. Presbycusis
7. Acoustic neuroma
8. Drug ototoxicity

ELECTROCARDIOGRAM

1. Mitral stenosis
2. Left ventricular enlargement
3. Heart block—1°, 2°, 3°, Wencke-Bach's phenomenon
4. Atrial fibrillation
5. Atrial flutter
6. Digitalis poisoning
7. Hypokalemia
8. Hyperkalemia
9. Hypocalcemia
10. Hypercalcemia
11. Myxedema
12. Infarction—anterior, anterolateral, inferior
13. Pulmonary embolism
14. Pericarditis
15. Bundle branch blocks

HEMATOLOGY

1. Iron deficiency
2. Hemolytic disease of the newborn
3. Lead poisoning
4. Infectious mononucleosis
5. Megaloblastic anemia—peripheral smear
6. Megaloblastic anemia—bone marrow
7. Acute leukemia—bone marrow
8. Lupus erythematosus cell
9. Sickle cell anemia
10. Thalassemia major
11. Spherocytosis
12. Idiopathic thrombocytopenic purpura (ITP)—bone marrow
13. Ovalocytosis
14. Bone marrow neuroblastoma
15. Sternberg-Reed cells (bone marrow)
16. Auer rod in acute myeloblastic leukemia
17. Pernicious anemia
18. Multiple myeloma

DERMATOLOGY AND PHOTOGRAPHS

1. Psoriasis
2. Primary and secondary syphilis
3. Rosacea
4. Measles
5. Rocky Mountain spotted fever
6. Chicken pox
21. Dermatitis herpetiformis
22. Melanoma
23. Poison ivy
24. Scabies
25. Tinea capitis, cruris
26. Acanthosis nigricans

7. Stevens-Johnson's syndrome
8. Erythema nodosum
9. Lupus erythematosus
10. Scleroderma
11. Dermatomyositis
12. Von Recklinghausen's disease, neurofibromatosis
13. Adenoma sebaceum (tuberous sclerosis)
14. Sturge-Weber's syndrome
15. Peutz-Jegher's syndrome
16. Hereditary telangiectasia
17. Cellulitis
18. Pemphigus
19. Atopic dermatitis
20. Drug eruptions—fixed
27. Chancroid and chancre
28. Condyloma acuminatum and lata
29. Zoster
30. Impetigo
31. Pityriasis rosea
32. Seborrheic dermatitis
33. Herpes progenitalis and labialis
34. Gonococcal arthritis—dermatitis syndrome
35. Lymphogranuloma venereum
36. Congenital syphilis
37. Klinefelter's syndrome
38. Turner's syndrome
39. Down's syndrome

ELECTROENCEPHALOGRAM

1. Petit mal
2. Brain tumor
3. Stroke—intracranial hemorrhage
4. Epilepsies
5. Head injury—hematomas

PATIENT MANAGEMENT PROBLEMS

Overview

A patient management problem (PMP) is an erasure test of clinical competence in which a series of clinical situations extracted from various stages of a simulated patient's course are presented. PMPs are basically situation type multiple choice questions with responses partially covered by the latent image overlay. When the examinee makes a choice, he erases the overlay with a latent image developer pen. Once developed, the uncovered latent image responses cannot be covered again. The examinee receives a penalty for erasing incorrect responses as well as for not erasing correct responses.

In the PMP, the examinee decides his choices by erasure. When he chooses his courses of action, he erases the choices; when he decides not to choose particular courses of action, he does not erase these choices. The examinee's decision to erase or not to erase will result in either correct or incorrect responses, as shown in Table 9.

Table 9. The Decision Model.

	RESULT	
DECISION	Correct Response	Incorrect Response
Erase	Correct response erased	Error of commission
Not to erase	Error of omission	Incorrect response avoided

As shown in Table 9, the examinee can make two types of errors: errors of commission, in which the examinee chooses incorrect (harmful or irrelevant) courses of action; and errors of omission, in which the examinee fails to select the correct (essential or useful) courses of action. The decision to erase can be depicted as a positive act $(+)$, and the decision not to erase can be depicted as a negative act $(-)$; the correct response can also be depicted as a positive instance $(+)$, and the negative response as a negative instance $(-)$. Thus the table can be simplified into Table 10.

Table 10. The Decision Outcome.

Decision	Response	
	$(+)$	$(-)$
Erase $(+)$	$+\ +$	$+\ -$
Not to erase $(-)$	$-\ +$	$-\ -$

The examinee will be credited for both the true positive $(+\ +$; erasing the correct response) and the true negative $(-\ -$; not erasing the incorrect response), and will be penalized for both the false positive $(+\ -$; the error of commission, in which the incorrect response is not avoided) and the false negative $(-\ +$; the error of omission, in which the correct response is not erased).

Decision Strategy

To gain high scores, the examinee should pay attention to both "what to erase" and "what not to erase." The decision strategy is:

1. To maximize:
   (a) True positives (erasing all correct responses).
   (b) True negatives (not erasing any incorrect responses).

2. To minimize:
   (a) False positives (not erasing any incorrect responses).
   (b) False negatives (erasing all correct responses).

The examinee usually realizes that when he erases correct choices (true positive) he receives positive scores; however, he should also remember that when he does not erase incorrect choices (true negatives), he also gains positive scores. The examinee usually understands that when he erases incorrect choices (false positive; errors of commission) he will receive negative marks; however, he should also recognize that when he does not erase correct choices (false negatives; errors of omission), he will also lose points.

In consideration of the above discussions, the examinee is advised to establish a balanced erasing pattern. Following two erasing patterns commonly found is not recommended.

1. Shotgun approach. The examinee indiscriminately makes a large number of erasures. The examinee will be able to select the majority of useful and essential courses of action; however, at the same time he will select many harmful, contraindicated, or unnecessary options. The examinee makes few errors of omission but commits many errors of commission.
2. Gun-shyness approach. The examinee erases only a few choices for fear of making mistakes, to allow for cost containment of the medical care, or to take an "efficient" short cut in making a clinical decision. The examinee will be able to avoid the majority of harmful or unnecessary courses of action, but at the same time he may omit beneficial and necessary choices. This examinee is making few errors of commission; however, he is committing many errors of ommission.

Useful Approach

1. Proceed in a logical, systematic, and organized manner.
2. Answer easy PMPs first. Easy PMPs are those which the examinee has worked previously, PMPs in the examinee's area of expertise, or PMPs familiar to the examinee through reading or preparation. Reserve time to deliberate the answering strategy for difficult PMPs.
3. Analyze the lead-in stem (i.e., the initial paragraph of the opening sentence) very carefully to identify the situation: the time and place the patient is seen (e.g., office or hospital), the epidemiological characteristics of the patient (e.g., "typical patient"), and the role the examinee is assigned to play (e.g., the patient's family physician).
4. Study the entire PMP and formulate possible diagnostic hypotheses (two or three initial hyposstheses) through examining a list of the diagnoses, available therapeutic modes, suggested laboratory and diagnostic procedures, and the display of historical and physical items.
5. For each clinical situation, read all the options listed: first eliminate all unnecessary and harmful options, then list all useful options and prioritize. Erase options according to the priority heirarchy, stop when information is adequate for subsequent action.
6. After every erasure, review all latent image answers already erased to confirm or modify the tentative diagnostic hypothesis generated to make further appropriate decisions (i.e., decide whether to continue to erase according to the priority list or stop).
7. When in doubt, review all the available information and consider the probability of correct responses—if it is greater than 0.5, erase; if it is less than 0.5, don't erase.
8. When appropriate responses have been erased, do not rub out other responses out of curiosity.

Specific Erasing Hints

In PMPs, the examinee is usually requested to engage in the following clinical tasks.

1. Obtaining an adequate clinical history.
2. Performing an appropriate physical examination.
3. Ordering necessary diagnostic studies and procedures.
4. Developing plausible diagnostic hypotheses.
5. Prescribing effective therapy.
6. Carrying out satisfactory follow-ups.

For each of the above specific clinical situations, the useful erasing hints are discussed below.

History taking

1. Erase organic history first, psychosocial and family history next, and then move to sexual history when this is specifically indicated.
2. In emergency or acute situations, erase only the most pressing questions (such as the location of abdominal pain); in the stable condition, more thorough historic items can be erased.
3. Search for symptoms that yield the greatest amount of information; with each erasure, try to reduce problem spaces (unknowns) in order to zero in on the differential diagnosis.
4. Erase current medication history, allergy history, and past medical and surgical history, usually in that order.

Physical examinations

1. In emergency or acute situations, erase only pertinent and limited examination items and avoid erasing unnecessary examinations which may cause discomfort (such as pelvic examination for a patient with acute myocardial infarction). In stable conditions, more thorough physical examinations should be erased.

2. In emergency situations, first erase vital signs, mental status, pupil signs, and cardiopulmonary functions.
3. Erase the options in a problem-oriented fashion rather than in a random fashion (as listed in the PMP). For example, a female patient with sore throat is listed with rectal examination, pelvic examination, examination of the lungs, and examination of the pharynx. The examinee is advised to erase the examination of the pharynx first, then examination of the lungs. Pelvic and rectal examinations are to be erased when the clinical situation warrants.

Diagnostic procedures

1. Order sensitive tests (which are likely to identify diseases) first, then order specific tests (which are likely to exclude diseases) for confirmation of the diagnosis.
2. Start with laboratory tests which yield specific information immediately, which cost less, and which cause less discomfort and less risk to the patient.
3. Order less invasive tests first (such as routine laboratory tests, including hemoglobin and urinalysis), then order invasive tests for confirmation of the diagnosis.
4. In serious or emergency situations, laboratory tests are often relied upon to make the diagnosis, and bold erasures can be performed. When the patient is in stable condition, laboratory tests are often employed to confirm the diagnostic hypothesis generated by the history and physicals; thus the examinee should be more selective in erasing. In the office (or ambulatory clinic) setting, the physician should avoid a "shotgun approach" even with routine laboratory tests and should be selective. Upon admission, many routine laboratory tests (such as CBC) can be ordered if the clinical syndrome is not clear (such as multiple cultures in a patient with a fever of unknown origin).
5. The latent image answers often do not offer any clues and may report that the test was done, scheduled, or requested. The examinee should not rub out other answers because of a lack of confidence.

Diagnostic hypotheses

1. Gather clues from the list of diagnostic procedures and therapeutic measures, epidemiological characteristics of the patient, the presenting symptoms, and the list of historic and physical items.
2. Formulate the disease cluster (such as pulmonary infections) first. Verify its existence by associated and specific findings from the history, physical, and laboratory test results. Differentiate it from other disease entities (e.g., mycoplasmal versus pneumococcal pneumonia) in the same disease cluster through discriminating and specific findings obtained from the history, physical, and laboratory test results.
3. Accept unexpected abnormal findings obtained from the history, physical, and laboratory studies and formulate new diagnostic hypotheses, or add to or modify previously generated hypotheses.

Therapeutic measures

1. In a life-threatening situation, therapeutic measures are often required immediately and should be erased, while in nondistressed situations, it is better to await the establishment of a definite diagnosis through information obtained from the history, physical, and laboratory test results.
2. Comprehensive management should be provided, including medications, patient and family education, change of life style (such as stopping smoking), diet therapy (such as a low-salt diet for hypertensive patients), marital or family counseling, high-risk analyses, routine screening procedures (such as cervical Papanicolaou smear), and rehabilitation services. Continuous care is required for the majority of patients and includes regular follow-ups, as in well child care, and the routine care of chronic illness. Preventive services, such as immunizations and prenatal care, are advisable. However, a shotgun approach to therapy is to be avoided.
3. Start with specific therapeutic measures yielding a high success rate (including high compliance) with reasonable cost and little discomfort. Unless specifically indicated, avoid ordering dangerous and toxic drugs for initial therapy.

4. Be aware of the side-effects of the medications prescribed and of complications following therapeutic measures (such as postpartum hemorrhage).

5. Be sure not to treat the patient with drugs to which he is allergic; be cognizant of the possible drug interactions.

6. In multiple problems, all problems are to be treated. If there is urgency in one problem (say, subacute endocarditis), treat that problem first. When the problem becomes stable, other problems (such as monilial vaginitis) can be treated.

7. Consultation and referral should be done after the basic work-ups have been completed.

8. The latent image answers may indicate only that the therapy was given, ordered, or started. However, sometimes the answer may say that the patient has not improved, has deteriorated, or has even died. If the examinee has erased the appropriate answers, he should be confident enough not to rub out other answers.

CLINICAL SET PROBLEMS

Similar to the patient management problems, the clinical set problems are also used to assess the examinee's clinical problem solving ability. In patient management problems, the invisible ink statements are used to construct the test questions; however, in clinical set problems, the modified multiple true-false type question format is adopted. The approaches outlined for the patient management problems are also applicable in answering clinical set problems.

As in the patient management problems, the clinical set problem is constructed from simulated case studies which often include the following patient management processes: history, physical, laboratory, diagnosis, treatment, and follow-up. Other relevant data of the clinical problems can also be included in the test items such as pathophysiology, high risk factors, preventive measures, etiological factors, cost consideration, facility and manpower needs. In most clinical set problems, two or more clinical aspects of the simulated cases are selected to form a "clinical set."

At the begining of each "clinical set," initial information (such as symptoms, signs, situation, laboratory and clinical findings) is provided to describe a clinical setting. Following this clinical framework, there are two or more (mostly three or four) test items presented. Each test item is constructed by the modified multiple true-false question format. Each test item consists of the lead-in stem and two or more (mostly five or six) numbered options. Each test item consists of a clinical aspect of the simulated case and often is represented by a question or an incomplete statement. With available information (often not complete) from the initial clinical presentations and the description in the stem, the examinee is asked to decide the truth or falsity of the numbered options listed following the stem. These options are listed randomly and are not listed according to priority or any orderly sequence. All options may be true and all options may be false. The examinee is asked to answer "T" if the option is essential and important in the total management of the patient or family; and to answer "F" if the option is irrelevant or inappropriate in the total management of the patient or family. To determine the truth of each option, the examinee should follow the basic principle of family medicine including comprehensive (e.g., psycho-social and preventive care) and continuous (e.g., follow-ups) total health care for the patient and family. Although rare and uncommon clinical problems in daily practice may appear in the clinical set problems, the examinee needs to be thoroughly familiar with common clinical problems seen in family practice.

REFERENCES

1. Bhardwaj, V.B.; Yen, Y.T. *Specialty Board Review: Family Practice.* New York: ARCO, 1977.
2. Yen, Y.T.; Bhardwaj, V.B. *Medical Examinations: A Preparation Guide.* 2nd edition. New York: Appleton-Century-Crofts, 1984.
3. Hubbard, J. *Measuring Medical Education,* 2nd edition. Philadelphia: Lea & Febiger, 1978.
4. Yen, Y.T. *Review and Assessment in Family Practice.* New York: Appleton-Century-Crofts, 1980.
5. Yen, Y.T.; Bhardwaj, V.B., "Patient Management in Primary Care Problems and Case Studies." Medical Examination Publishing Co., 1981.

Chapter 1

Psychiatry

Directions: Each of the questions or incomplete statements below is followed by five suggested answers or completions. Select the BEST answer in each case.

1. When the supermarket checker forgets to charge for a package of chewing gum which the child keeps in his hand, the parents are delighted. The parents' attitude is that of

   A. superego lacunae
   B. reaction formation
   C. undoing
   D. intellectualization
   E. regression   (1:136)

2. Of the following, prognosis in the treatment of homosexuals depends most on the

   A. type of treatment
   B. environmental situation
   C. motivation
   D. ability to relate to the opposite sex
   E. parental relationships   (4:146)

3. Many males have concern over penis size. The size of the penis is important for which *one* of the following reasons?

   A. A small penis provides insufficient stimulation to the female during intercourse.
   B. A large penis cannot be easily accommodated by female genitalia in the aroused state.
   C. Penis size is directly related to body size.
   D. Penis size has important psychological implications.

E. Penis size in the nonerect state is directly related to penis size in the erect state.
                                   (1:128)

4. Vaginal and clitoral orgasms are distinguished in the female by the following

   A. Vaginal and clitoral orgasms cannot be distinguished.
   B. Vaginal orgasm can occur only from vaginal stimulation but not from clitoral and labial stimulation.
   C. The subjective experience of orgasm is more intense in vaginal responses.
   D. In vaginal orgasm there is contraction of the pelvic floor musculature and of the uterus.
   E. The physiological response derived from clitoral orgasm is more intense than that from vaginal orgasm.   (1:566)

5. Impotence in males is most commonly due to

   A. phimosis
   B. psychological factors
   C. vitamin A deficiency
   D. vasectomy
   E. contraceptive use by the female partner
                                   (1:267)

6. Three times in the past month, a 32-year-old married white woman has arrived unexpectedly for consultation after-hours at her family physician's office. She has complained of chest pain, but no specific physical findings can be discovered. She has also complained

17

about the arrogance of the receptionist. The next time she arrives to see the doctor when he is working alone in the evening, he should

A. tell her firmly that there is nothing wrong with her and that she should see a psychiatrist
B. point out that she needs careful, thorough evaluation and give her the next available appointment during scheduled office hours
C. ask her to call the office next morning
D. sit down and have a good, long, heart-to-heart talk with her
E. drive her out of the office   (5:296)

7. Primary prevention programs

A. work to lower the incidence of psychiatric disorders
B. are planned for early identification of schizophrenics
C. minimize the handicapping effect of mental illness
D. operate for adolescents in jail
E. intend to build more mental hospitals
                                        (1:1013)

8. To make a legally acceptable will the person making the will must fulfill all of the following criteria *except* that he need not

A. know that he is making a will
B. know the nature and extent of his property
C. know the natural objects of his bounty
D. know what he is doing when he signs it
E. be able to read and write   (3:859)

9. Three weeks after her three-year-old son was killed in an auto accident, a previously well 28-year-old mother is suffering from waves of somatic distress, is irritable and unfriendly toward her husband, accuses herself unjustly of negligence, is unable to attend to her housework, and is preoccupied with visual images of her son in which she sees him calling her. The situation is probably

A. a normal grief reaction
B. acute psychotic depression
C. psychoneurosis
D. a paranoid state
E. toxic psychosis   (3:181)

10. As part of the adjustment reaction of adolescence, all of the following symptoms may be present *except*

A. school failure
B. delinquency
C. depression
D. sexual impulse
E. paranoid delusions   (1:972)

11. A 35-year-old housewife is very anxious about being at home alone when her husband is away. She states that she is afraid someone may break into the house at night, and says, "I don't see anything wrong with that. None of the women I know like to be alone at night." To facilitate her statement, you should say,

A. "Well, it is reassuring to know you have the same anxieties that other housewives have."
B. "First let us try to understand your feelings and what these feelings do to you."
C. "You are right, nothing is wrong with that."
D. "You mean that most of your friends like to be alone in the daytime."
E. "When you say 'alone' perhaps you are worried about sexual attack."   (3:187)

12. When a patient encourages a physician to assume a directive position and then procrastinates in following the physician's suggestions, he is most likely to be

A. displaying a weak ego
B. trying to compensate for low self-esteem
C. malingering
D. expressing hostility with passive rebellion
E. afraid of the physician   (1:495)

13. Separation anxiety in early childhood may be associated with

A. hospitalization
B. school phobia
C. maternal deprivation
D. transient normal reaction
E. all of the above   (1:929)

14. A child with school phobia

A. requires tranquilizers
B. should be hospitalized to observe how he functions when separated from his family

C. should remain at home until he gets over it
D. should be sent back to school immediately, and then the underlying problem worked out
E. should go to school part-time   (3:472)

15. Adjustment reactions are characterized by

A. transient reactions
B. symptomatic reaction to the current situation
C. symptomatic reaction to emotional conflict
D. relief when the situation is corrected
E. all of the above   (3:538-540)

16. Which of the following statements about anxiety is false?

A. Anxious people usually complain of bodily discomfort which they believe to be actual physical illness.
B. Diarrhea is frequently the chief complaint for which the anxious patient seeks medical care. It is best not to treat the diarrhea symptomatically until its psychological cause is identified.
C. Fatigue and irritability are common symptoms of chronic anxiety.
D. The physician's calm encouragement and reassurance often have strong curative powers.
E. The more acute the anxiety, the better the success of treatment; chronic low-grade anxiety has a poor prognosis. (1:420)

17. A young female patient gives a history of aching anterior chest pain interspersed with sharp stabs. She also complains of palpitations, difficulty in breathing, light-headedness, tingling of the extremities, and exhaustion, and you note that she sighs frequently. Physical examination is negative. The most likely diagnosis is

A. hyperventilation syndrome
B. metabolic alkalosis
C. respiratory acidosis
D. asthma
E. anemia   (1:426)

18. Hysterical patients often develop

A. manic-depressive psychosis
B. schizophrenia
C. involutional melancholia
D. paranoid state
E. obsessive-compulsive neurosis   (3:498)

19. In treating an acute combat neurosis, which of the following is appropriate?

A. Handle the soldier in the front-line station with brief, firm support and temporary sedation.
B. Return the soldier to his home country for retraining.
C. Remove the soldier immediately to the base hospital for intensive psychotherapy.
D. Order the soldier to remain in front-line duty and take disciplinary action.
E. Send the soldier to a military court.
    (1:148)

20. Common fantasies preceding suicidal acts include

A. fantasies of identification
B. fantasies of a reunion
C. fantasies of destroying a "bad" part
D. fantasies of rebirth
E. all of the above   (3:118)

21. The treatment of stuporous patients who have taken barbiturates in suicidal attempts include all of the following except

A. continuous observation of vital signs
B. maintaining an open airway
C. gastric lavage of the ingested drug
D. measurement of urinary output
E. administering intravenous fluids   (1:704)

22. The most frequent cause of death in acute barbiturate poisoning is

A. renal failure
B. hepatotoxicity
C. thromboembolic phenomena
D. gastric hemorrhage
E. respiratory depression   (1:404)

23. Treatment of a "bad trip" precipitated by hallucinogens, particularly LSD, is usually best carried out by

A. administering phenobarbital
B. supportive, repetitive reassurance and orientation
C. arm and leg restraints
D. intravenous administration of Valium (diazepam)
E. none of the above   (3:668)

24. A morphine addict, having developed tolerance to 2 g of morphine per day, undergoes forced abstinence and loses his tolerance. His

reaction to a subsequent 2 g dose of morphine may best be described as

A. unreactive
B. mildly stimulative
C. mildly euphoric
D. strongly euphoric
E. potentially lethal   (1:498)

25. Disulfiram (Antabuse) causes unpleasant effects after ethanol ingestion by

A. preventing the oxidation of ethanol to acetaldehyde
B. inhibiting the oxidation of acetaldehyde formed from ethanol
C. increasing the sensitivity of nerve cells to ethanol
D. increasing the rate of absorption of ethanol
E. enhancing the central action of ethanol
                                             (1:409)

26. Good results in achieving abstinence with alcoholics are obtained by

A. phenothiazine medication
B. vitamin B injections
C. membership in Alcoholics Anonymous
D. long-term hospitalization at mental hospitals
E. imprisonment   (1:537)

27. Methadone is an opiate that

A. does not produce habituation
B. blocks the euphoric effects of other opiates
C. causes no withdrawal symptoms when stopped
D. is a morphine antagonist
E. has no analgesic effect   (1:508)

28. A clinical picture like that of paranoid schizophrenia is seen in patients who habitually take

A. barbiturates
B. heroin
C. marijuana
D. morphine
E. amphetamines   (1:319)

29. Which one of the following classes of drugs is considered the most appropriate in the treatment of anxiety?

A. barbiturates
B. phenothiazines

C. tricyclic antidepressants
D. benzodiazepines (e.g., Librium [chlordiazepoxide], Valium [diazepam])
E. morphine   (1:800)

30. Cannabis and LSD may cause all of the following except one. Select that one.

A. acute panic reaction
B. euphoria
C. fragmentation of thought
D. prolonged enhancement of sexual drive
E. paranoid behavior   (1:513)

31. The premorbid personality of a patient who has an involutional depressive reaction is most likely to have been

A. hypochondriacal
B. passive-dependent
C. compulsive
D. cyclothymic
E. contented   (3:596)

32. What type of psychiatric disorder is frequently associated with carcinoma of the pancreas or large bowel?

A. paranoid reaction
B. phobic state
C. depressive reaction
D. schizophrenia
E. antisocial personality   (3:436)

33. A suicidal patient frequently will exhibit subtle signs of depression. Which of the following feelings is least indicative of depression?

A. paranoia
B. sense of worthlessness
C. guilt
D. sadness
E. hopelessness   (3:405)

34. A 17-year-old white male was seen by you for a laceration wound in his hand. He told you that bad guys wanted him and injured his hand because he was an important person in the school. He also told you about his homosexual desires and that he planned to leave his girlfriend for her promiscuity. You are possibly dealing with a case of

A. involutional depression
B. juvenile delinquency
C. adjustment reaction

D. paranoid state
E. psychoneurosis   (3:453)

35. A response to the proverb "Two heads are better than one," of "A person with two heads could think better" is characteristic of

A. a hysterical disorder
B. good abstraction
C. a schizophrenic reaction
D. severe mental retardation
E. an organic psychotic reaction   (1:317)

36. In the development of schizophrenia, an important process is

A. introjection
B. regression
C. reaction-formation
D. depression
E. sublimation   (3:385)

37. The patient exhibits stiffness, tremor, and an expressionless face. The medication he has been taking for his anxiety is most likely

A. barbiturates
B. Tofranil (imipramine)
C. Thorazine (chlorpromazine)
D. Valium (diazepam)
E. Miltown (meprobamate)   (1:780)

38. Electroshock therapy is frequently modified by the use of succinylcholine to prevent certain complications. The most common complication is

A. temporary hypotension with cerebral hemorrhage
B. dislocation of the hip
C. compression fracture of the midthoracic vertebra
D. rupture of the aorta
E. permanent hypotension with cerebral hemorrhage   (1:612)

39. Jaundice during chlorpromazine therapy is characterized by

A. acute yellow atrophy
B. cirrhosis of the liver
C. serum hepatitis
D. cholestasis
E. hepatolenticular degeneration   (3:823)

40. Pick's disease

A. typically shows symptoms of apathy

B. is more common in men than in women
C. is more common than Alzheimer's disease
D. typically affects the occipital lobe
E. is characterized by senile plaques
                                     (3:244-246)

41. A patient with acute myocardial infarction is admitted to the coronary care unit (CCU). He is extremely anxious. You would

A. prescribe diazepam (Valium)
B. start corticosteroid continuous infusion
C. tell the patient the truth that he will die soon
D. reassure the patient that he has no illness
E. promise the patient that you will discharge him in the morning   (109:202)

42. Thomas is a frequent visitor to the family practice center, where he presents himself as a helpless person who feels he is not being adequately taken care of by the staff there. He is probably

A. passive-aggressive
B. a schizophrenic, hebephrenic type
C. an obsessive-compulsive neurotic
D. a drug addict
E. a phobic neurotic   (5:613)

43. A 35-year-old housewife has had three episodes of chest pain during the past two weeks. Each time she has visited the emergency room, with normal EKG and isoenzymes. Today she visited your office complaining of chest pain of one hour's duration. Results of physical examination and EKG are essentially normal. You would now

A. prescribe digitalis
B. prescribe dobutamine
C. prescribe hydralazine
D. provide psychotherapy
E. give IV morphines   (110:382)

44. A 30-year-old housewife has been afraid of snakes and heights since childhood. During the past six months she has experienced repeated panic attacks whenever she drove the automobile across the downtown area. The treatment of choice is

A. benzodiazepines (Valium)
B. phenothiazines (Thorazine)
C. imipramines (Tofranil)

D. phenobarbital
E. propranolol (Inderal)   (106:129-131)

45. The most dramatic responses to treatment of neuroleptics are generally seen with

A. severely depressed individuals
B. withdrawn and apathetic schizophrenics
C. manic and hypomanic individuals
D. agitated paranoid schizophrenics
E. chronic organic brain syndromes
          (39:625-628)

46. A 70-year-old male living alone was brought to your office by his neighbor for irritability and confusion. He appears emaciated and his tongue is reddish and swollen, with atrophy of papillae and ulcerations. His skin is dry, scaly, and hyperpigmented. The treatment of choice is

A. mycostatin
B. amphotericin B
C. ascorbic acid
D. nicotinamide
E. tetracyclines   (39:806)

47. The most commonly abused drug is

A. Thorazine
B. ampicillin
C. morphine
D. demerol
E. ethyl alcohol   (111:345-360)

48. Lithium may cause

A. central diabetes mellitus
B. central diabetes insipidus
C. nephrogenic diabetes insipidus
D. peripheral diabetes insipidus
E. nephrogenic diabetes mellitus   (111:195)

49. Steepling is most commonly indicative of

A. sadness
B. contemplation
C. defensiveness
D. suspicion
E. confidence   (112:125-134)

50. Olfactory hallucinations most often occur in

A. amphetamine abuse
B. a tumor at the frontal lobe
C. depressive illnesses
D. a patient with phobic state
E. chiasma lesions   (76:2150)

51. A patient tells you that her husband wants her to engage in "unnatural sexual activity." She feels it is wrong but doesn't know what to do and asks your help. You can:

A. call in the husband and tell him to respect his wife's sensitivities.
B. tell the wife that she should try to satisfy her husband's sexual needs; otherwise he might look for gratification elsewhere.
C. suggest she come in with the husband and try to refer them for sex counseling.
D. attempt to clarify the wife's sexual attitudes and her reasons for feeling the activity is wrong, and give her some preliminary guidance.
E. tell her that sex is dirty and not in the realm of family practice.   (102)

52. A husband complains of his wife's being overweight, her sloppiness, and her improper training of the children. He is embarrassed to be seen with her and mentions a miserable childhood with an obese mother he was ashamed of. His wife was thin prior to marriage, but gradually gained considerable weight during the child-bearing and childrearing years. The wife, although wishing she were thin, dismisses her husband's concern about the problem and feels it indicates his lack of understanding of the pressures she is under. You should now:

A. point out to the husband that he is overreacting to the wife's appearance because of his experience with his mother
B. point out to the wife the fact that she may be jeopardizing the marital relationship and offer help with dieting
C. discuss with both the apparent seeds of a serious problem in the marriage, pointing out that this could lead to more serious difficulty which might eventually jeopardize the marriage, and say that professional help should be seriously considered
D. tell the couple that their problems are not in the realm of family practice
E. refer the couple to a psychiatrist immediately since this is a psychiatric emergency
          (100:480-497; 50:276)

53. The prime responsibility for providing emotional support for the terminally ill patient rests with:

A. the head nurse on the ward
B. the social worker

C. the patient's friends
D. the oncologist
E. the attending family physician   *(3:181)*

54. You are called by the police to examine a patient for alcoholism after an accident. The patient refuses to be examined. You then proceed:

A. to examine the patient
B. to draw blood from the patient for determination of alcohol concentration
C. to call for physician assistants to restrain the patient
D. to refuse to examine the patient
E. to inject diazepam intravenously to calm the patient, then examine the patient at your ease   *(33:218)*

55. In the absence of a special contract, the family physician:

A. may guarantee a cure
B. should guarantee that the treatment will benefit his patient
C. is under obligation to exercise ordinary degrees of skill, care, and judgment, as exercised by members of his profession practicing in the same or a similar locality in the light of the present state of medical and surgical science
D. who is practicing in sparsely settled areas must have the same degree of skill and judgment as a physician practicing in urban areas
E. is required by law to exercise an extraordinary degree of special care for his own patients to show physicians' benevolence   *(33:1-2)*

56. Mr. A. has been your patient for a number of years and you know he has a serious cardiac condition. He is married, has seven children, drives a school bus for a living. You have pleaded with him to quit driving the bus, but he has adamantly and consistently refused to do so. His reason for refusing is that he knows he will be unable to find another job, and without work his family will undergo severe economic hardship. His employer, the school board, does not require a physical examination for the job; consequently there is no method by which they can find out about Mr. A.'s condition independently. The following statements are true:

A. as his physician you are legally bound to inform the school board of Mr. A.'s condition
B. as his physician you are bound by your professional code of ethics to keep the information in confidence
C. as his physician you are bound by your professional code of ethics to inform the school board of his condition
D. you should gossip with the mother of a school child who boards your patient's bus
E. none of the above   *(33:385)*

57. Of the following, the causal factor most clearly established in monogolism is:

A. advanced maternal age
B. exposure to radiation
C. maternal anoxia
D. virus infection in the first trimester of pregnancy
E. consanguinity   *(3:739)*

58. For the child, which of the following tests will give the most pertinent information regarding the degree of mental retardation?

A. electronencephalogram
B. psychological examination
C. roentgenograms of the skull
D. blood chemistry
E. pneumoencephalogram   *(3:717)*

Directions: Each group of numbered words or phrases is followed by a list of lettered items. MATCH the lettered item most closely associated with the numbered word or phrase.

Questions 59 to 61
59. Paranoid psychotic reactions
60. Hypertensive crisis precipitated by cheese
61. May exacerbate acute intermittent porphyria

A. Monoamine oxidase (MAO) inhibitor
B. Barbiturates
C. Amphetamines   *(3:444)*

Questions 62 to 65
62. Flight of ideas
63. Sleep disturbance
64. Psychomotor retardation

65. Problems with food intake

    A. Mania
    B. Depression
    C. Both
    D. Neither   (1:714)

Questions 66 to 69
66. Intellectualization
67. Stereotypy
68. Neologism
69. Projection

    A. Schizophrenia
    B. Manic state
    C. Paranoid state
    D. Obsessive-compulsive neurosis   (1:317)

Questions 70 to 73
70. Flight of ideas
71. Word salad
72. Confabulation
73. Circumstantiality

    A. Schizophrenia
    B. Manic state
    C. Korsakoff's psychosis   (1:715)

Questions 74 to 78
74. Sodium chloride
75. Librium
76. Lithium bicarbonate
77. Imipramine (Tofranil)
78. MAO inhibitor

    A. Delirium tremens
    B. Manic state of manic-depressive psychosis
    C. Bromide intoxication
    D. Endogenous depression   (1:388)

Questions 79 to 81
79. Infantile autism
80. Mental retardation
81. Involutional melancholia

    A. Dejection
    B. Confabulation
    C. Mutism
    D. Delayed speech development
    E. Waxy flexibility   (3:693-694)

Questions 82 to 86
82. "I don't know why everything happens to me."

83. "Will you be able to help me, Doctor?"
84. "I know I shouldn't feel this way, but. . ."
85. "How can I get my mind off my problem?"
86. "I know what you are trying to do, Doctor; you're trying to make me angry."

    A. Obsessive-compulsive personality
    B. Hysterical personality
    C. Phobic personality
    D. Depressed personality
    E. Paranoid personality   (1:475)

Questions 87 to 90
87. Hysterical vomiting
88. Globus hystericus in adults
89. Anorexia nervosa
90. Chronic alcoholism (the patient is sober and in good physical condition)

    A. Electroconvulsive therapy
    B. Insulin shock therapy
    C. Prefrontal lobotomy
    D. Psychotherapy
    E. Psychotherapy in conjunction with medical treatment   (4:89, 109, 181)

Questions 91 to 95
91. Alcoholism
92. Anorexia nervosa
93. Hyperkinesis
94. Involutional melancholia
95. Claustrophobia

    A. Panic reaction
    B. Psychosis
    C. Personality disorder
    D. Psychophysiological disorder
    E. Minimal brain dysfunction
                           (4:71, 107, 172, 204)

Questions 96 to 98
96. False fixed belief
97. Misinterpretation of perceptual stimulus
98. Symbolically acts out in reverse something unacceptable that has already been done

    A. Delusion
    B. Illusion
    C. Undoing   (4:34, 37, 60)

Questions 99 to 102
99. Intolerable external reality is removed from awareness

100. Unacceptable strivings, thoughts, and impulses are excluded from awareness
101. Deliberate forgetting of disturbing feelings or ideas
102. Separation of an unacceptable impulse from the memory origin

A. Repression
B. Isolation
C. Denial
D. Suppression   (4:51-60)

Questions 103 to 106
103. WAIS
104. TAT
105. Bender-Gestalt
106. MMPI

A. Test of organicity
B. Projective test
C. Intelligence test
D. Personality profile   (3:205-214)

Questions 107 to 110
107. Test for criminal responsibility
108. Test for insanity
109. Understanding of right and wrong
110. Unable to control the act committed

A. M'Naghten Rule
B. Irresistible impulse
C. Both
D. Neither   (1:1031)

Questions 111 to 114
111. Ambitious, tense, hard-pushing, repressed aggression
112. Passive, hostile, immature
113. Striving with ambivalence about dependency and achievement
114. Cyclothymic, repressed hostility

A. Ulcerative colitis
B. Peptic ulcer
C. Essential hypertension
D. Asthma   (1:598)

Questions 115 to 116
115. Turmoil and identity crisis
116. Initial major period of social integration

A. Ego (adaptive capacity)
B. Superego (conscience)

C. Id
D. Latency
E. Adolescence   (4:15; 5:575)

Questions 117 to 121
117. Sexual energy and drive
118. Pleasure principle
119. Reality principle
120. Conscience
121. Highest personal goal

A. Id
B. Ego
C. Ego-ideal
D. Superego
E. Libido   (1:136)

Questions 122 to 125
122. IQ
123. Personality
124. Localizing brain lesion in all cases
125. Aids in neuropsychiatric evaluation

A. WISC
B. Rorschach test
C. Both
D. Neither   (3:218,220)

Questions 126 to 129
126. Used for adults
127. Personality
128. Intelligence
129. Liver function

A. MMPI
B. WAIS
C. Both
D. Neither   (5:250-252)

Questions 130 and 131
130. Mutism
131. Gradual deterioration is inevitable

A. Catatonic schizophrenic reaction
B. Chronic brain syndrome associated with arteriosclerosis
C. Both
D. Neither   (1:314)

Question 132
132. Beneficial to discuss suicidal thoughts

A. Patient going into depression

B. Patient coming out of depression
C. Both
D. Neither   (1:704)

Questions 133 and 134
133. Terminal crescendo tremor
134. Static and kinetic tremor

A. Parkinsonism
B. Hyperthyroidism
C. Tardive dyskinesia
D. Cerebellar disease
E. Hepatic coma   (76:97-99)

Questions 135 to 137
135. Today a 20-year-old excited man states that the date is 1776, everything appears distorted, and colors are vivid. He hears music in his head.
136. Today a 47-year-old man states the day is June, 1985. His wife states that he recently bought her expensive gifts but now feels he was imprudent and faces financial ruin.
137. Today an 18-year-old man appearing somewhat more disheveled than his current peers states that he does not know the dates. He is concerned that some friends have misplaced objects at his apartment to trick him and are now laughing at his plight.

A. Depression
B. Manic-depressive
C. Organic brain syndrome (presenile or senile dementia)
D. Schizophrenia
E. Toxic psychosis   (3:132)

Directions: For each of the incomplete statements below, ONE or MORE of the numbered completions is correct. In each case select
  A. *if only 1, 2, and 3 are correct*
  B. *if only 1 and 3 are correct*
  C. *if only 2 and 4 are correct*
  D. *if only 4 is correct*
  E. *if all are correct*

138. The characteristics of schizoid personality include

  1. suspicion and withdrawal
  2. overdependence
  3. homosexuality
  4. hypersensitivity   (4:121)

139. The schizophrenic will usually preserve the following mental functions:

  1. affect
  2. intelligence
  3. association
  4. memory   (1:309)

140. Visual hallucination is most commonly caused by

  1. toxic psychosis
  2. trance state
  3. acute brain syndrome
  4. schizophrenia   (5:73)

141. The side-effects of phenothiazines include

  1. blurred vision
  2. loss of ejaculation
  3. fainting
  4. jaundice   (1:773)

142. Psychotic symptoms are *least* often the presenting complaints in

  1. parathyroid adenoma
  2. porphyria
  3. thyrotoxicosis
  4. rheumatoid arthritis   (3:196-205)

143. Patients with postpartum depression

  1. usually have it again with subsequent pregnancies
  2. are often helped by hormone therapy
  3. may need antidepressants
  4. have a much better prognosis than do patients with other forms of depression
                                          (1:380)

144. Onset is most common in adolescence or early adulthood in which of the following?

  1. manic-depressive psychosis
  2. schizophrenia
  3. drug addiction
  4. involutional depressive reaction   (3:359)

145. Involutional melancholia

  1. occurs most often at or about the climacteric
  2. seldom occurs in persons with passive-aggressive personality
  3. is more common in women
  4. requires no treatment   (1:144)

146. The mental disorder(s) in which suicide attempts are most frequent is (are)

1. psychoneurosis
2. manic-depressive illness
3. schizophrenia
4. involutional depression   (4:182,189)

147. Paranoid behaviors may be described as

1. delusions of grandeur
2. litigiousness
3. delusions of persecution
4. violence   (1:479)

148. A favorable prognosis in schizophrenia is suggested by

1. acute onset of the illness
2. catatonic reaction
3. severe precipitating factors in the environment that can be modified
4. acute symptomatology   (4:220)

149. Opiate ingestion is frequently suggested by

1. needle marks
2. miosis
3. urine test
4. abstinence syndrome   (1:505)

150. Youths who abuse and become dependent on amphetamines are likely to have a history of

1. school failure
2. treated hyperkinesis
3. alienation from society
4. gang behavior   (1:515)

151. With continued administration, tolerance often develops to therapeutic effects of

1. meperidine
2. chlorpromazine
3. amphetamine
4. ergotamine   (1:575)

152. Addiction has been associated with the prolonged use of

1. morphine
2. meprobamate (Equanil, Miltown)
3. pentobarbital (Nembutal)
4. chlorpromazine (Thorazine)   (1:575)

153. The following drugs will cause physical dependence:

1. alcohol
2. barbiturates
3. heroin
4. marijuana   (1:575)

154. Frequent complications in comatose patients with acute barbiturate intoxication include

1. pneumonia
2. acute renal insufficiency
3. circulatory failure
4. acute splenic infarct   (5:437)

155. The symptoms of barbiturate withdrawal include

1. insomnia
2. hallucination
3. restlessness
4. convulsions   (1:519)

156. To control a strict superego, gratification should come from

1. self-respect
2. antisocial behavior
3. pride in one's own effort
4. hostility over the accomplishments of one's peers   (3:67)

157. Dyspareunia is frequently associated with

1. sexual satisfaction
2. frigidity
3. anxiety-free status
4. inexperienced women   (5:278)

158. Mary and John have heard about a sensitivity training group (T-group) which is sponsoring a marathon group therapy session. They come to you for advice about such groups and are curious about the possibility of attending. In offering such advice, you would want to determine which of the following?

1. the emotional integrity of the couple
2. the mental illnesses suffered by the couple, if any
3. the qualification and the training of the sponsoring group staff
4. the reasons for attending   (1:758)

159. Which of the following statements are true about masturbation?

1. it does not occur in a marriage in which problems exist in the relationship
2. increased interest in masturbation in elderly patients is often an early sign of senility
3. it is uncommon in children under six
4. it is practiced by males and females at all ages, both married and single   (1:561)

160. The incidence of suicide is higher in

1. advanced age
2. males than females
3. peacetime than in wartime
4. physicians   (*1:706*)

161. Meprobamate (Equanil, Miltown)

1. has less potent tranquilizing activity than does chlorpromazine
2. induces barbiturate-like addiction
3. blocks flexor reflexes
4. releases central stores of norepinephrine   (*1:814*)

162. Treatment of the hyperventilation syndrome includes

1. sedation
2. rebreathing CO_2
3. breathing O_2
4. taking a detailed history of the onset of symptoms in relation to current events in the patient's life   (*1:620*)

163. A 24-year-old woman complains of a sudden onset of weakness which causes her to fall to the floor without loss of consciousness and which develops when she is suddenly surprised or frightened. Which of the following symptoms is *not* likely to be a part of the clinical picture?

1. nocturnal hallucinations
2. sleep paralysis
3. sudden attacks of irresistible sleepiness
4. migraine headaches   (*1:676*)

164. Motives for suicide include

1. a need for self-punishment
2. a wish to join a dead parent
3. revenge
4. psychosis   (*1:707*)

165. A housewife confides in you that her husband is putting pressure on her to consider "switching," or even the possibility of a group marriage. You would now

1. advise the patient that the marriage has no chance for survival
2. advise the patient to conform to her husband's suggestions
3. advise her to seek care elsewhere
4. offer family counseling to explore the situation   (*101:1-43*)

166. A husband and wife complain bitterly of each other's lack of consideration or concern for the other. They are engaged in active feuding, including withholding of money by the husband and refusal to prepare meals by the wife. Each one's complaints center on the refusal of the other to behave in a fashion that would convey caring and consideration about the other. The husband is very worried about money and is enraged that his wife won't economize. The wife states that her husband's worries are exaggerated, that he has always been a miser, and that she can't live as if the wolf were constantly at the door. You would

1. side with the husband in demanding that the wife prepare meals for him
2. provide family counseling to help them work together in less destructive ways
3. provide reassurance for the wife that this quarrel is commonplace in marriage
4. help both parties to clarify expectations   (*100:498-551*)

167. Adaptation stages of a dying patient usually include

1. denial
2. anger
3. depression
4. acceptance   (*111:131-132*)

168. Pseudodementia

1. may increase suicidal risk
2. often shows rapid onset
3. may show cognitive deficit
4. is commonly seen in adolescents   (*109:328*)

169. A patient with grand-mal has been well controlled by phenytoin (Dilantin) for the past five years. During the routine visit, physical examination is unremarkable and he has no specific complaints. The only abnormal blood chemistry finding is the low serum phosphate level of 2 mg/dl. You would now

1. perform lymph node biopsy
2. order intravenous urography
3. order upper gastrointestinal barium studies
4. prescribe vitamin D   (*73:2158*)

170. A working mother brings to your office her seven-year-old boy who has had chronic constipation and recently has frequently soiled his clothes with feces. You would

1. advise the removal of the boy from school
2. advise continuous use of enemas
3. advise the mother to punish the boy whenever fecal soiling occurs
4. start a bowel training (behavioral modification) program   (12:90)

171. A young schizophrenic patient was controlled with chlorpromazine (Thorazine) for a year without any problems. In recent weeks, he has developed tremors, dyskinesia, akathesia, and torticollis. You would now

1. discontinue the drug
2. decrease the dosage
3. switch to a thioridazine (Mellaril)
4. substitute with imipramine (Tofranil)   (73:2004)

172. A 27-year-old male complains of premature ejaculation. His history, physical, and laboratory work-ups are essentially normal. You would now

1. tell the patient the truth, that nothing can be done for him
2. administer depo-testosterone
3. explain the use of coitus interruptus
4. reassure the patient that the condition can be reversed   (73:2030)

173. Seizures may be caused by

1. hyponatremia
2. phenothiazine usage
3. hypoglycemia
4. alcohol usage   (78:1237)

174. A 23-year-old male with heroin overdose has developed pulmonary edema. His blood gases show a pH of 7.47, a Pco_2 of 33 mmHg, and a Po_2 of 44 mmHg. Following the administration of 35% oxygen, his blood gases are expected to be

1. $Pco_2 = 70$ mmHg
2. $Pco_2 = 60$ mmHg
3. $Po_2 = 84$ mmHg
4. $Po_2 = 46$ mmHg   (76:1363)

175. Depression may occur with which of the following medications?

1. alpha-methyldopa
2. propranolol
3. alcohol
4. oral contraceptives   (39:656)

176. Doxepin (Sinequan)

1. has a good sedative effect
2. should be taken with alcohol
3. may not produce desirable effects for three weeks
4. is also useful for glaucoma   (39:631-633)

177. Amitriptyline intoxications are treated with

1. gastric lavage
2. the use of active charcoal
3. physostigmine administration
4. IV atropine   (39:1014)

178. Obesity may be caused by

1. administration of butyrophenone (haloperidol)
2. craniopharyngiomas
3. Cushing's syndrome
4. anorexia nervosa   (78:948-949)

Each of the questions or incomplete statements below is followed by four suggested lettered options. For each of these lettered options, indicate "T" if the option is true, or indicate "F" if the option is false.

179. A patient consults you because he says that he does not know what to do—his wife has expressed much dissatisfaction with him and is currently engaged in an extramarital affair which she makes little attempt to hide from him. The patient says everyone is telling him to leave her. Your contact with the wife reveals her to be unconcerned about her husband's feelings and she openly states that if she could find someone else she would leave him. They have one 13-year-old child. You should:

A. tell the husband that the wife doesn't seem to care much about him and that he should seriously consider separation
B. talk with the wife about the advantages of trying to keep the family together and the destructive effect of her behavior on her husband and son
C. suggest to the husband that perhaps if he stands by, his wife will realize that any relationship has its disappointments and she will then be ready to work on the marriage

D. tell the husband that while you do not object to giving advice, it is obvious that he is deeply unhappy over his wife's behavior and yet he is neither capable nor desirous of leaving her (otherwise he would). Suggest that it would be helpful for him to talk to someone who may be able to help him find a less taxing way of dealing with the situation (whether he stays or goes)   (100:539-543)

180. Which of the following statements is true for the relationship between the physician and patient?

A. it is consensual
B. the physician is bound to render professional service to every patient who applies
C. it may be contractual
D. when a physician obtains a state license to practice medicine, he has to practice medicine immediately   (33:1)

181. Conditions that do not constitute abandonment are those in which the:

A. physician's answering service refuses to call the physician
B. physician and patient mutually agree to terminate the relationship
C. physician accuses the patient of his ignorance and then suddenly refuses to see him
D. patient terminates the relationship   (33:11)

182. Which of the following statements are true concerning the physician's liability for negligence of third person?

A. a family physician who is practicing in a three-man-partnership is liable for the actions of the partners
B. a physician is not responsible for the negligence of a substitute if he uses reasonable care in his selection and the substitute is not in his employment or associated with him as a partner
C. a surgeon who operates at a hospital not owned or controlled by him and who is assisted in an operation by nurses provided by the hospital is not responsible for the mistakes or negligence of such nurses
D. a physician is not responsible for the carelessness of a nurse who gives an erroneous sponge count during a hysterectomy so that a sponge is left inside the abdomen

183. Which of the following statements is/are true about informed consent?

A. the physician's duty is fulfilled when the disclosure is sufficient to enable the patient to make an intelligent choice as to whether or not he desires to have the procedure performed
B. in a medical emergency where the patient is in no condition to make an intelligent determination for himself, disclosure of collateral risks may not be required
C. when an explanation of every attendant risk may result in unnecessarily alarming the apprehensive patient, the disclosure can be limited to relevant facts
D. the physician has no duty to make a full disclosure to the patient of collateral risks and dangers inherent in the suggested treatment or procedure   (33:45)

184. A mother complains that her three-year-old is shy with strangers, tends to cling to her, and does not respond positively to other children. In giving a history, the mother described the child as always having been a "difficult" child—her schedule was never regular, every new situation was met with resistance, she cried easily, etc. The mother is wondering whether her own anxiety—this is her first child—and the negative feelings she sometimes experiences played a role in the child's difficulties, and whether she should get treatment for herself, the child, or both. You will tell the mother that:

A. it is very commendable that she is willing to look at her own reactions, it is possible that her negative feelings have perhaps caused her to be overprotective and to interfere with the child's separation from her, and treatment for her might be an excellent idea
B. she should get treatment for the child since she is bound to have difficulties when she starts school
C. the child will get through the difficulty eventually so there is no reason for her to worry, and that neither she nor her child needs counseling or guidance
D. some children are from birth much more

"difficult" than others, may require special handling, and are bound to heighten any mother's anxiety; and that it might be worthwhile for her to get some help in dealing with the issues that arise, or you could try to help her with it
(52:75-84)

185. A family has a child with cystic fibrosis (CF). The parents seek your guidance concerning the possibility of other children being born with the disease and whether they should have other children. You should now:

A. reassure them that the chances are only one in four that the next child will be born with the illness

B. tell them they owe it to the unborn children not to bring them into the world if there is a chance they will have this disease, because the chances of unhappiness for them and an affected child are overwhelming; suggest adoption if they want more children

C. tell them that much has been done to prolong life expectancy in CF, and perhaps by the time their children reach adolescence, a cure will have been found

D. help them think through how much they want children and consider the risks— what it would mean for a child and for them   (12:1998; 98:118-119, 99:VII-XIII)

186. You are called in because a 15-year-old has made a suicide attempt. She claims that her parents don't love her and are too restrictive, but her parents claim that her behavior shows poor judgment and could get her into serious trouble. You will now:

A. discuss with both the girl and the parents the fact that they have not found a way of living together that meets all their needs, and that they should seek professional help to see if matters could be made more comfortable for all of them

B. suggest that the youngster receive treatment since she needs help both in relation to the behavior and because of the possibility of another suicidal attempt

C. suggest that they let her do what she wants so she will learn from the consequences of the behavior

D. suggest that since the parents are having a difficult time controlling their daughter,

they request a PINS petition (Person In Need of Supervision) from the family court, which will put the power of the court behind them without giving the youngster a record   (96:140-141)

187. A mother complains bitterly that her teenage daughter is secretive, consorts with kids who drink, is irresponsible about household chores, and is sullen when she tries to talk to her about it. She asks whether you could talk to the daughter and get her to behave differently. You do talk to both of them and find that a vicious cycle has been escalating between them in which the parents are more and more restrictive in relation to the girl's social life while the youngster is vacillating between anger at her parents. You also find that they are right in some of their complaints. You will now:

A. reassure the mother that you have known the girl since she was a baby and you are sure that she can't be doing anything wrong, and that many teenagers go through periods like this

B. refer both of them for intensive psychotherapy

C. help the mother (parents) become less restrictive so that a break is made in the cycle of punishment and further defiance

D. tell the daughter how much her mother has done for her and that she should show appreciation by being more cooperative   (97:87-88)

Directions: This part of the test consists of a situation followed by a series of incomplete statements. Study the situation and select the best answer to complete each statement that follows.

John, a five-year-old boy, is referred by his kindergarten teacher for aggressive and destructive behavior in the classroom. He has been a severe behavior problem since birth, showing aggressivity towards his older sister and older brother. His sleeping and eating patterns are erratic. He is described by his mother as always being excitable, overreactive with poor attention, and accident-prone, and he "refuses to listen or learn."

188. Based upon the history, the diagnosis is most likely

A. autism
B. childhood schizophrenia
C. normal child
D. attention deficit syndrome
E. undisciplined child   (1:723)

189. John's developmental history, including neuromuscular maturation and speech development, would likely indicate

A. normal development
B. rapid development
C. erratic and/or delayed development
D. mental retardation
E. that he was a fast learner in nursery or kindergarten   (1:723)

190. John's parental history would most likely show

A. history of mental illness
B. history of epilepsy
C. history of psychosis
D. no significant pathology
E. mental retardation   (2:161-190)

191. Based upon the history and clinical observations, the approximate estimate of intelligence would likely be

A. severely retarded
B. normal
C. borderline
D. superior
E. moderately retarded   (3:205)

192. Which of the following helps confirm your diagnosis?

A. patient's history
B. positive neurological "hard signs"

C. abnormal skull x-rays
D. IQ below 20
E. trisomy 21   (1:723)

193. The hyperactive reaction is usually diagnosed by the following symptoms:

A. hyperactivity
B. irritability
C. short attention span
D. distractibility
E. all of the above   (1:723)

194. The major treatment approaches for John will most likely be

A. parental counseling for the management of the behavioral difficulties
B. special education
C. medication
D. child guidance and follow-up
E. all of the above   (3:814)

195. In terms of your drug treatment, the medication of choice is

A. Benadryl (diphenhydramine)
B. Atarax (hydroxyzine)
C. Valium (diazepam)
D. Quide (piperacetazine)
E. Ritalin (methylphenidate)   (3:815)

196. John's mother is very concerned about the prognosis. You will tell her that in late childhood John will

A. become more hyperkinetic
B. stay the same
C. become less hyperkinetic
D. possibly decrease his intelligence
E. possibly become psychotic   (1:723)

Answers and Explanations

1. **(A)** Superego lacunae allows the individual to act without feelings of guilt. It usually reflects the hidden impulses in the parents which they subtly encourage the child to act out. Children may learn from parental examples.

2. **(C)** The prognosis depends mostly on how motivated the homosexual is to change and the condition of the deviation. The homosexual frequently possesses the ability to relate to the opposite sex (bisexuality).

3. **(D)** Penis size varies in a range fairly constant in the normal male. However, the concern over the size of the penis is practically universal among men. The size of the penis is in the range of 7-11 cm in the flaccid state and 14-18 cm in the erect state. The size of penis bears no direct relationship to the body size and the flaccid dimension bears little relation to the erect dimension. The female genitalia have a wide adaptability to penis size.

4. **(A)** Female orgasm is a unitary concept and experience which cannot be separated into vaginal and clitoral responses. Anatomically and physiologically, there is only one type of orgasm: the rhythmic contractions of the outer third of the vaginal barrel.

5. **(B)** Psychological factors are the greatest cause of impotence. In over 90% of cases, impotence can be traced to conflict between the sexual impulse and its expression because of fear, anxiety, anger, or moral prohibition. The common causes of impotence due to organic factors include diabetes, castration, and multiple sclerosis.

6. **(B)** The therapeutic distance can be maintained by seeing the patient during office hours with attendance of the nurse. To have a long talk with the patient after office hours will increase intimacy and may hamper the doctor-patient relationship. A seductive patient needs comprehensive medical and emotional care in a professional milieu by a family physician before calling for psychiatric consultation.

7. **(A)** Primary prevention programs exist to prevent maladaptation or malfunctioning from ever occurring. Programs for early detection and treatment of the diseases are programs for secondary prevention, while tertiary prevention limits or reduces the handicapping effect of the disease process.

8. **(E)** A person's competency to make a will is known as testamentary capacity. The person signing a will must know clearly what he is doing when he signs it. This means that he knows that he is making a will, and he knows the nature and extent of his property and the natural objects of his bounty (i.e., the members of his family, his warm friends, the institutions he is interested in).

9. **(A)** Grief reactions in mothers who lose small children are commonly severe, with a duration of four to six weeks.

10. **(E)** Adjustment reaction is a temporary, transitional period of maladaptation in response to unusual stresses. Adjustment disturbance in adolescence is usually the rule rather than the exception. An adolescent with paranoid delusion should be suspected as psychotic until proved to be otherwise.

11. **(B)** In order to secure the optimum rapport and maximum information, the physician must be flexible and the interview must be characterized by spontaneity. The patient usually feels that he is understood and his point of view appreciated if the physician permits him to tell his own story. To facilitate further communication, physicians should be nonjudgmental, with no presuppositions.

12. **(D)** This patient is passive-aggressive in personality. He expresses hostile wishes through covert and passive means. Subtle resistances are likely to be masked under a facade of conformity to the therapeutic ritual and the physician is frequently blamed for changes in the patient's life situation. In the face of overt acting-out behavior, realistic limit-setting by the physician may become necessary.

13. **(E)** The separation anxiety in early childhood is the child's fear and apprehension upon being removed from the parent or parent figure. This also happens in children who change foster homes too frequently. To avoid separation anxiety, the mother's overnight stay with her preschool child in the hospital is a valuable supportive measure.

14. **(D)** The child should be engineered back to school as quickly as possible. The parents may accompany the child to school, but should not remain. The teacher must cooperate to keep the child in the classroom. The parents must avoid interest in the child's physical complaints and be firm in preparing the child for school attendance. Family therapy has been tried for severe cases and hospital therapy is only reserved as a last resort.

15. **(E)** Adjustment reactions in infancy are symptomatic responses of the infant to separation from the mother and include developmental delay. Adjustment reactions of childhood are usually manifested in simple repetitive activities, such as nailbiting, thumbsucking, enuresis, masturbation, and temper tantrums. Adjustment reactions of adolescence are largely indicative of the youth's struggle for identity.

16. **(B)** Anxiety is usually successfully treated without intensive psychoanalysis to reconstruct the psychogenesis. Minor tranquilizers often help to alleviate anxiety and make the patient more amenable to psychotherapy, if needed. Relieving the patient's distress (e.g., diarrhea) will enhance the therapeutic relationship.

17. **(A)** One of the most common complaints of anxious patients is difficulty in breathing. Patients often demonstrate this by deep sighs. They frequently complain of fainting, light-headedness, or tingling of the extremities, which are due primarily to a decrease in blood carbonate (a respiratory alkalosis). The diagnosis is often confirmed by asking the patient to hyperventilate, which reproduces the light-headedness, tingling, and faintness. This will also reassure the patient.

18. **(B)** Manic-depressive psychosis is usually found in cyclothymic patients, involutional melancholia is found in obsessive-compulsive patients, and paranoid state is usually found in patients with paranoid personality. Many hysterical patients often display a basically schizoid personality and eventually develop schizophrenia following years in mental hospitals.

19. **(A)** The soldier with an acute combat neurosis should be treated promptly and firmly with strong psychological support, temporary sedation as needed, and early return to duty, if possible. Withdrawal from duty and hospitalization a distance away from the front line tends to accentuate or perpetuate emotional disability.

20. **(E)** Fantasies precede suicidal acts. Family physicians who encounter patients with any of the fantasies mentioned should ask patients about thoughts of suicide. The suicide threat from a patient should call for immediate management.

21. **(C)** Gastric lavage is only advisable in con-

scious patients who have ingested drugs recently. A comatose or markedly confused patient may develop bronchial aspiration during gastric lavage. Intravenous fluids are usually in the form of 5% glucose in water and saline to maintain renal function. Urinary catheterization is usually done to measure the urinary output. Hemodialysis is sometimes indicated. The airway is kept open by intubation; tracheostomy is often required.

22. **(E)** The most frequent cause of death from barbiturate intoxication (accidental ingestion or suicidal attempt) is usually shock due to cardiovascular and respiratory failure. Respiratory failure is more frequent than cardiovascular failure as a cause of death. Artificial respiration should be started for comatose or seriously ill patients.

23. **(B)** "Talking down" is usually the only treatment required for bad trips from hallucinogens. Reality is repeatedly defined by indicating that the frightening experience and the perceptual distortions are caused by the drug. The patient's orientation can be maintained by advising him of his identity, that of those who are with him, and his location, and by helping him to identify concrete objects. If anxiety is very severe and the behavior is uncontrollable, then chlorpromazine given intramuscularly may be indicated. Phenobarbital will further confuse the patient, and restraints may cause the patient to injure himself in panicky attempts to get free. Valium is of little value in patients with acute psychosis.

24. **(E)** The patient has already lost his tolerance to morphine; thus the safe dose for morphine would be 120 mg oral or 30 mg parenteral.

25. **(B)** Ethanol is first oxidized to acetaldehyde and then further oxidized to acetate with the presence of the enzyme aldehyde dehydrogenase. Disulfiram competes with coenzyme NAD for active centers of the enzyme aldehyde dehydrogenase, and thereby reduces the rate of oxidation of acetaldehyde, which then accumulates to cause the unpleasant symptoms, including headache, vomiting, and hypotension. Disulfiram is contraindicated in patients with heart or liver disease.

26. **(C)** Alcoholics Anonymous (AA) is a loosely organized voluntary fellowship of alcoholic persons. The largest identifiable group of abstinent former alcoholics are current or former AA members.

27. **(B)** Although methadone is used for morphine addiction, it is a morphine substitute rather than an antagonist. Methadone will produce the same therapeutic effect (i.e., analgesia) as other opiates, but not the euphoria of other similar substances. It will produce habituation and similar withdrawal symptoms which are milder and more prolonged than those of heroin.

28. **(E)** Amphetamine intoxication usually causes symptoms similar to paranoid schizophrenia. Patients with amphetamine intoxication are often beset by paranoid delusions and fear of attack or harm to themselves. Barbiturates, heroin, marijuana, and morphine may cause schizophrenia-like symptoms; however, schizophrenics can become addicted to any of them.

29. **(D)** Benzodiazepines are called anxiolytic drugs (minor tranquilizers). The major tranquilizers (phenothiazines) and tricyclic antidepressants are no more effective as antianxiety agents, and they commonly produce many side-effects. Barbiturates and opiates produce greater depressant effects on the respiratory system and are more likely to be abused, with risk of suicide.

30. **(D)** The long-term use of cannabis and LSD will cause apathy, lack of drive, lack of libido, and job instability. An acute reaction is fragmentation of thought, euphoria, paranoid behavior, and acute panic reaction, which may lead to suicide and violence. The acute intoxication is usually treated with psychotherapy (talk-down) and phenothiazines.

31. **(C)** In a significant number of cases of the involutional depressive reaction, the patient's previous personality often was compulsive, inflexible, rigid, and superego-dominated. Involutional depression often evolves out of a marked neurosis of earlier life.

32. **(C)** Depressive reactions are frequently en-

countered in carcinoma of the pancreas or large bowel. Symptoms of depression, anxiety and premonition of serious illness are among the most common presenting complaints of patients with carcinoma of the pancreas.

33. **(A)** Depression is the most common precursor of suicide, and the depressed patient who exhibits the following symptoms in severe forms should be regarded as a serious risk: guilt, worthlessness; hopelessness; withdrawal; loss of appetite for food, sex, sleep, and activity; extreme agitation; and an intense wish for punishment.

34. **(D)** The characteristics of the paranoid state are hyperalertness, oversuspiciousness, reality distortion, and jealous, erotic, grandiose, persecutory, and litigious delusions. The paranoid psychotic often engages in homosexuality and is overly jealous toward the partner. The stress is often aggravated by injury.

35. **(C)** One of the characteristics of schizophrenia is the disturbance of thinking. Patients with organic brain lesions will tend to omit important items, but schizophrenics think and reason in their own autistic terms, according to their own intricate private rules of logic.

36. **(B)** By the mechanism of regression, the personality may suffer loss of some of the development already attained and revert to a lower level of integration, adjustment, and expression. The stronger the fixations which may have been established during the course of development, the more readily will frustrating and conflicting situations be evaded by regression to those fixations. Extreme forms and degrees of regression result in a serious disorganization of personality and thus constitute an important element in schizophrenia.

37. **(C)** The neuroleptic triad of parkinsonism, dystonia, and aleathisia may occur with phenothiazine therapy. If symptoms are distressing or disabling, a reduction in dose or an antiparkinsonian medication may be indicated. However, minor tranquilizers are often used for anxiety therapy instead of the major tranquilizers (phenothiazines).

38. **(C)** Muscle relaxants are used to prevent fractures during the convulsion by the electroshock. Curare was discontinued because of fatality due to central effect. Succinylcholine is used most frequently. Patients with deficiency of the enzyme succinylcholinesterase may die from prolonged apnea. A short-acting intravenous barbiturate is often used as premedication to anesthetize the patient.

39. **(D)** Jaundice usually appears from the second to the eighth week after the institution of chlorpromazine therapy in approximately 4% of cases. There is no evidence of damage to the hepatic parenchyma; the jaundice is cholestatic in origin. The drug should be discontinued if jaundice appears.

40. **(A)** Pick's disease is an uncommon chronic brain syndrome. It occurs much less frequently than does Alzheimer's. This affliction occurs twice as frequently in women as in men. Typically, the patient shows apathy, loss of memory, and inability to deal with new situations. Aphasia gradually develops, along with the established dementia. The brain areas involved are mainly the frontal and temporal lobes. Senile plaques, frequently found in senile dementia, are rarely found in Pick's disease.

41. **(A)** Patients admitted to the CCU are frequently suffering from CCU neurosis, which may include profound anxiety and deep depression due to pain, fear of death, uncertainty, confinement, cerebral hypoxia, sleep disturbances, and the frightening features of the environment. The defense mechanism of denial is commonly seen and may be beneficial for the patient. The family physician should deal with the patient with honesty and compassion.

42. **(A)** People with passive-aggressive personality show both passivity and aggressivity. The aggressiveness is usually expressed in such passive ways as obstructionism, pouting, procrastination, clinging, indecisiveness, and helplessness. These patients are often manipulative and are sometimes very annoying to the medical staff. A progressively wider spacing of appointments is frequently employed.

43. **(D)** Cardiac neurosis is characterized by chest pains, shortness of breath, a sense of tightness in the chest, faintness, and weakness. The patient perceives the impending heart attack and an emergency room visit is prompted. Prescription of diazepam (Valium) and reassurance usually result in subsequent recurrences. Psychotherapeutic intervention is necessary to identify the precipitating factors (friends with cardiac problems, fantasies, stresses) and to assist the patient in gaining insights.

44. **(C)** Agoraphobia is characterized by fear of going out into the open, into closed spaces, or into streets and crowds. Spontaneous panic attack will develop with extreme fearfulness, feelings of impending doom, and cardiorespiratory symptoms (pounding heart and dyspnea). Confrontation with the avoided object or activity is needed to eliminate the patient's anxiety. Imipramine (Tofranil, Imavate) and phenelzine (Nardil, a monoamine oxidase inhibitor) are the drugs of choice due to their antipanic effects.

45. **(D)** Common neuroleptics include chlorpromazine (Thorazine), trifluoperazine (Stelazine), thioridazine (Mellaril), thiothixene (Navane), and haloperidol (Haldol). The best response to neuroleptics is seen in acute schizophrenia, when agitation, paranoid delusions, and hallucinations are present. Response in withdrawn, apathetic, or chronic schizophrenics is less favorable. Neuroleptics are also useful for the immediate management of a manic episode and for the treatment of psychotic organic brain syndromes to reduce confusion. They are also used as adjunct drugs to antidepressants in the treatment of involutional melancholia.

46. **(D)** Pellagra is often seen in patients with alcoholism, liver cirrhosis, chronic diarrhea, diabetes mellitus, tuberculosis, thyrotoxicosis, malignant carcinoid, and neoplasia.

47. **(E)** Although heroine addiction attracts the most attention, alcohol remains the most widely used drug of abuse. This is partly due to the easy availability of alcohol and its ready social acceptance. Alcoholism is the most common cause of drug abuse and hospitalization and is a common problem encountered in family practice offices.

48. **(C)** Lithium is used for mania and depression in manic-depressive illness. Its side-effects include nausea, vomiting, diarrhea, tremor, hypothyroidism, and nephrogenic diabetes insipidus (polyuria, polydipsia, and concentration defects).

49. **(E)** In steepling, the patient joins his hands with his fingers extended and his fingertips touched. This often indicates confidence and assurance. When the patient is sad, the hands are droopy and flaccid and the feet move in a slow, circular pattern. In contemplation, the hand is at the chin, stroking the chin or beard. In the defensive position, the arms are crossed, the legs are crossed, and the head is drawn back. A suspicious person often puts his hands in his pockets or behind his back and does not show open palms.

50. **(C)** Olfactory hallucinations are often central in origin, usually caused by lesions on the inferior and medical surface of one temporal lobe in or near the uncus; the seizure it produces is therefore called uncinate. Olfactory hallucination is commonly caused by patients with depressive illness or schizophrenia. In these patients olfactory sensations are intact and the disagreeable smelling odors are delusions.

51. **(D)** There is much the family physician can do before deciding that the sexual difficulty is serious enough to warrant referral for sex therapy. The patient's raising this question with the physician indicates that she trusts him or her enough to be receptive to his or her gradual suggestion that sexual satisfaction is "a continuum of experience with each position on the continuum equally important in and of itself," as opposed to the notion that only orgasm achieved through vaginal penetration is normal. The patient's reactions to sexuality can be briefly explored, with emphasis on helping her think of what would make the sexual experience more pleasurable for her. The couple can then be helped to communicate more effectively concerning each other's needs. The husband can be asked to come in, but at a time and in a way so that he will not perceive it as an occasion for chastisement.

52. **(C)** The problem presented by this couple

contains the seeds of serious marital difficulty. The husband seems to be a compulsive character who cannot tolerate the disorganization that is attendant on family living. He sees raising the children as the wife's responsibility rather than a shared one, and is asking for something that may be quite impossible to achieve in this family: a wife and children who are compulsive in the same areas he is. The wife is rebelling against the husband's putting all responsibility on her, and her overweight may be a way of getting back at him. This only widens the gulf between them. It is important to help this couple get counseling, since otherwise they will either remain together with more and more friction and conflict or the marriage might break up.

53. **(E)** The dying patient arouses very uncomfortable feelings in the physician, death reminds him of his own mortality. All too often, the dying patient for whom nothing else can be done is neglected by the attending physician and the nursing staff. This should never be allowed to happen, as terminally ill patients suffer from extreme loneliness and hopelessness and must receive emotional support from the attending family physician.

54. **(D)** If a physician is called upon to examine the individual as a patient who is in need of treatment, he can proceed with all the freedom granted by the rules of his profession, provided that the patient does not object to the examination. If the patient objects, the physician should make a note that medical attention was refused and should not examine the patient; treatment without consent can become assault and battery.

55. **(C)** The liability of a physician's cure is compared with the careful and skillful physicians practicing in a similar community or in accordance with his school of medicine.

56. **(E)** Principles of medical ethics provide that a family physician may not reveal the confidences entrusted to him in the course of medical attendance, or the deficiencies he may observe in the character of patients, unless he is required to do so by law or unless it becomes necessary to do so to protect the welfare of the individual or of the community. The family physician is the judge of the need for disclosure, except when commanded to speak by a court.

57. **(A)** Late maternal age has been related to the birth of children with Down's syndrome. Nondisjunction of chromosomes is typically related to the older mother.

58. **(B)** The degree of mental retardation is best measured through psychological examination for eventual social adjustment. The level of mental retardation is frequently determined by the intelligence quotient (IQ).

59. **(C)** Amphetamine psychosis is characterized by vivid visual hallucination and paranoid reaction (persecutory delusions and ideas of reference). Food stuffs containing tyramine (e.g., cheese, beer, wines, chicken liver, and pickled herring) used concurrently with MAO inhibitors will cause severe hypertensive crisis. Barbiturates are absolutely contraindicated in patients with acute intermittent porphyria, as they can precipitate an acute attack.

60. **(A)**

61. **(B)**

62. **(A)**

63. **(C)**

64. **(B)**

65. **(C)** Flight of ideas is characteristic of mania; psychomotor retardation (slowness, tiredness, or lack of outward initiative) is characteristic of depression. The depressed patient usually has poor appetite and low food intake, while the manic patient may eat voraciously or be too active to eat adequately. The manic patient may be so active that he never gets to bed or is no sooner in bed than he is up; the depressed patient usually can get to sleep but tends to awaken early and stay awake.

66. **(D)**

67. **(A)**

68. **(A)**

69. **(C)** Neologism refers to the coinage of new words, usually by condensing several other words, each of which has a special meaning for the patient. Stereotypy is the constant repetition of any speech pattern or action; both are characteristics of schizophrenia. Projection is the attribution to another person or object of thoughts, feelings, motives, or desires which are really one's own disavowed and unacceptable traits, mostly seen in the paranoid state. Intellectualization is a state of brooding or anxious pondering about abstract theoretical or philosophical issues which is frequently seen in adolescents as a reaction to the emerging sexual impulses and is also seen in obsessive-compulsive neurosis.

70. **(B)**

71. **(A)**

72. **(C)**

73. **(A)** Word salad is usually seen in schizophrenia; it is a type of speech in which neologisms or incoherent words or phrases that lack logical meaning are used exclusively. Circumstantiality is a disorder of association in which too many associated ideas come into consciousness because of too little selective suppression. The circumstantial patient eventually reaches his goal after many digressions. Excessive detail is employed to describe simple events, at times to an absurd or bizarre degree. Circumstantiality is seen in schizophrenia and organic brain disease. Flight of ideas is a nearly continuous high-speed flow of speech. The patient leaps rapidly from one topic to another, with each topic being more or less related to the preceding topic or to environmental stimuli, but progression of thought is illogical and the goal is never reached. This is characteristic of an acute manic state. Confabulation is an unconscious filling in of gaps in memory by imagined experiences. These recollections change from moment to moment and are easily induced by suggestion. It is characteristic in Korsakoff's psychosis.

74. **(C)**

75. **(A)**

76. **(B)**

77. **(D)**

78. **(D)** Elimination of bromide in bromide intoxication is hastened by the administration of sodium chloride by mouth or by intravenous infusion of physiological saline. Paraldehyde is used for delirium tremens along with Thorazine (chlorpromazine). Lithium carbonate is used for manic episodes of the manic-depressive psychosis. Tricyclic antidepressants (e.g., imipramine) and monoamine oxidase inhibitors (e.g., phenelzine [Nardill] are used for endogenous depression.

79. **(C)**

80. **(D)**

81. **(A)** Mutism is a form of negativism characterized by refusal to speak for conscious or unconscious reasons. Children with infantile autism usually fail to use language for the purpose of communication and are obsessively fascinated by objects, forming poor interpersonal relationships. However, the intellectual potential is preserved and speech development is not usually delayed, although these children cannot communicate meaningfully. The mentally retarded usually show delayed development, including that of speech. Dejection is the key symptom of involutional melancholia (depression). Waxy flexibility is the maintenance of imposed postures, as when a limb remains passively in the position in which it is placed. This phenomenon is characteristic of catatonic schizophrenia.

82. **(B)**

83. **(C)**

84. **(A)**

85. **(D)**

86. **(E)** Hysterical patients are usually egocentric, helpless, attention-seeking, and manipulative. Phobic patients usually express a magical wish along with fear that the wish will not be granted. Obsessive-compulsive patients will often use the defense of intellectualization. The depressed patient is pre-

occupied with worries. Paranoid patients frequently show suspiciousness and mistrust.

87. (D)

88. (D)

89. (E)

90. (E) Hysterical vomiting usually occurs in children, and globus hystericus (the sensation of having a lump in the throat) usually occurs in adults. The somatic symptoms are frequently converted from the anxiety which arises out of some conflictual situation. Psychotherapy is the usual treatment. Anorexia nervosa is a psychophysiological reaction characterized by extreme emaciation caused by loss of appetite. The treatment must include a combined medical and psychiatric approach. The treatment of chronic alcoholism often requires the use of medication (e.g., Librium) and psychotherapeutic approaches.

91. (C)

92. (D)

93. (E)

94. (B)

95. (A) Alcoholism is a personality disorder characterized by excessive use of alcohol to the point of habituation, overdependence, or addiction. Anorexia nervosa is a form of psychophysiological disorder characterized by marked, prolonged appetite loss with accompanying marked weight loss (psychogenic malnutrition), frequently seen in young people. Hyperkinesis is usually caused by minimal brain dysfunction with overactivity, restlessness, distractibility, and short attention span. Involutional melancholia is a psychotic reaction with initial onset in the involutional period (late middle life), characterized by depressive affect or paranoid mentation. Claustrophobia is the persistent obsessive fear of closed (confined) places, a form of neurosis.

96. (A)

97. (B)

98. (C) Delusions are false fixed beliefs that are not in keeping with the individual's cultural or educational level. Delusions are observed in psychotic reactions. Illusions are misinterpretations of real external sensory experiences (usually optical or auditory). These are frequently normal. Undoing is a primitive defense mechanism in which some unacceptable past behavior is symbolically acted out in reverse, usually repetitiously (symbolic atonement); it is frequently seen in obsessive-compulsive neurosis.

99. (C)

100. (A)

101. (D)

102. (B) Denial is an unconscious mechanism wherein one behaves as if the problem does not exist, but lying is a conscious process. Denial is the simplest form of ego defense and is closely related to rationalization. Repression, the motivated unconscious forgetting, is the earliest and one of the most commonly employed defense mechanisms; it is the cornerstone of psychodynamics. Suppression is conscious forgetting, is not a true defense, and is a commonly employed coping mechanism of normal personalities. Isolation can remove the emotional charge associated with the original memory. This mechanism is commonly used by obsessive-compulsive persons.

103. (C)

104. (B)

105. (A)

106. (D) TAT (Thematic Apperception Test) is a semistructured projective test consisting of 20 drawings of persons engaged in various activities. The patient is asked to make up a story for each drawing. Bender-Gestalt test is a test of organic involvement which measures an individual's ability to remember and reproduce complex geometric designs. WAIS (Wechsler Adult Intelligence Scale) is an individual test to measure intelligence by means of verbal and performance tests. MMPI (Minnesota Multiphasic Personality Inventory) consists of 550 questions designed to construct the personality profile of the subject.

107. **(C)**

108. **(D)**

109. **(A)**

110. **(B)** The M'Naghten rule defines criminal responsibility, which concerns the ability of the defendant to know he was doing wrong. It is not a test of sanity and is not formulated as such; rather, it is a test of legal responsibility for acts. This M'Naghten rule is supplemented by the irresistible impulse rule, which states that the accused cannot be held responsible for his behavior if he was unable to resist acting as he did.

111. **(C)**

112. **(A)**

113. **(B)**

114. **(D)** These illnesses are called psychophysiological disorders. Ulcerative colitis is usually associated with patients who are sensitive to rejection or hostility. Peptic ulcer is usually associated with patients struggling between conflicting desires and independence. Hypertension is commonly seen in patients with repressed aggression. Although there are wide variations of personality disturbances among asthmatics, classic asthmatics are those with cyclothymic personalities.

115. **(E)**

116. **(D)** The latency period is the period of middle childhood from the fifth through the ninth years. During the latency period, the child turns away from the restricted family constellation toward other, outside relationships. This is the initial major period of social integration. The period of adolescence is that between puberty and young adulthood (approximately ages 12 to 20), which is marked by a great surge of physical develop-

ment and major social and psychological adjustments. Emotional turmoil and identity crisis are frequently seen.

117. **(E)**

118. **(A)**

119. **(B)**

120. **(D)**

121. **(C)** Libido is the sexual instinctual forces and drives. Id is composed of all the instinctual drives, including sexual (libido) and nonsexual, and is bound by the pleasure principle. Ego is motivated primarily by logical secondary process thinking, which makes possible the delay of gratification through the reality principle. Ego-ideal is the idealized self-image, the private personal optimal goal. Superego is the conscience part of the personality, derived largely from significant relationships in which standards and models, good and bad, have been set.

122. **(A)**

123. **(B)**

124. **(D)**

125. **(C)** WISC (Wechsler Intelligence Scale for Children) is an intelligence test which aids in evaluating the impact of pathology on the intellectual and cognitive capacities of children. The Rorschach test is designed to deduce personality traits of individuals from an analysis of spontaneously produced visual images stimulated by indeterminate stimuli: a set of inkblots. The test is useful in making neuropsychiatric diagnoses. Both WISC and Rorschach tests are too nonspecific to date to localize the brain lesion in common clinical practice.

126. **(C)**

127. **(A)**

128. **(B)**

129. **(D)** MMPI (Minnesota Multiphasic Personality Inventory) is a personality test for adults

and adolescents aged 16 and up. It can be administered and scored by a relatively untrained person, with the final interpretation done by experienced professionals. WAIS (Wechsler Adult Intelligence Scale) is an intelligence test used for ages 16 years and over.

130.   **(A)**

131.   **(D)** The prognosis for both diseases is not always hopeless. The prognosis for the duration of chronic brain syndrome associated with arteriosclerosis is somewhat in excess of four years, on average. However, the mental state is characterized by episodic disease with intervening plateaus often lasting considerable periods of time. Mutism is characteristic of catatonic schizophrenia, the withdrawn type. The prognosis of catatonic schizophrenia is more favorable than that of other types of schizophrenia.

132.   **(C)** Depressed patients have a short attention span and the initial interview must be brief. However, the depressed patient is at high risk for a suicide attempt, particularly coming out of and going into the depression. The possibility of suicidal preoccupation should be approached directly. Many patients feel relieved to be able to talk to a confidant about such thoughts. Verbal expression may lessen the need to take action.

133.   **(D)**

134.   **(B)** Parkinsonism is characteristic for resting tremor (pill-rolling tremor), bradykinesia, mask face, loss of associated movements, and decreased range of movement and can be treated by giving L-dopa. Tardive dyskinesia is caused by phenothiazine administration; athetosis is the predominant character of tremor. "Flapping tremor" (asterixis) is a nonrhythmic asymmetric lapse involuntary sustained posture of the extremities; this is seen in hepatic encephalopathy but not in hepatic coma. The tremor of hyperthyroidism is best seen with the arms extended and the fingers spread apart. It represents an abnormal accentuation of physiologic static-kinetic tremor and therefore predominantly involves the flexion-extension movements, is small in amplitude, and occurs at a rate of about 10-12 Hz. A terminal crescendo tremor

is a hallmark of disorders of the outflow pathway of the cerebellum (from dentate nucleus) and its connections in the midbrain and thalamus.

135.   **(E)**

136.   **(B)**

137.   **(D)** Toxic psychosis can be caused by the use of hallucinogens (LSD), amphetamines, or alcohol. The reply "1776" is facetious. Hallucinogens often distort perceptions and may also cause hallucinations with vivid color images. The manic-depressive person is characterized by a recent high and current depression; during the manic cycle he may overspend while in the depression cycle he may feel impending bankruptcy. Schizophrenics are so preoccupied with paranoid delusions that the date is unimportant to them any way.

138.   **(E)** People with schizoid personality often become schizophrenic in later life. Schizoid personality includes shyness, oversensitivity, seclusiveness, avoidance of close or competitive relationships, and often eccentricity. Autistic thinking and daydreams are common, and such people are often unable to express hostile and aggressive feelings. They often become homosexuals.

139.   **(C)** Schizophrenia is characterized by the disturbance of association, affect, and activity; however, the function of intelligence and memory is usually spared.

140.   **(A)** Schizophrenia is usually characterized by auditory hallucination. Visual hallucinations, which are common among primitive peoples during trance states, are benign in nature and disappear with the termination of the trance. Colorful and vivid visual hallucinations are found in acute brain syndromes, including acute infectious diseases and lesions in the visual cortex. Visual hallucinations are frequently experienced by amphetamine and LSD users. In delirium tremens, the visual images tend to be terrifying.

141.   **(E)** The side-reactions of phenothiazines include pseudoparkinsonism, blurred vision, inhibition of ejaculation, postural hypotension, and jaundice.

142. **(D)** Although uncommon, psychotic symptoms do occur in patients with hyperparathyroidism owing to adenomatosis. Usually the presenting picture has been that of acute brain syndrome (delirium) or behavioral change expressed with depressive or paranoid psychosis. In many untreated patients with thyrotoxicosis, paranoid psychosis may occur. Psychotic hallucinatory and delusional experiences frequently occur in patients with porphyria. Patients with rheumatoid arthritis often demonstrate suppressed grief and hostility rather than psychotic symptoms.

143. **(B)** Postpartum depression carries a prognosis similar to that of other forms of depression. It is liable to recur with subsequent pregnancies at a rate of 15-25%. Antidepressants and electroconvulsive therapy are useful in treatment; hormonal therapy is not helpful.

144. **(A)** Schizophrenia frequently begins in adolescence or early adult life, as does drug addiction. Onset of manic-depressive psychosis is usually between the ages of 15 and 40. Involutional depressive reaction usually begins at climacteric (late adulthood).

145. **(B)** Involutional melancholia occurs three to five times more commonly among women and usually occurs between ages 40 and 65 (at the climacteric). It occurs more commonly in people with the obsessive-compulsive or passive-aggressive personality. If untreated, the prognosis is very poor. With treatment by electroshock therapy and antidepressant medication, the recovery rate is excellent.

146. **(C)** Involutional depression presents the greatest suicide risk of all mental disorders; however, the physician also has to keep in mind the possible danger of suicide among patients with manic-depressive illness, particularly during the initial and final phases of the depressive episode.

147. **(E)** The characteristic paranoid behaviors are jealousy, eroticism, grandiosity, litigiousness, and persecution. The most frequent and the most important behavior is the delusion of persecution, which often leads the patient to believe that he is threatened, causing him to take violent action in self-defense.

148. **(E)** In general, the prognosis of schizophrenia is guarded. However, the following signs are considered to be favorable: sudden onset with conspicuous precipitating factors; presence of affective (depression or elation), catatonic, or confusional symptoms; marriage; a well-adjusted premorbid social life.

149. **(E)** Bluish phlebitic scars and needle marks may indicate that the patient has used opioids in the past. The presence of miosis and some degree of drowsiness would suggest that the patient is under the influence of opioids at the time of examination. A characteristic abstinence syndrome (yawning, pupillary dilatation, muscle twitching, abdominal cramps, vomiting, hypertension, and sweating) can be elicited by withdrawal of the opioids. If the patient has used opioids in the previous 24 hours, their presence in the urine can be demonstrated by chemical or chromatographic tests.

150. **(E)** Drug-dependent youths have used drugs in an attempt to solve their maladaptive behavior problems, such as school failure and alienation from society. However, the therapeutic use of amphetamines for hyperkinesis and narcolepsy of childhood may also lead to dependence on the drugs without careful monitoring. Some youths become addicted to earn respect from peers.

151. **(B)** Meperidine (Demerol) and amphetamines will cause tolerance to therapeutic effect. Tolerance often develops to the sedative effect (not the main therapeutic effect) of chlorpromazine and other phenothiazines over a period of days or weeks (one to two weeks). Usually tolerance does not develop to the antipsychotic effects (main therapeutic effect of chlorpromazine) of phenothiazines.

152. **(A)** Narcotics (e.g., morphine) and barbiturates (e.g., pentobarbital) will cause both psychological and physical dependence. Meprobamate will cause psychological dependence and also physical dependence in higher dosage over a prolonged period. Chlorpromazine does not appear to be addicting.

153. **(A)** Physical dependence refers to physical symptoms that appear when the drug is withdrawn. Symptoms of withdrawal are re-

ferred to as the abstinence syndrome and are the result of addiction to morphine, heroin, methadone, barbiturates, and alcohol; thus they will produce physical dependence. Nicotine, cocaine, marijuana, LSD, caffeine, and amphetamines will cause emotional dependence. Minor tranquilizers (e.g., Miltown, Librium, Valium) in large doses will often cause abstinence syndrome.

154. **(A)** The frequent complications of acute barbiturate intoxication, which often lead to death, include cardiovascular failure, respiratory distress, renal insufficiency, and pulmonary pathology resulting from immobilization, including acute pulmonary edema, atelectasis, and pneumonia. Pneumonia is the most frequent complication, and prophylactic antibiotics are often instituted.

155. **(E)** The earliest sign of barbiturate withdrawal is insomnia accompanied by weakness, restlessness, sweating, and shakiness occurring within 24 hours of cessation. Postural hypotension, muscular twitching, vomiting, anxiety, delirium, and hallucination also occur. Convulsions usually appear after 15 hours of withdrawal; psychotic symptoms begin between the third and the seventh days. Withdrawal symptoms rarely last more than one week.

156. **(B)** An inflexible, strict superego will usually lead to unhappiness and neurosis; however, a defective superego will encourage hostile and antisocial behaviors without guilt. When ego functioning is evaluated as striving toward or achieving the ideals and goals, the superego will facilitate pleasurable satisfactions to prevent strict inflexibility. Thus gratification comes from self-respect, personal integrity, pride in effort or accomplishment, or self-righteousness.

157. **(C)** Dyspareunia is painful or difficult sexual intercourse in the female. It is usually present in patients with severe or chronic frigidity, but it may also be present in young or inexperienced women. Dyspareunia and vaginismus are usually the consequence of anxieties and fears that impair sexual satisfaction in women.

158. **(E)** A sensitivity training group seeks to develop self-awareness and an understanding of group processes rather than to gain relief from emotional disturbances. The emotionally disturbed person should not be referred to the T-group with the expectation that he will thereby achieve relief of his illness. Mentally ill individuals should not be referred to the T-group, which will only increase the psychiatric casualties. The staff members of the encounter group have to be trained to deal with difficult complications of group encounters and to select the members carefully to be useful in the group dynamic process. The motives of the couple are also important considerations.

159. **(D)** Research by Kinsey into the prevalence of masturbation indicated that nearly all men and three-fourths of all women masturbate at some time during their lives. Sexual self-stimulation is very common in infancy and childhood. Masturbation becomes more frequent in adults to whom intercourse is not available; thus it is common among the elderly.

160. **(E)** Suicide is the tenth most prevalent cause of death in the United States. The suicide rate is higher in peacetime than in wartime, and it is four times higher for men than for women. The incidence of suicide increases with increasing age. Physicians have ten times higher suicide risk than the general populace. The suicide rate is also higher for single, divorced, and widowed adults.

161. **(A)** Meprobamate is different from chlorpromazine in that it is only useful for neurosis and of little value for psychosis. The pharmacological effects of meprobamate are very similar to those of barbiturates, are undistinguishable from amobarbital, and will produce tolerance and addiction. Withdrawal symptoms include convulsion, coma, and psychotic behavior. Meprobamate has muscle relaxant activity and will depress the flexor and patellar reflexes in decerebrate cats.

162. **(C)** Rebreathing CO_2 by means of placing a paper bag over the nose and mouth will restore the imbalance caused by the decreased blood carbonate due to respiratory alkalosis in the hyperventilation syndrome. The exploration of life events at the time of onset of symptoms will form the basis of psychotherapy to treat the anxiety underlying the hyperventilation syndrome.

163. **(D)** The symptoms cited are characteristic of narcolepsy, which is a pathology of sleep. It includes overwhelming sleep attacks, together with cataplexy (sudden loss of tone), sleep paralysis (total inability to move the body while in a state of relative mental alertness and orientation on awakening from sleep), and hypnagogic hallucinations (very vivid imagery that occurs on falling asleep and on awakening). Narcolepsy is a disorder of REM (rapid eye movement) sleep, or dreaming sleep.

164. **(E)** Suicide frequently occurs in psychotics, associated with delusions or hallucinations; it is also common in depressed patients. Some patients commit suicide out of revenge against a loved person. The act of dying by suicide is often perceived by the patient as a pleasurable reunion with a dead person, frequently the parental figure. A need for self-punishment in patients is usually associated with failure at work.

165. **(D)** Sexual behavior has changed rapidly, with many lifestyles being tried which in the past would not have been considered. In studies of couples engaged in switching or those entering group marriages, it has been found that these steps are much more frequently an attempt to cope with and save a marriage which has some problems in it than a first step toward the dissolution of a marriage. A family counseling session is needed to explore the true meaning of "switching" for the husband, and support should be offered for the couple to work through the problems (including sexual problems) they have had.

166. **(C)** The marriage apparently is in serious trouble and it is likely that without professional help from their family physician they will be unable to modify their malignant interaction. In providing family counseling, the family physician is advised to refrain from siding with either party until the situation is clarified. Even if there is reality in the husband's concern about the finances, it is obvious that this couple is dealing with the stresses confronting them by attacking each other and trying to change each other, rather than by finding some way of working together in a way that would take each one's needs and differences into consideration. The spouses have by now perceived each other as enemies who make life hard to bear. The family physician can point out what each is doing and the consequences of their actions; he can tell them that if they continue this way, the situation will probably continue to deteriorate. The family physician can help them clarify whether the relationship is salvageable and whether a somewhat less destructive way of living together can be found. If the situation gets worse, the couple can be referred to an experienced family counselor for further assistance.

167. **(E)** Kübler-Ross has postulated five stages of dying: denial, anger, bargaining, depression, and acceptance. The family physician providing care for dying patients needs to offer support and to radiate realistic hope for the patient. The dying patient is badly in need of comprehensive and continuous care.

168. **(A)** Pseudodementia is seen in the elderly person with rapid onset who complains of cognitive deficit and memory impairment. In the interview, the patient often responds with the answer, "I don't know." The patient appears sad, depressed, preoccupied, anxious, and may show the symptom of self-accusation with increased suicidal risk. The patient often has a previous history of depression or mania.

169. **(D)** Long-term use of Dilantin may be associated with hyperplasia of the gums, folate-responsive megaloblastic anemia, peripheral neuropathy, osteomalacia, hypophosphatesemia, and lymphoma. The early sign of osteomalacia includes low phosphate, normal calcium, elevated alkaline phosphatase, bone pain (low back pain), and muscular weakness. Vitamin D (in large doses) and phosphate (milk is rich in phosphorus) can be administered.

170. **(D)** Encopresis is often associated with chronic constipation, fecal impaction, overflow incontinence, and psychogenic megacolon. It usually represents unconscious anger and defiance of the parents' punitive responses. A thorough understanding of parent/child psychodynamics is required and the fecal impaction needs to be removed. The behavioral modification program of bowel training is then started. The child should not be removed from the school, and chronic use of enemas and laxatives is to be avoided.

171. (A) Extrapyramidal side-effects can be managed by discontinuation of drugs, reduction of dosage, substitution with a different neuroleptic, or addition of anti-Parkinsonian agents. Thioridazine (Mellaril) is noted for its low incidence of extrapyramidal side-effects; however, it possesses anticholinergic activities. Trihexyphenidyl (Artane), 2-10 mg/day, is added for its anti-Parkinsonian effect. In acute dystonic reactions, intramuscular injections of Benadryl can be used.

172. (D) Premature ejaculation is the most common male sexual dysfunction and is often associated with teenage exposure to prostitutes, exclusive reliance on heavy petting and coital simulation, and the practice of coitus interruptus. The "squeeze technique" or "stop-start technique" offer success for most individuals. The cooperation of the female partner is of paramount importance; the female partner practices the "squeeze technique" when ejaculation is imminent by placing her thumb on the frenulum and her second fingers on the dorsal surface of the penis (above and below the coronal ridge); pressure is applied by her for 3 to 5 seconds.

173. (E) Seizures may be caused by severe birth trauma (anoxia), metabolic effect (hypoglycemia, hyponatremia, hypocalcemia, uremia), infection (encephalitis, meningitis), brain tumors, intracranial hemorrhages, lead poisoning, and drugs (alcohol, barbiturates, steroids, phenothiazines, and change in anticonvulsants). Taking a detailed history is the initial work-up for a patient suffering from seizure disorder.

174. (D) Due to alveolar filling with edema fluid, oxygen cannot reach the alveolar-capillary membrane and shunting occurs; thus blood in the pulmonary circulation is not oxygenated. In this instance, increasing the inspired oxygen concentration from 21% (room air) to 35% has relatively little effect on the Po_2. Even the administration of 100% oxygen may only increase the Po_2 to 60 mmHg. To correct the severe hypoxemia, positive end-expiratory pressure (PEEP) needs to be used to open alveoli.

175. (E) Reserpine gives the classic example of drug-induced depression. Many other drugs may also induce depression, and this should be detected early. These medications include corticosteroids, oral contraceptives, antihypertensives (alpha methyldopa, guanethidine, clonidine, propranolol), alcohol, opiates, benzo-diazepines, disulfiram, and digitalis.

176. (B) Doxepin is a tertiary amine which inhibits the reuptake of serotonin. Doxepin possesses good sedative effects and can be taken in a single bedtime dose to improve the sleep pattern of the patient. Alcohol itself may cause depression and is best avoided. If alcohol is used, the dose needs to be increased because of increased catabolism of the drug. The dose can be started at 50-75 mg/day. Without toxicity, the dose can be brought up to 150 mg/day at the end of the first week by an increment of 25 to 50 mg a day. It takes about two weeks to reach a blood level plateau (effective plasma level is 100 ng/ml), and three to four weeks (or even six weeks) may be needed to obtain desirable effects. Doxepin has anticholinergic effects and should not be used in patients with glaucoma.

177. (A) Amitriptyline (Elavil) is a tricyclic antidepressant which may be abused. Overdoses cause tachycardia, heart block, congestive heart failure, paralytic ileus, hypotension, delirium, toxic psychosis, and convulsion. Treatments include gastric lavage, emesis, and catharsis to remove ingested drugs. Physostigmine is used to treat severe anticholinergic effects. Propranolol or procainamide is used for arrhythmias, and diazepam is used to control convulsions.

178. (A) Obesity is easy to diagnose but difficult to treat. The most common cause of obesity is overeating with inadequate physical activity; however, many patients are noncompliant in eating less and in exercising more. Some patients become obese due to underlying medical conditions, including craniopharyngioma, adiposogenital dystrophy (early childhood obesity and genital hypoplasia), Prader-Willi syndrome (obesity, hyperphagia, short stature, hypotonia, hypogonadism, small hands and feet, mental retardation), Cushing's syndrome, and adiposis dolorosa (Dercum's disease—peripheral neuropathy, generalized obesity, and painful subcutaneous fat). Causes of iatrogenic obesity include the use of phenothiazines, butyrophenones, tricyclic antidepressants, corticosteroids, oral contraceptives, and cyproheptadine (Periactin).

179. **A-F, B-F, C-F, D-T**
There is no harm in the physician (or any other professional helper) giving advice, making recommendations, educating, etc. However, it is important to know when it will be helpful and when harmful. When the person is in deep conflict and is struggling to find relief by trying to move one way or another, it is most helpful initially to recognize the dilemma the person is confronting. The intention here must be to avoid pushing the patient toward one or another course of action, but to legitimate his right to feel in conflict and to offer help to see if the distress can be relieved in some way. Referral could be the initial action. Somewhat later, as the man makes some progress (perhaps in being more assertive and less tolerant of his wife's behavior), the wife could become involved and the marital problem could become the focus of treatment.

180. **A-T, B-F, C-T, D-F**
The relation of the physician and patient is usually consensual; the patient knowingly seeks the assistance of the physician, and the physician knowingly undertakes to act in this relation. The relationship may be contractual (oral and written) and the physician may be bound by it. A physician is not bound to render professional service to every person who applies; he may decide whether he will accept a patient. When a physician whose custom is to treat only patients who come to his office has the right to refuse to continue treatment away from his office.

181. **A-F, B-T, C-F, D-T**
The general rule of abandonment makes it clear that a physician undertaking to treat a patient generally must give such continued attention as the condition requires unless he is discharged by the patient, or unless he gives the patient reasonable time in which to obtain the services of another physician.

182. **A-F, B-F, C-F, D-T**
The physician is only responsible for the negligent actions of his employee (be has the power to select, discharge, direct, or control his assistants); he is not responsible for the actions of fellow employees.

183. **A-T, B-T, C-T, D-F**
The relationship of physician and patient is consensual. A physician who undertakes to treat someone without his expressed or implied consent is guilty of an unlawful act for which he may be held liable in case of damage. The reason for disclosure of the collateral risks is to give the patient a basis for accepting or rejecting the proposed treatment.

184. **A-F, B-F, C-F, D-T**
Parents' anxiety can be quite great with such "difficult" children since they do not appear to have the coping ability of the "easier" children. Instead of reaching out to new experiences, they pull back; playing with other children can be a considerable strain for them. Their schedules are much less regular and they react with greater intensity and discomfort to inner and outer stimuli. These children generally need considerable support and cushioning from their environment. Demands should be made only in moderation and the child should not be pushed to conform to what might otherwise seem to be age-appropriate behavior. Parents can sometimes benefit from assistance in handling these children, since the interaction of the child's difficulties and the parents' anxiety and guilt can more readily lead to problems then with easier children. The family physician is sufficiently familiar with the emotional needs of these children and he can offer such help, although referral is sometimes necessary.

185. **A-F, B-F, C-F, D-T**
The knowledge that they can pass on a disabling and potentially fatal condition to their children throws a family into tremendous conflict. They will tend to cope with that tragedy and the decisions it forces upon them as they do other difficult life decisions they face. They might tend to act impulsively, utilize denial, blame each other, feel this might not have happened if they were married to someone else, etc. The decision about having other children is bound to be

fraught with conflict and requires careful thinking through in a way that does not minimize the risks and also permits the hopeful aspects to be considered; the family doctor should offer to help the family do this. If referral is made, it should not be on the basis that "they need counseling," but rather that they are faced with a difficult decision with which anyone could use help. This approach avoids the pitfall of implying that they need counseling because they cannot handle their own decision, and also avoids the implication that they will be turning the decision over to someone else.

186.   A-T, B-F, C-F, D-F
A suicide attempt is a serious matter. The girl must have been feeling desperate to be pushed to such an extreme. The extent and seriousness of her pathology is at this time not clear, but the fact that she has a set of well-organized complaints is a good sign. It would be much more serious if she complained that she did not want to live because she was hurting the people she loved, or if she appeared disoriented and confused. In any of the latter situations she would need to be referred for psychiatric evaluation immediately, and the possibility of hospitalization would have to be considered. Given the problem as it is presented, psychiatric referral is indicated so that the onus is not put on either side of the conflict. The family physician can briefly explore some of the most pressing complaints and get the parents to ease off on some of the restrictions.

187.   A-F, B-F, C-T, D-F
Improvement can sometimes be brought about in a situation like this without long-term help. The girls's response indicates that her relationship with the parents is not disrupted. The parents need to be told that their restrictive and punitive measures are only serving to alienate her further and that they should perhaps remove some of the restrictions. Where the girls is getting into situations that they think might be dangerous, they should discuss with her how to deal with them, since going against the peer group can present considerable difficulty; restrictions should be based on safety rather than on principle or punishment. If at all possible, parents should make less of an issue of chores. The girl can be told that the

parents do want to work something out and are willing to meet her halfway. Frequently parents put much pressure on teenagers because of their anxiety that otherwise teenagers will somehow not develop a sense of responsibility; their way of doing this, however, often undermines the teenager's self-esteem by conveying the message that the youngster is irresponsible and a disappointment.

188.   (D) Hyperkinetic reaction is characterized by overactivity, restlessness, distractibility, and short attention span. Although a normal child may show this behavior at times to some degree, in the hyperkinetic child it is almost unceasing and is not outgrown until much later in his development. The undisciplined child may show this behavior at times, but in the hyperkinetic child it is continuous and is not affected by discipline alone.

189.   (C) The development pattern of the hyperkinetic child is usually erratic and/or delayed. However, the hyperkinetic child is rarely retarded and is capable of strong, healthy, open attachment. His oversensitivity to stimulation makes it impossible for him to attend to more than one stimulus at a time, and he is unable to reject a stimulus. This leads to continual distractibility, which causes difficulty in learning.

190.   (D) The parental history is usually normal without significant mental pathology, although the hyperkinetic syndrome is associated with the course of the mother's pregnancy and the child's birth. Common factors encountered include C-section, twin birth, the onset of a prediabetic condition, poor prenatal care, toxemia, placenta previa, premature separation of placenta, and breech delivery.

191.   (B) The hyperkinetic disorder is primarily a physiological condition with impairment of fine movements and coordination, deficits in attention and affect, perceptual and memory faults, and central sensory impairment. However, the intelligence quotient is usually in the range of 90-95.

192.   (A) The diagnosis is primarily based on the patient's history (excitability, distractibility, difficulty in learning, perseveration, erratic sleeping and eating patterns, and accident proneness) and "soft" neurological signs (minor defects of coordination and laterality). Fifty percent of hyperactive children may show abnormal EEG changes.

193. **(E)** Hyperactive children are unusually active, overly energetic, impulsive, and accident-prone. Although his intelligence is normal or may even be above average, the hyperactive child has difficulty concentrating and is very distractible, which causes difficulty in learning and is frequently the reason for referral from the schoolteacher.

194. **(E)** Treatment combines the pharmacological approach with therapy for the child and parental guidance. Both the parents and the child should recognize where he may compete with peers equally, where he may be required to limit participation, and where he may best act as an observer. The environment is structured so as to allow the development of the child's best personality characteristics and assets.

195. **(E)** Quide (piperacetazine) is used for psychosis. Ritalin (methylphenidate) is the most widely used drug in the treatment of hyperkinesis. The most likely mechanism of action of Ritalin is an "alerting" action which enhances the central adrenergic mechanism. Children with abnormal EEG changes are very responsive to Ritalin therapy. Other stimulants used include amphetamines and 2-dimethylaminoethanol. When stimulants do not work, a trial of a phenothiazine or chlordiazepoxide (Librium) is indicated.

196. **(C)** Although hyperkinetic children are at a higher risk for developing depression, antisocial behavior, and academic retardation in adolescence, the physiological disorder of hyperkinesis is usually outgrown between the ages of 12 and 18. The improvement of hyperkinesis is possibly due to maturation of physiological functions and better social acceptance from relatives and friends.

Chapter 2

Surgery

1. The following conditions are all precancerous *except*

    A. senile keratosis
    B. junctional nevus
    C. blue nevus
    D. arsenic hyperkeratosis
    E. Bowen's disease   (30:514)

2. A child has suffered an injury to the distal phalanx of his right index finger. Twenty-four hours later he has developed swelling, redness, pain, and semiflexion of the right index finger. The most likely diagnosis is

    A. acute tenosynovitis
    B. felon
    C. acute paronychia
    D. carbuncle
    E. flexor tendon injuries   (30:2081)

3. Which of the following is the most common presenting symptom of renal carcinoma in the adult?

    A. severe flank pain
    B. hematuria
    C. abdominal mass
    D. frequency of urination
    E. cachexia   (31:860)

4. Complication(s) of parathyroidectomy include(s)

    A. hypoparathyroidism
    B. hemorrhage
    C. recurrent laryngeal nerve damage
    D. recurrent disease
    E. all of the above   (30:1576)

5. A solitary, firm, smooth, discrete, and freely movable breast lesion in a 28-year-old female is probably

    A. carcinoma
    B. chronic cystic mastitis
    C. fibroadenoma
    D. ductal papilloma
    E. sclerosing adenosis   (30:536)

6. A 25-year-old young man suddenly notes chest pain and dyspnea. Vocal and tactile fremitus is reduced, breath sounds are diminished, and the chest film shows absent lung markings on the left side. The most probable diagnosis is

    A. atelectasis of left lung
    B. spontaneous pneumothorax
    C. pulmonary tuberculosis
    D. emphysema
    E. pulmonary embolism   (29:83)

7. A 50-year-old heavy smoker is found by routine chest x-ray to have a coin lesion in the right-upper lung field. The physical examination is within normal limits and the PPD is negative. The management of choice is

    A. antibiotics
    B. thoracotomy

C. observation
D. reassurance
E. chemotherapy   (30:694)

8. Which of the following combinations is most consistent with unilateral renal artery stenosis as a cause of systemic arterial hypertension?

A. proteinuria, red cell casts in the urinary sediment, increased serum creatinine, and an intravenous pyelogram that shows small renal shadows of unequal size
B. increased excretion of aldosterone, a normal intravenous pyelogram, and a normal blood renin level
C. increased serum potassium, decreased serum sodium, and an intravenous pyelogram that shows nonvisualization of one kidney with a normal kidney on the other side
D. decreased serum potassium, increased serum sodium, a low blood renin level, and an intravenous pyelogram that shows renal shadows of unequal size
E. a mild elevation of the blood renin level and an intravenous pyelogram that shows renal shadows of unequal size   (30:1008)

9. In traumatic arteriovenous fistula, which of the following is least likely to happen?

A. increase in venous pressure distal to the fistula
B. increase in diastolic pressure
C. decrease in systolic pressure
D. increase cardiac output
E. elevated pulse rate   (30:932)

10. A 40-year-old female with a history of rheumatic mitral stenosis suddenly complains of pain and numbness over the left leg. The physical examination reveals an absence of pulsation over the pedis dorsalis and an increase of pulsation over the common femoral pulse. The most likely diagnosis is

A. thrombophlebitis obliterans
B. occlusion of popliteal artery
C. embolism of femoral artery
D. thrombosis of femoral artery
E. thrombosis of aorta   (30:924)

11. A 50-year-old male executive complains of claudication in the left leg with walking, with the pain subsiding at rest. Examination finds a normal pulse in the common femoral artery but absent popliteal and pedal pulses. The surface skin of the left leg is normal. The possible diagnosis is

A. phlebothrombosis
B. femoral artery occlusion
C. Leriche's syndrome
D. Raynaud's disease
E. occlusion of the popliteal artery   (30:922)

12. A 40-year-old teacher suddenly develops abdominal pain. She has been on an ulcer therapy for five years. Physical examination reveals a board-like rigidity of her abdomen. The most likely diagnosis is

A. acute pancreatitis
B. acute cholecystitis
C. ectopic pregnancy
D. perforated peptic ulcer
E. rupture of appendiceal abscess (29:145-146)

13. The most common cause of intestinal obstruction is obstruction secondary to

A. neoplasm
B. adhesive bands
C. hernia
D. intussusception
E. volvulus   (30:1045)

14. A 60-year-old male who has had cholelithiasis without surgery develops progressive jaundice with palpable gallbladder. Occult blood is found in steatorrheic stools. The most likely diagnosis is

A. pancreatic head tumor
B. stone in the common bile duct
C. tumor of the ampulla of Vater
D. cancer of the gallbladder
E. chronic cholecystitis   (30:1361)

15. A 60-year-old diabetic man is found to have dull abdominal pain and progressive jaundice with palpable gallbladder. The most likely diagnosis is

A. common bile duct stone
B. chronic cholecystitis
C. hydrops of the gallbladder
D. carcinoma of the pancreatic head
E. stone in the gallbladder   (30:1361)

16. The following features are part of Peutz-Jeghers syndrome except

A. intestinal polyposis
B. hematoma
C. familial disease
D. association with melanin pigmentation of the lips and oral mucosa
E. recurrent colicky abdominal pain   *(30:1155)*

17. The following statements are true for familial polyposis of the colon *except* that

A. total colectomy is recommended
B. it is a hereditary disease
C. it will usually develop into colorectal carcinoma
D. a large number of adenomatous polyps will appear in the colon and rectum
E. cancers of familial polyposis are all polypoid cancers   *(30:1194)*

18. A male newborn infant is found to have respiratory distress. He drools saliva excessively, becomes cyanotic, and often chokes and regurgitates. The most likely diagnosis is

A. esophageal atresia
B. respiratory distress syndrome
C. hypertrophic pyloric stenosis
D. aortic vascular rings
E. aspiration pneumonia   *(30:1643)*

19. A full-term infant, born after an uncomplicated pregnancy and delivery, required resuscitation and continued to have labored respiration. Heart sounds were best heard to the right of the midsternal line. No breath sounds were heard in the left chest. The most likely diagnosis is

A. dextrocardia
B. diaphragmatic hernia
C. atelectasis
D. hyaline membrane disease
E. transposition of the great vessels   *(30:1078)*

20. Carcinoid is most frequently found in

A. sigmoid colon
B. ovary
C. ileum
D. appendix
E. jejunum   *(31:623)*

21. A patient with head injury was brought to your office. You would now

A. order a skull CT scan
B. start an IV line
C. establish an airway
D. administer corticosteroids
E. order cerebral angiography   *(30:1762-1766)*

22. A 35-year-old workaholic executive complains of severe rectal pain awakening him in the middle of the night. The most likely diagnosis is

A. proctalgia fugax
B. amaurosis fugax
C. rectal carcinoma
D. dysentery
E. ulcerative colitis   *(30:1236)*

23. A 45-year-old farmer has experienced claudication of both lower legs after walking for a few blocks. The patient also complains of coldness of the legs and impotence. On physical examination, the femoral and the pedal pulses are absent. The blood pressure is 140/90 mmHg. The most likely diagnosis is

A. Leriche's syndrome
B. Raynaud's disease
C. Buerger's disease (thromboangitis obliterans)
D. sexual dysfunction
E. diabetes mellitus   *(30:898)*

24. A 10-year-old boy has just gotten a small abrasion on his forearm. The best course of action is

A. systemic administration of antibiotics
B. topical application of corticosteroids
C. topical application of antibiotics
D. systemic administration of corticosteroids
E. infiltration of local anesthetics   *(106:121-125)*

25. A 27-year-old ballet dancer has suddenly developed crampy abdominal pain associated with nausea and vomiting. She has had obstipation and has been unable to pass flatus. Three months ago she underwent a prophylactic appendectomy. Physical examination reveals a distended abdomen without definite tenderness. The most likely diagnosis is

A. acute cholecystitis
B. perforated peptic ulcer
C. mechanical small bowel obstruction
D. ectopic pregnancy
E. paralytic ileus   *(31:590)*

26. The *least* likely cause of mechanical large bowel obstruction is

    A. volvulus
    B. fecal impaction
    C. adhesions
    D. diverticulitis
    E. carcinoma   (30:1037)

27. What percentage of colorectal carcinomas are within reach of the sigmoidoscopic examination?

    A. 0
    B. 1
    C. 5
    D. 10
    E. 35   (30:1197)

Directions: For each of the incomplete statements below, ONE or MORE of the numbered completions is correct. In each case select:
    A. if only 1, 2, and 3 are correct
    B. if only 1 and 3 are correct
    C. if only 2 and 4 are correct
    D. if only 4 is correct
    E. if all are correct

28. Which of the following statements concerning pheochromocytoma are correct?

    1. It may cause paroxysmal hypertension.
    2. It causes a decrease in urinary catecholamines.
    3. Surgical removal of the tumor is the treatment of choice.
    4. Phentolamine (Regitine) will cause a rise in blood pressure during the normotensive phase of the disease.   (28:207-208)

29. Tracheostomy may be of value in acute respiratory distress, since it

    1. increases tidal air
    2. decreases the dead space of the respiratory tree
    3. improves vital capacity
    4. facilitates aspiration of bronchial secretions   (30:595)

30. A 50-year-old man suddenly develops severe abdominal pain. Findings upon physical examination are within normal limits. Thirteen hours later the pulse rate increases, the blood pressure falls, and the abdomen is distended with rigidity. The most probable diagnosis is

    1. mesenteric embolism
    2. acute appendicitis with perforation
    3. mesenteric thrombosis
    4. acute hemorrhagic pancreatitis   (30:1433)

31. A young patient complains of crampy abdominal pain, vomiting, constipation, and abdominal fullness. On physical examination, the peristalsis wave is visible and the abdomen is distended with resonant note. The bowel sounds are increased in both pitch and frequency. An upright plain film of the abdomen may show which of the following?

    1. a gas bubble in the stomach
    2. nothing in the colon and rectum
    3. centrally placed small bowel loops with air-fluid levels
    4. absence of any gas pattern in the entire film   (29:159)

32. Pneumoperitoneum is frequently seen in which of the following conditions?

    1. perforated peptic ulcer
    2. perforation of the colon
    3. residual postoperative air
    4. acute appendicitis   (29:146-147)

33. Treatment of Hirschsprung's disease includes

    1. strictly medical treatment
    2. total excision of the hypertrophic dilated part
    3. continuous frequent dilatation of the anus
    4. resection of the distal narrow part of the gut   (30:1213)

34. A patient with congenital hypertrophic pyloric stenosis usually has

    1. recurrent vomiting starting the first one or two days of life
    2. bile-stained vomitus
    3. acidosis
    4. a palpable tumor in the right-upper abdomen   (30:1648)

35. Common complications of the untreated indirect inguinal hernia include

    1. incarceration
    2. testicular atrophy
    3. strangulation
    4. thickening of transverse fascia   (31:669)

36. Following an automobile accident in which he sustained a steering wheel injury, a young patient is brought to the emergency room. He is conscious, but restless. The physical examination shows faint heart sounds and a narrowing of the pulse pressure. The neck and the arm veins are visible. The EKG and the chest x-rays are within normal limits. Which of the following procedures should be done at once?

    1. abdominal paracentesis
    2. thoracocentesis
    3. cardiac catheterization
    4. pericardiocentesis   (30:205)

37. Post head trauma syndrome may include which of the following?

    1. headache
    2. insomnia
    3. personality changes
    4. restlessness   (78:1331)

38. A 40-year-old engineer has had a 15-year history of peptic ulcer disease. In the past four weeks, he has noted increasing ulcer pains. During the past two days, he has developed anorexia, vomiting, and ulcer pains which were not relieved by antacids. The vomitus contained ingested food and was bile-free. The laboratory findings may reveal

    1. hypochoremia
    2. hyperchoremia
    3. alkalosis
    4. acidosis   (31:461)

39. A ruptured abdominal aortic aneurysm will usually present with

    1. back pain
    2. abdominal pain
    3. a pulsatile mass in the abdomen
    4. disappearance of lower extremity pulses   (31:706)

40. A 7-year-old girl complains of abdominal pain. You would

    1. order a plain film of the abdomen
    2. order a CBC
    3. type and cross-match the blood
    4. perform H & P   (73:1579-1582)

41. Bank blood has

    1. an increased concentration of potassium
    2. an increased concentration of sodium
    3. a decreased concentration of platelets
    4. a decreased concentration of ammonia   (78:525)

Directions: Each set of lettered headings below is followed by a list of numbered words or phrases. For each numbered word or phrase select:
    A. if the item is associated with A only
    B. if the item is associated with B only
    C. if the item is associated with both A and B
    D. if the item is associated with neither A nor B

Questions 42 to 46

    A. Cancer of the left colon, early case
    B. Cancer of the right colon, early case
    C. Both
    D. Neither
42. Anemia
43. Obstruction
44. Adenocarcinoma
45. Bowel change
46. Weight gain   (31:678)

Questions 47 to 51

    A. Acute pancreatitis
    B. Acute appendicitis
    C. Both
    D. Neither
47. Decrease of serum calcium
48. Rectal tenderness
49. Pneumoperitoneum
50. Leukopenia
51. Cholelithiasis   (30:1246, 1350)

Questions 52 to 55

    A. Rupture of the liver
    B. Rupture of the spleen
    C. Both
    D. Neither
52. Left shoulder pain
53. Infectious mononucleosis
54. Blunt trauma
55. Only observation on the surgical ward is needed   (30:1263, 1378)

Directions: Each group of numbered words or phrases is followed by a list of lettered statements. MATCH the lettered statement(s) most closely associated with the numbered word or phrase.

Questions 56 to 59

56. Duodenal obstruction of the newborn
57. Intussusception
58. Imperforate anus
59. Congenital megacolon

   A. Barium enema
   B. Plain film of the abdomen taken in the upright position
   C. Plain film of the abdomen taken in the inverted position
   D. Upper GI series   *(29:181)*

Questions 60 to 62

60. Portal hypertension
61. Renovascular hypertension
62. Cushing's syndrome

   A. Splenoportography
   B. Adrenal venogram
   C. Renal arteriogram   *(30:1376, 1513)*

Questions 63 to 65

63. Glomus tumor of the finger
64. Hemorrhagic nevus in the back of the foot
65. Lymphangitis of the lower extremities

   A. Total excision
   B. Antibiotics
   C. Irradiation   *(30:169, 513)*

Questions 66 to 68

66. First degree burns
67. Second degree burns
68. Third degree burns

   A. Painless
   B. Erythema
   C. Lichenification   *(31:233)*

Directions: The following clinical set problem consists of clinical information presented in the format of questions or incomplete statements followed by a group of the numbered options.

Indicate "T" if the option is true; indicate "F" if the option is false.

A 34-year-old female executive complained of abdominal pain of 12-hour duration. The pain started at the epigastrium which shifted to the right lower abdomen. The patient reported that she was anorexic and constipated; she also experienced nausea but vomiting did not occur. At this time, you would:

69. order EKGs
70. refer to a surgeon
71. order complete blood count
72. order barium enema
73. order urinalysis

Acute appendicitis was diagnosed and appendectomy was performed that evening. Next morning, she suddenly developed a fever of 102°F with tachycardia and tachypnea. A few posterior basal rales were heard at the base other physical examinations were unremarkable. Chest x-rays were essentially normal. The appropriate treatment options include:

74. absolute bed rest
75. Tylenol with codeine (35 mg) 3 tablets q 2h p.o.
76. gentamycin 1gm I.V. q 6h
77. immediate laparotomy
78. erythromycin 500 mg q 6h p.o. *(30:1246-1255)*

Answers and Explanations

1. **(C)** The blue nevus is rarely the source of melanoma, while junctional nevus is frequently implicated as the source of malignant melanoma. Senile keratosis is potentially a precancerous lesion. Arsenic hyperkeratosis frequently becomes malignant. Bowen's disease is usually a precancerous lesion of basal cell carcinoma.

2. **(B)** Felon is infection of the digit pulp at the distal phalangeal level. Erythema, pain, and tenderness are characteristic findings. The pulp space should be incised for drainage.

3. **(B)** Painless gross hematuria is the most common symptom in adults with renal carcinoma. Abdominal mass is the most common symptom in children with renal malignancy, but is usually found late in the adult. Pain is usually a late manifestation; symptoms of metastasis (weight loss, anemia, bone pain, or pathological fracture) may be the presenting complaints.

4. **(E)** Primary hyperparathyroidism (due to parathyroid adenomas, hyperplasia, or carcinoma) is usually treated surgically. Postoperative complications consist of hypoparathyroidism (hypocalcemia, tetany), hemorrhage, recurrent laryngeal nerve damage, and recurrent disease (because of failure to excise enough parathyroid tissue).

5. **(C)** Fibroadenomas are most common in persons aged 20-35. They present as lobular but not scattered masses with a firm, rubbery consistency and sharply defined edges. Most commonly solitary, they may occasionally be multiple. They are differentiated from cancer by the smooth rather than irregular lobulations and by the age group in which they occur. Biopsy is usually required for definite diagnosis.

6. **(B)** Although pneumothorax can be caused by tuberculosis or trauma, the most common type is spontaneous pneumothorax in a healthy young person who suddenly develops chest pain, dyspnea, and decreasing breathing sounds. Diagnosis is usually made by chest film showing the collapsed lung. Severe progressive dyspnea in a patient with a collapsed lung means tension pneumothorax. Treatment consists of inserting a large-bore needle into the pleural space and connecting the open end of the needle with tubing to a water bottle on the floor. This will suffice until a chest tube can be inserted.

7. **(B)** Often a small mass in the lung is discovered on roentgenographic examination in a person with no pulmonary symptoms. The age of the patient, where he has lived, the history and physical examination, skin tests, and laboratory tests may point toward a statistically likely diagnosis. In the older adult who is a heavy smoker, excision of a coin lesion is usually indicated, because a high percentage are carcinomas.

8. **(E)** Hypertension with small kidneys ("Goldblatt's kidney") is usually caused by un-

ilateral pyelonephritis, radiation fibrosis, posttraumatic fibrosis, and congenital hyperplasia without renal arterial stenosis. Patients with hypertension, low serum potassium, high serum sodium, and low renin activity are suspected for primary aldosteronism due to hyperplastic adrenal glands (adenoma or rarely cancer). Unilateral renal artery stenosis usually causes a decrease in renal length greater than 1.5 cm, as compared with the contralateral kidney, on rapid-sequence excretory urography. The blood renin level is usually moderately elevated.

9. **(B)** The immediate effects of arteriovenous fistula include a decrease in blood flow to tissues distal to the lesion and an increase in venous pressure. The peripheral vascular resistance is lowered as a result of blood flowing directly through the newly created arteriovenous shunt. This results in a decrease in systolic and diastolic blood pressure, an increase in heart rate, and an increase in cardiac output.

10. **(C)** The five Ps of acute occlusion—pain, paralysis, paresthesia, absent pulses, and pallor—are the principal clinical features in arterial embolism. The most common underlying heart diseases are mitral stenosis, atrial fibrillation, and myocardial infarction. The emboli ejected from the heart lodge in the arteries of the bifurcation of the common femoral artery and the bifurcation of the popliteal artery. The pulse proximal to the site of the embolus may be increased. The treatment is immediate embolectomy.

11. **(B)** Occlusion of the femoral artery produces claudication in the leg with moderate exercise but is usually asymptomatic at rest. Occlusion of the popliteal artery develops into severe claudication or rest pain associated with trophic changes in the foot, ultimately resulting in ulceration and gangrene.

12. **(D)** Sudden onset of severe abdominal pain, past history of an ulcer, absolute abdominal rigidity, and the presence of free air under the diaphragm all point to perforated ulcer. A stomach tube should be inserted to avoid further peritoneal soilage, and prompt surgery is in order.

13. **(B)** Probably about 20% of surgical admissions for acute abdomen are for intestinal obstruction. Adhesive bands are the most frequent cause of obstruction for all age groups combined. Strangulated groin hernia is the second most frequent cause, and neoplasm of the bowel is third. These three etiological agents account for more than 80% of intestinal obstructions. Hernia is the most common cause of obstruction in childhood. Colorectal carcinoma and diverticulitis coli are prominent etiological agents in the older age group. The mortality rate for intestinal obstruction is around 10%.

14. **(C)** Tumor of the ampulla of Vater frequently occurs in males in their sixties and seventies. Cholelithiasis has also been implicated as a contributing factor in carcinoma of the gallbladder, but with lower frequency. Rapid onset of jaundice, weight loss, palpable liver, and a gallbladder that is smooth and nontender favor the diagnosis of malignancy in the ampulla of Vater. Anemia with evidence of upper gastrointestinal bleeding (occult blood) and steatorrhea are often seen.

15. **(D)** Carcinoma of the pancreatic head is frequently found in diabetic males over 60 years of age. The patient may be pain-free but usually complains of dull aching confined to the midepigastrium; weight loss and progressive jaundice are common and the liver and gallbladder are usually palpable. Chronic cholecystitis is associated with discrete attacks of epigastric or right-upper quadrant pain with jaundice or fever; the gallbladder is rarely palpable. If the cystic duct remains obstructed when the acute cholecystitis subsides, the gallbladder may become distended with clear mucoid fluid to form hydrops of the gallbladder, which will usually cause pain without jaundice. Asymptomatic gallstones are rare, and cholelithiasis is usually manifested by chronic cholecystitis. Choledocholithiasis is usually accompanied by colicky pain and progressive jaundice. In contrast to patients with neoplastic obstruction of the common bile duct or ampulla of Vater, the gallbladder is usually not distended because of associated inflammation (Courvoisier's law).

16. **(B)** Peutz-Jeghers syndrome is an uncommon familial disease manifested by intestinal polyposis (the colon and rectum are also involved in one-third of cases and the stomach in about

one-fourth) and brown pigmentation of the skin and mucous membranes. There has been no proved case of malignancy in any Peutz-Jeghers polyp with hematoma. Recurrent colicky abdominal pain caused by transient intussusception is the most frequent symptom. Surgical treatment is polypectomy.

17. **(E)** Familial polyposis is a rare hereditary disease characterized by the appearance, early in life, of large numbers of adenomatous polyps in the colon and rectum. Carcinoma of the colorectum will develop in essentially 100% of patients; thus total colectomy and cutaneous ileostomy have been advocated. The cancers developed are not all polypoid cancers, however; polypoid, ulcerating, and scirrhous cancers occur in the same proportions as idiopathic colonic cancer.

18. **(A)** The diagnosis of esophageal atresia should be considered in any newborn infant with respiratory distress, excessive salivation, or cyanosis. Inability to pass a small, relatively rigid rubber catheter through the esophagus into the stomach usually establishes the diagnosis. One to three milliliters of water-soluble contrast medium is introduced into the tube and an x-ray is taken with the infant in the upright position. This will define the level of the blind proximal pouch, and the presence of air in the stomach and gastrointestinal tract will confirm communication between the distal esophagus and the trachea. Direct anastomosis is the treatment of choice.

19. **(B)** Usually an infant with diaphragmatic hernia (foramen of Bochdalek) presents in a state of acute respiratory distress with cyanosis and markedly increased respiratory rate and effort. The affected hemithorax is usually dull to percussion, and there is evidence of shift of mediastinal structures to the opposite side. The diagnosis is almost always apparent on standard roentgenogram of the thorax, which often clearly demonstrates gas-filled intestines. Immediate surgical repair is indicated.

20. **(D)** The most common site of carcinoid tumors is the appendix, followed by the small bowel (mostly the ileum). Carcinoid arises from argentaffin cells in the crypts of Lieberkuhn and forms yellowish, firm nodules in the submucosa. The carcinoid syndrome consists of cutaneous flushing, diarrhea, bronchoconstriction, skin rash, and right-sided cardiac valvular disease due to collagen deposition. Urinary 5-hydroxyindoleacetic acid (5-HIAA, a metabolite of serotonin) is usually increased. This is a malignant neoplasm in slow motion.

21. **(C)** The most important initial step in the management of any severe trauma is the establishment of an airway. This is especially true with head injuries. Acute respiratory embarassment alone can cause massive brain swelling and worsening of an existing brain injury. Following the establishment of an airway, the level of consciousness, the condition of the pupils, and vital signs (particularly pulse rates and the blood pressure) should be evaluated and bleeding sites should be identified and controlled. IV lines are kept open to initiate a diagnostic test in evaluating for possible intracranial hemorrhage. Intracranial hematomas are readily diagnosed and accurately localized by CT scan. The lateral cervical spine film is ordered to rule out the fracture dislocation of the cervical spine. In an office setting, following the stabilization of the patient's acute condition, further evaluation (such as CT scan) should be carried out at the hospital if the condition warrants.

22. **(A)** Proctalgia fugax is a severe spasmodic rectal pain lasting a few minutes. The cause is unknown, but it is associated with patients who are over-worked and anxious. Sigmoidoscopy is performed and reasurrance is offered with application of analgesic suppositories, heat pads, and warm baths. Diazepam (Valium) may be found to be useful.

23. **(A)** Leriche's syndrome (aortoiliac occlusive disease) is an ischemic syndrome resulting from occlusion of the abdominal aorta due to atherosclerosis. It is characterized by claudication and impotence. The physical examination usually discloses absence or diminution of the femoral pulses combined with absence of the popliteal and pedal pulses. Aortography can establish the diagnosis as well as the extent of the occlusive disease. The aortic occlusion may be corrected by directly removing the obstruction by a thromboendarterectomy or by insertion of a prosthetic bypass (Dacron or Teflon) graft.

24. **(C)** Minor skin traumas (such as minor cuts, scratches, and abrasions) can be treated by the immediate application of topical antibiotics to prevent secondary infections. Most common skin infections are caused by *Staphylococcus aureus* and *Streptococcus pyogenes.* Neomycin is effective against staph, bacitracin is effective against strep, and neomycin and polymyxin cover less common infections caused by Gram-negative organisms. An ointment containing neomycin-bacitracin-polymyxin preparation is the drug of choice for preventing secondary infections, including subsequent poststreptococcal glomerulonephritis. Contact dermatitis and allergic sensitization may rarely occur.

25. **(C)** Acute small bowel obstruction is most commonly due to adhesions acquired from abdominal operation. Simple mechanical obstruction without vascular compromise often presents with nontenderness on palpation. The absence of tenderness does not rule out the diagnosis of acute bowel obstruction. The more proximal the obstruction, the less the distention and the more the vomiting. Paralytic ileus is usually secondary to pancreatitis, peritonitis, renal calculi, or pneumonia. Ectopic pregnancy is a possibility, and further differentiation may be required.

26. **(C)** Large bowel obstruction is commonly caused by carcinoma of the bowel, volvulus of the sigmoid colon, and stenosing diverticulitis. However, the most common cause is fecal impaction in the elderly; this may be associated with dietary habit, frequent constipation, and inadequate fluid intake. Although adhesion is the most common cause of small bowel obstruction, it is relatively rare in large bowel obstruction. Abdominal pain and abdominal distention are the prominent pictures. Vomiting may not occur until late in the course, with fecal character. Peritonitis may occur following cecal perforation.

27. **(E)** Fifty years ago, 75% of the colorectal cancers are within reach of sigmidoscopic examinations; now 35% of the colorectal carcinomas are still within reach of rigid sigmoidoscope.

28. **(B)** Paroxysmal hypertension is the most characteristic symptom of pheochromocytoma and is due to sudden release of catecholamines, sometimes caused by pressure on the adrenals or postural change. Headache, palpitations, sweating, nausea and vomiting, pallor, dilated pupils, and tachycardia may follow. However, the usual symptoms are persistent hypertension associated with retinopathy, mottling of the skin, tingling, and pyrexia. Glycosuria is frequently seen in extra-adrenal pheochromocytomas. Urinary excretion of catecholamines or their metabolite, vanillylmandelic acid (VMA), is increased. The histamine provocative test (rarely used) will increase the blood pressure during the normotensive phase, while the 5 mg IV phentolamine blocking test will decrease the blood pressure (a fall of 35 mmHg systolic and 25 mmHg diastolic pressure) during the hypertensive phase. The treatment of choice is surgical removal.

29. **(C)** The value of tracheostomy as a route for removal of excessive recurrent bronchial secretions is well established. Frequently a tracheostomy permits better artificial ventilation of the lungs in the patient who has sustained extensive chest trauma or has severe respiratory or cardiovascular insufficiency. Tracheostomy may cause coughing and *Pseudomonas* infections of the lungs. Proper care is needed.

30. **(B)** Acute occlusion of the superior mesenteric artery may be caused by either embolism or thrombosis. It usually presents itself as intestinal obstruction with a less acute onset. The patient may have a prior history of repeated episodes of cramping abdominal pain following the ingestion of food (intestinal angina). The most striking symptom is extreme abdominal pain that is unresponsive to narcotics and minimal physical findings. Later, bloody diarrhea, shock, and abdominal distention and rigidity may develop. Abdominal tapping may be useful for diagnosis, and the treatment is immediate surgical intervention.

31. **(A)** Within a few hours of the onset of intestinal obstruction, x-ray studies of the abdomen reveal an abdominal gas pattern. Both the supine film and the upright film should be ordered together and should include both the pelvis and the diaphragm. The left-lateral decubitus film may be substituted for the upright film if the patient is too ill to stand or sit. Air-fluid levels are easy to detect on an upright film and indicate small bowel ob-

struction in patients with characteristic symptoms of crampy pain, obstipation, distention, and vomiting. In small bowel distention, the loops are centrally placed with feathery appearance, while in colonic distention the loops are usually located in the periphery of the abdomen and show a puckered, sacculated appearance.

32. **(A)** The most common cause of pneumoperitoneum is the perforated peptic ulcer. Perforation of the colon causes massive pneumoperitoneum, and the residual postoperative air may last up to three weeks. Subphrenic abscess also causes pneumoperitoneum. Appendicitis is rarely a cause of pneumoperitoneum. An erect abdominal film or left-lateral film will demonstrate the free air.

33. **(D)** Hirschsprung's disease is a congenital absence or agenesis of the mesenteric parasympathetic nerve ganglia in a segment of distal colon. The dilated segment of colon is not the primary cause, and the Swenson operation includes the excision of the distal aganglionic narrow segment of colon. The disease is often diagnosed by rectal biopsy.

34. **(D)** Congenital hypertrophic pyloric stenosis is an abnormality of the pyloric musculature which results in mechanical obstruction of the distal portion of the stomach. It usually occurs in first-born male children, with familial predisposition. Projectile vomiting usually is manifested within three to five weeks of birth. The content of the gastric vomitus is bile-free. Waves of gastric peristalsis passing from the left-upper quadrant over to the right are usually observed. A firm, olive-shaped mass is frequently palpable in the right-upper abdomen in 70-97% of cases. A metabolic alkalosis with hypochloremia may develop. The Fredet-Ramstedt pyloromyotomy is frequently performed.

35. **(B)** The two most common complications of indirect inguinal hernia (less likely for direct hernia) are incarceration and strangulation. When an inguinal hernia becomes incarcerated, emergency surgery is usually indicated except for high-risk patients. When the diagnosis of strangulation is made, patients usually require immediate surgery.

36. **(C)** With a combination of arterial hypoten-

sion and venous hypertension, with or without shock from an automobile steering wheel injury, blunt chest trauma, or stab wounds in the left anterior chest, cardiac tamponade should be suspected. The suspicion should be confirmed by prompt needle aspiration of the pericardium, both to confirm the diagnosis and to institute therapy.

37. **(E)** From 12 to 18 months may be needed to judge the ultimate prognosis for patients who have had a significant head injury. Residual behavioral sequelae are associated with the severity and the extent of the neurological deficits. Many patients complain of headache, dizziness, and insomnia. As these symptoms subside, the patient may become irritable, restless, insecure, anxious, or depressed. Reassurance and supports are offered and mild tranquilizers are used to speed recovery. Physical therapy and job retraining help patients to return to an active social life, particularly young patients.

38. **(B)** A pyloric obstruction secondary to chronic ulcer disease presents with bile-free emesis and hypochloremic alkalosis. When the condition persists, the dehydration and hypovolemia become paramount and a metabolic acidosis supervenes.

39. **(A)** A ruptured abdominal aneurysm is characterized by sudden severe abdominal pain radiating into the back. Faintness or syncope follows. The pain may improve and faintness disappears after the first hemorrhage, only to reappear and progress to shock later. A discrete, pulsatile, exquisitely tender abdominal mass can be felt and immediate surgery is required. A ruptured abdominal aortic aneurysm only rarely occludes one or both iliac arteries. Thus absence of peripheral pulses in such a circumstance more probably indicates either profound shock and low perfusion or pre-existing occlusive vascular disease.

40. **(D)** Abdominal pain is a common symptom requiring systematic differentiation. The basic decision is to differentiate medical versus surgical abdomen. The history will provide a diagnosis in the majority of cases, and physical examination will aid in the direction of the diagnosis. The most productive physical is the examination of the abdomen. The subjective complaint (character and nature) of ab-

dominal pain should be corroborated by objective findings—tenderness, guarding, spasm, and bowel sound. Laboratory studies are primarily for confirmatory purposes. Moreover, psychogenic causes of abdominal pain should not be overlooked—elaborate diagnostic studies may further aggravate anxieties and abdominal pain may persist.

41. **(B)** Bank blood has increased Hgb, potassium, and ammonia levels, but platelets, factor V, and factor VII are essentially not available. The concentration of sodium is only slightly decreased. Thus, in patients receiving large quantity of potassium and in infants undergoing exchange transfusion, fresh blood is usually used.

42. **(B)**

43. **(A)**

44. **(C)**

45. **(A)**

46. **(D)** Colonic cancer is usually adenocarcinoma. Carcinoma of the left colon is usually annular, characterized by the symptoms of obstruction due to the smaller size of the lumen and the solidity of the contents. A change in bowel habits may be the first symptom noted, with a progressive decrease in the caliber of the stools. Blood and mucus is seen in or on the stool. Cancer of the right colon is usually characterized by persistent dull, nagging, right-lower quadrant pain, anemia, and a mass in the right abdomen. Colonic cancer on either side will frequently cause weight loss. Late cases of colonic cancer on both sides will cause anemia and obstruction.

47. **(A)**

48. **(B)**

49. **(D)**

50. **(D)**

51. **(A)** Acute pancreatitis and appendicitis are both characterized by acute abdominal pain. Pelvic appendicitis is usually manifested by rectal tenderness. Acute pancreatitis is associated with cholelithiasis, alcoholism, mumps,

hyperparathyroidism, and intra-abdominal operations. Moderate leukocytosis (10,000-30,000/cu mm), elevated serum lipase (normal 0-1.5 Cherry-Crandall units), hyperamylasemia (300 Somogyi units), and lowered serum calcium level (7.5 mg/100 ml) are frequently helpful in the diagnosis of acute pancreatitis. Acute appendicitis will cause moderate leukocytosis (10,000-18,000/cu mm). Pneumoperitoneum is characteristic of perforated peptic ulcer and is rarely seen in acute appendicitis or pancreatitis.

52. **(B)**

53. **(B)**

54. **(C)**

55. **(D)** The spleen is the organ most commonly injured in blunt trauma, followed by the intestine and the liver. Traumatic rupture of the liver usually causes shock, abdominal pain, spasm, and rigidity, while rupture of the spleen causes generalized abdominal pain with radiation to the left shoulder, although shock may occur in splenic rupture. Often the patient is asymptomatic at first. Spontaneous splenic rupture may happen in patients with infectious mononucleosis, mostly during the second to fourth weeks of the course. The treatment of splenic and hepatic rupture is immediate surgery.

56. **(B)**

57. **(A)**

58. **(C)**

59. **(A)** An upright plain film of the abdomen will show characteristic double bubble (air in the stomach and duodenum) in duodenal obstruction of the newborn. Barium enema will demonstrate a filling defect in the ascending colon in intussusception—previously healthy infants 3 to 11 months of age with this defect suddenly develop severe crampy abdominal pain with bloody stool and palpable abdominal mass. In congenital megacolon (newborn or later age), barium enema reveals a dilated colon and narrowed aganglionic segment. A plain film taken in the inverted position for a patient with imperforate anus shows a colonic pouch filled with air. There is the possibility

of the existence of fistulas connecting to urinary or reproductive organs.

60. **(A)**

61. **(C)**

62. **(B)** Transhepatic cholangiography is used to differentiate between pancreatic carcinoma and cholelithiasis. Carcinoma produces a smooth, tapering, complete obstruction, but calculi cause a typical convex deformity. Since hemorrhage and bile peritonitis may occur, transhepatic cholangiography should only be done when the patient is prepared for surgery. Splenoportography affords a method of determining the pathological features of the portal circulation. lt provides graphic demonstration of the site of obstruction—i.e., intrahepatic or extrahepatic. Renal arteriography is the best screening test for renovascular hypertension and to determine the stenosis of a main or segmental renal artery. Arteriograms or venograms of the adrenal circulation have been utilized to localize adrenal tumors or to demonstrate adrenal hyperplasia in Cushing's syndrome. Adrenal venography may cause adrenal hemorrhage and thrombosis, so adrenal angiography is more frequently utilized.

63. **(A)**

64. **(A)**

65. **(B)** The glomus tumor is a rare, benign, and extremely painful small neoplasm of the skin and subcutaneous tissue occurring on the extremities, particularly in the nailbeds of the hands and feet. The tumor is derived from the glomic end-organ apparatus consisting of arteriovenous anastomoses, which functions normally to regulate the blood flow in the extremity to control the temperature. Total excision is indicated, since the tumor is radioresistant. The following characteristics of any pigmented nevus are indications for excision: change in color or pigment distribution, development of erythema, change in size and consistency, change in surface characteristics (bleeding, erosion, oozing), pain, burning, or lymphadenopathy. Lymphangitis, an inflammation of lymphatic pathways manifested by tenderness and streaking erythema of the skin, is frequently caused by hemolytic streptococci and is often associated with swelling of the regional lymph nodes. Treatment is with appropriate antibiotics sensitive to causal organisms.

66. **(B)**

67. **(B)**

68. **(A)** First degree burns cause erythema and pain, second degree burns cause erythema and blistering, and third degree burns result in pale or charred skin, thrombosed superficial vessels, and insensitivity to touch or painful stimuli.

69. **(F)**

70. **(F)**

71. **(F)**

72. **(F)**

73. **(F)**

74. **(F)**

75. **(F)**

76. **(F)**

77. **(F)**

78. **(F)**

Acute appendicitis is basically an clinical diagnosis; its diagnosis is usually based on detailed history information and physical findings. Localized tenderness at RLQ, particularly at the McBurney's point with rebound tenderness is suggestive of acute appendicitis. Laboratory tests are used for confirming the suspicion, moderate leukocytosis with predominant neutrophils is the most frequent finding and can aid in the diagnosis. Urine is usually normal but may show WBCs or RBCs. Plain film of abdomen may show distended loops of small intestine in the RLQ, gas-filled appendix, fecalithes in the RLQ, increases soft tissue density, altered right flank stripe. Barium enema may show non-filling of the appendix. Twenty-five percent of patients receiving abdominal surgery may develop atelectasis. Treatment consists of clearing the airway by chest percussion, coughing, or nasotracheal suction.

Chapter 3

Gynecology

Directions: Each of the questions or incomplete statements below is followed by five suggested answers or completions. Select the BEST answer(s) in each case.

1. During her fourth month of pregnancy, the patient comes for follow-up prenatal care. You find that the uterus is enlarged to the level of the umbilicus. You may suspect that the patient has

   A. twins
   B. myoma uteri
   C. ectopic pregnancy
   D. hydramnios
   E. hydatidiform mole   (8:313)

2. A teenage girl comes to you for contraceptive advice. You would

   A. call her mother immediately
   B. refuse to see her
   C. tell her to behave herself and drive her out of the office
   D. encourage her by prescribing the "pills" without exploring the situation
   E. explore the situation to determine her need for contraceptives and be ready to support her in solving the problem
                                          (17:170-171)

3. A 27-year-old single female requests contraceptive advice. She has had three induced abortions during the past two years. You would

   A. accuse her of manslaughter
   B. refuse to see her

C. discuss the effectiveness and safety of each contraceptive method
D. advise her not to use any contraceptives and to resort to induced abortions when she becomes pregnant
E. tell her to behave herself and to stop having intercourse   (17:170-171)

4. A 32-year-old woman complains of postcoital bleeding. On examination, a small, soft polypoid mass is found protruding from the cervical canal. What is the next step you would take?

   A. antibiotic treatment
   B. reassurance only
   C. irradiation
   D. acid douches
   E. excisional biopsy   (8:242)

5. Carcinoma in situ of the cervix uteri discovered in pregnancy at the fourteenth week of gestation should be treated as follows:

   A. Schiller staining of the cervix and total hysterectomy
   B. continuation of the pregnancy with biopsies and smears and postpartum reevaluation
   C. total hysterectomy with bilateral salpingo-oophorectomy
   D. amputation of the cervix and continuation of the pregnancy
   E. irradiation   (10:129)

6. Class IV suspicious Papanicolaou smear has

been found in a 28-year-old woman on routine physical examination. She probably needs

A. reassurance
B. repeat Papanicolaou smear and cervical biopsy
C. oral contraceptive pills
D. hysterectomy
E. estrogen vaginal cream for one month, then repeat smears   (16:571)

7. Postcoital bleeding with a small cervical ulcer in a pregnant woman requires

A. observation
B. vaginal cytology
C. punch biopsy
D. cone biopsy
E. cervical cauterization   (17:626)

8. A 25-year-old unmarried college student complains of severe vulvar pruritus and dysuria. Examination reveals a malodorous, frothy, yellow-green discharge. The laboratory study is most likely to show

A. multiple flagellate protozoa seen on the wet smear
B. multiple brown-black colonies growing on Nickerson's medium
C. Gram-negative intracellular diplococci on Gram stain
D. small Gram-negative rods
E. positive darkfield examination   (7:80-81)

9. A strawberry-like appearance of the vagina with the presence of small petechial lesions on the cervix strongly suggests the diagnosis of

A. streptococcal vaginitis
B. pelvic congestion
C. trichomonal vaginitis
D. monilial vaginitis
E. cervical polyp   (6:264)

10. A diabetic female patient complains of severe vulvar pruritis with discharge. Examination reveals fiery red mucosa with a patchy, curd-like white discharge. The laboratory examination will most likely show

A. mobile flagellate protozoa on wet smear
B. multiple brown-black colonies growing on Nickerson's medium
C. positive Thayer-Martin culture

D. Gram-negative intracellular diplococci
E. positive darkfield examination   (7:84)

11. The most appropriate therapy for monilial vaginitis is

A. aqueous penicillin 4.8 million units intramuscularly
B. oral Flagyl (metronidazole) 250 mg three times daily for the patient and two times daily for her sexual partner, for ten days
C. nystatin vaginal suppositories 100,000 units at bedtime for 14 days
D. Terramycin (oxytetracycline) vaginal tablets 250 mg inserted at bedtime for 10 days
E. reassurance that the condition will improve spontaneously in four days   (7:85-86)

12. A 35-year-old woman complains of dysuria and dribbling after urination. A small suburethral mass is found by digital examination. The compression of the anterior vaginal wall produces purulent discharge at the urethral meatus. The most likely diagnosis is

A. venereal urethritis
B. abscess of Skene's duct
C. carcinoma of the urethra
D. urethral diverticulum
E. Gartner's duct cyst   (16:662)

13. The most common tumor producing ascites in females is

A. cervical carcinoma
B. endometrial carcinoma
C. adenomyosis
D. ovarian tumor
E. adnexal tumor   (8:493)

14. Hydrothorax is often associated with the following:

A. serous cystadenoma of the ovary
B. bilateral polycystic ovaries
C. pseudomucinous cystadenoma of the ovary
D. ovarian fibroma
E. myoma uteri   (6:584)

15. The most frequent cause of amenorrhea in young female adults is

A. primary ovarian failure
B. hypothyroidism
C. pituitary failure

D. psychoneurosis

E. pregnancy   (6:735)

16. Pseudomyxoma peritonei is associated with

   A. cervical carcinoma
   B. myoma uteri
   C. metastatic carcinoma of the uterus
   D. gonococcal tubo-ovarian abscess
   E. ovarian cystadenoma   (17:663)

17. Stein-Leventhal syndrome is characterized by acquired amenorrhea, obesity, and occassional hirsutism. The ovaries show

   A. atrophy
   B. multiple corpora lutea
   C. cortical fibrosis and multiple follicular cysts
   D. germinal-cell hyperplasia and capillary engorgement
   E. cortical stromal hyperplasia   (16:650)

18. Six months ago, a 35-year-old female patient was accidentally found to have a small, movable pelvic mass during a routine physical examination without any complaints. Now she suddenly experiences excruciating pain in the right-lower abdomen. The most likely diagnosis is

   A. acute pyelonephritis
   B. acute appendicitis
   C. torsion of an ovarian cyst
   D. myoma uteri
   E. diverticulitis   (6:564-565)

19. Myomas are usually asymptomatic. Which of the following types of uterine myomas do frequently cause symptoms?

   A. intramural
   B. submucous
   C. subserous
   D. pedunculated
   E. cervical   (6:428)

20. The treatment of choice for symptomatic adenomyosis in a 40-year-old woman with three children is

   A. hormonal therapy
   B. total hysterectomy
   C. total hysterectomy and bilateral oophorectomy
   D. psychotherapy only
   E. repeated curettage   (7:225)

21. The most frequent complications of simple uterine retroversion include

   A. backache
   B. irregular menstruation
   C. leukorrhea
   D. constipation
   E. none of the above   (6:367)

22. A 35-year-old unmarried nulliparous woman complains of lower abdominal pain over both sides just prior to menstruation. She has also noted bleeding from the rectum associated with the menses. On pelvic examination, a small, hard, fibrotic nodule is found. The most likely diagnosis is

   A. rectal carcinoma
   B. myoma uteri
   C. cervical carcinoma
   D. endometriosis
   E. adenomyosis   (8:336-341)

23. A nulliparous woman complains of postmenopausal bleeding. She is a diabetic. The physical examination reveals obesity and hypertension. Pelvic examination shows normal vulva and cervix, but the uterus is slightly enlarged. The most likely diagnosis is

   A. cervical polyp
   B. cervical cancer
   C. endometrial carcinoma
   D. myoma uteri
   E. ovarian tumor   (6:411)

24. Fixed uterine retrodisplacement is commonly associated with

   A. appendicitis
   B. diverticulitis
   C. endometriosis
   D. cervical polyp
   E. monilial vaginitis   (6:625)

25. The treatment of choice for an abscess of Bartholin's gland is

   A. antibiotics
   B. sitz baths
   C. incision and drainage
   D. marsupialization
   E. gentian violet painting   (17:564)

26. In a case of chronic pelvic inflammatory disease, the sudden onset of hyperpyrexia, shock, and tachycardia usually indicates

A. intestinal obstruction
B. torsion of an ovarian cyst
C. rupture of a pelvic abscess
D. acute appendicitis
E. ectopic pregnancy   (7:292-293)

27. The preferred treatment of a ruptured tubo-ovarian abscess is

A. cul-de-sac drainage
B. total hysterectomy and bilateral salpingo-oophorectomy
C. observation only
D. antibiotics only
E. antibiotics and observation   (8:255)

28. A young woman recently noted lower abdominal pain accompanied by chills and low-grade fever. On examination, the abdomen is spastic and tenderness is elicited by the manipulation of the cervix. Examination of the cervical discharge reveals the causative organism. The most likely diagnosis is

A. gonococcal salpingitis
B. ectopic pregnancy
C. tuberculous salpingitis
D. acute appendicitis
E. regional ileitis   (8:249)

29. A 25-year-old woman is seen for infertility. She has been married for two years. Your initial evaluation is within normal limits; you instruct her in the recording of basal body temperature and ask her to return in three months for further evaluative studies. The basal body temperature chart shows a biphasic curve in the first month and a sustained temperature elevation curve for the second and the third months. The patient possibly has

A. hyperestrogenism
B. estrogen insufficiency
C. pelvic inflammatory disease
D. pregnancy
E. Stein-Leventhal syndrome   (8:360)

30. The female patient who appears for her routine annual examination at a family physician's office should *not* receive the following procedures:

A. rectovaginal examination
B. breast examination
C. cytologic smear
D. percussion of the lung fields
E. none of the above   (6:136)

31. Endometrial biopsy shows secretory phase, indicating

A. preovulatory phase
B. that menstruation is in progress
C. that ovulation has occurred
D. proliferative stage
E. that no ovulation is possible   (6:79-82)

32. In a normal cycle of 34 days' duration, ovulation occurs

A. two weeks before menstrual flow
B. two weeks after onset of menstrual flow
C. at midcycle
D. not at all
E. the first day of menstruation   (6:841)

33. The most common cause of congenital female pseudohermaphroditism is

A. exogeneous androgen
B. chromosomal abnormality
C. ovarian agenesis
D. virilizing ovarian tumor
E. congenital adrenal hyperphlasia   (6:217)

34. A 16-year-old girl has a complaint of primary amenorrhea. On assessment of her work-up, you have obtained the following information: height, 5 ft 4 in; weight, 148 pounds; normal pelvic examination; normal 17-ketosteroids; normal visual fields; and negative pregnancy test. A normal menstrual period is induced by IM injection of 100 mg progesterone. This supports the following interpretation

A. she has adrenal cortical hyperplasia
B. she is producing adequate levels of estrogen
C. she has arrhenoblastoma
D. she has pituitary tumor
E. she has Turner's syndrome   (17:83-84)

35. A 26-year-old housewife has been taking the combination oral contraceptives for three years. Her withdrawal bleeding has progressively decreased over the past year, with the flow becoming scanty and lasting for only two days. During the last three cycles, she has developed amenorrhea. The best treatment is

A. the administration of testosterone
B. the discontinuation of the pill
C. the addition of more progestogen component

D. the addition of more estrogen component
E. reassurance   *(39:471)*

36. The *worst* choice of contraception for a woman with a history of ectopic pregnancy is

A. oral contraceptives
B. intrauterine device
C. diaphragm
D. condom
E. foam and jelly   *(16:736)*

Directions: For each of the incomplete statements below, ONE or MORE of the numbered completions is correct. In each case select:

A. if only 1, 2, and 3 are correct
B. if only 1 and 3 are correct
C. if only 2 and 4 are correct
D. if only 4 is correct
E. if all are correct

37. The after-supervision of patients with evacuated hydatidiform mole includes the following:

1. another pregnancy may not be permitted within a year
2. quantitative HCG titer is followed every one to two weeks until negative
3. persistent HCG titer requires dilatation and curettage (D and C)
4. persistent HCG titer with negative D and C does not require chemotherapy   *(10:31)*

38. Drugs used to treat choriocarcinoma include the following:

1. actinomycin D
2. mercaptopurine
3. methotrexate
4. rifampin   *(6:613)*

39. Methotrexate has which of the following side-effects?

1. bone marrow suppression
2. gastrointestinal disturbances
3. hepatitis
4. oral ulcers   *(6:683)*

40. Monilial vaginitis is frequently seen in women with

1. pregnancy
2. long-term systemic antibiotic therapy
3. diabetes
4. oral contraceptive use   *(7:83-84)*

41. Vesicovaginal fistulas are often caused by

1. repair of the cystocele
2. radiotherapy of cervical cancer
3. invasion of cervical cancer
4. radical hysterectomy   *(6:300)*

42. Urethrovaginal fistulas are often caused by

1. irradiation
2. repair of urethrocele
3. repair of cystocele
4. lymphogranuloma venereum   *(6:363)*

43. Rectovaginal fistulas may result from which of the following?

1. cervical cancer invasion
2. radiotherapy for cervical cancer
3. hemorrhoidectomy
4. lymphogranuloma inguinale   *(6:364)*

44. The following statements concerning diethylstilbestrol are true:

1. it is associated with clear-cell adenocarcinoma of the vagina of the offspring when given in pregnancy
2. stilbestrol ingested by the mother during pregnancy later may be related to vaginal adenosis in her daughter
3. it has been used for postcoital contraception
4. vaginal suppositories are often used for atrophic vaginitis   *(17:90,163)*

45. The following tumors may metastasize to the ovary:

1. cervical cancer
2. endometrial carcinoma
3. vulvar cancer
4. vaginal cancer   *(7:621)*

46. Clomid therapy is useful in patients with

1. Turner's syndrome
2. Stein-Leventhal's syndrome
3. Sheehan's syndrome
4. anovulatory conditions   *(17:85)*

47. The treatment of endometrial carcinoma consists of

1. hysterectomy and bilateral salpingo-oophorectomy in well-differentiated lesions
2. observation and follow-up
3. preoperative intracavital radium plus total hysterectomy and bilateral salpingo-

oophorectomy in poorly differentiated lesions

4. irradiation   (9:122)

48. The triad of adenomyosis includes

1. menorrhagia
2. dysmenorrhea
3. enlarging uterus
4. fever   (8:395)

49. Carcinoma of the cervix most frequently originates from

1. subcylindrical cells of the squamous columnar junction
2. squamous epithelium of the portio vaginalis (epidermoid carcinoma)
3. the cylindric epithelium of the cervical canal (adenocarcinoma)
4. uterine fundus   (6:252-263)

50. Endometriosis is frequently treated effectively by

1. pregnancy
2. oral contraceptives
3. surgery
4. intrapelvic injection of nitrogen mustard
                                  (10:166-168)

51. Women who develop cancer of the vulva have a higher than average incidence of pre-existing

1. pruritus vulvae
2. leukoplakia of the vulva
3. granulomatous venereal disease
4. kraurosis of the vulva   (8:514-517)

52. After menarche, an imperforate hymen may be associated with

1. hematometra
2. urinary retention
3. abdominal pain
4. hematocolpos   (6:199)

53. Which of the following statements are true with regard to venereal warts (condyloma acuminatum)?

1. they may be transmitted from husband to wife or vice versa
2. they are the manifestation of secondary lues
3. they are frequently associated with trichomoniasis or moniliasis of the vagina

4. they are caused by the same virus as lymphogranuloma venereum   (8:279-280)

54. Chronic gonorrheal pelvic inflammatory disease

1. is usually treated with antibiotics
2. is usually treated with mycostatin
3. which does not respond to one or two attempts at conservative therapy is treated by surgical resection
4. rarely results in infertility   (8:252-256)

55. Side-effects of IUD use include

1. leukorrhea
2. chronic endometritis
3. pelvic pain
4. hypermenorrhea   (8:597)

56. The following statements are *not* true about vaginal bleeding:

1. it can be associated with hypertension
2. dysfunctional uterine bleeding is a major cause
3. it can be a presenting symptom of idiopathic thrombocytopenic purpura
4. it is rarely the presenting complaint
                                  (10:95-96)

57. The following statements are true about vaginal bleeding:

1. postmenopausal vaginal bleeding is usually normal
2. in young children it is often due to a foreign body in the vagina
3. postcoital vaginal bleeding is usually psychogenic in origin
4. vaginal bleeding accompanying a missed period is likely to be miscarriage (10:95-96)

58. Which of the following are characteristic of oral contraceptives?

1. they increase the total thyroxine concentration in the blood
2. they increase the PBI
3. they increase the risk of thromboembolic disease
4. a high dose of estrogen and progestin alone may inhibit ovulation   (10:146-147)

59. A 23-year-old female requests oral contraceptives. Her brother died due to myocardial infarction at age 40. Her physical examina-

tions, including the Pap test, are essentially normal. You would now

1. prescribe D-thyroxine
2. prescribe combination contraceptive pills
3. prescribe cholestyramine
4. order serum triglycerides   (73:839)

60. A postmenopausal woman complains of chronic low back pain. The x-rays of the lumbar spine show generalized demineralization. You would now

1. encourage alcohol drinking
2. administer oral phosphate
3. institute desiccated thyroid
4. evaluate the risk of endometrial carcinoma
                                       (39:716)

61. The following features are commonly present in acute subdural hematoma of a young woman:

1. spastic hemiplegia
2. unequal pupil size
3. deterioration of consciousness
4. papilledema   (31:767)

62. A postmenopausal woman with breast carcinoma was maintained by means of estrogen therapy with satisfactory results. During a routine follow-up office visit, she complains of anorexia, nausea, vomiting, weakness, thirst, polyuria, and drowsiness. Now you would

1. offer reassurance
2. order a skull CT scan
3. prescribe vitamin E and vitamin D
4. order a serum calcium level test   (39:711)

Directions: Each set of lettered headings below is followed by a list of numbered words or phrases. For each numbered word or phrase select:

A. if the item is associated with A only
B. if the item is associated with B only
C. if the item is associated with both A and B
D. if the item is associated with neither A nor B

Questions 63 to 67

A. Contraceptive pills
B. IUD
C. Both

D. Neither
63. Prevent fertilization
64. Inhibit tubal peristalsis
65. Will not cause any side-effects
66. More effective
67. Suitable for use for mass programs in developing societies   (7:719-749)

Questions 68 to 71

A. Menarche
B. Climacterium
C. Both
D. Neither
68. Anovulatory cycle
69. Dysfunctional bleeding
70. Hot flashes
71. Monophasic BBT (basal body temperature)
                                       (6:129,798)

Questions 72 to 74

A. Estrogen
B. Progesterone
C. Both
D. Neither
72. Breast development
73. Secretory endometrium
74. Proliferative endometrium   (7:195-209)

Questions 75 to 78

A. Chronic pelvic inflammatory disease
B. Ectopic pregnancy
C. Both
D. Neither

75. Vaginal bleeding
76. Delayed menstruation
77. Abdominal pain
78. Culdocentesis of brownish-colored blood
                                       (6:478)

Questions 79 to 81

A. Endometrial polyp
B. Cervical polyp
C. Both
D. Neither
79. Vaginal bleeding
80. Associated with malignancy
81. Excision   (6:293,389)

Questions 82 to 84

    A. Arrhenoblastoma
    B. Granulosa cell tumor
    C. Both
    D. Neither
82. Menorrhagia
83. Enlargement of the clitoris
84. May become malignant   *(9:181-185)*

Questions 85 to 89

    A. Estrogen-dominant birth control pills
    B. Progestin-dominant birth control pills
    C. Both
    D. Neither
85. Depression
86. Gastric disturbances
87. Amenorrhea
88. Fluid retention
89. Weight gain   *(17:181-185)*

Directions: Each group of numbered words or phases is followed by a list of lettered terms. MATCH the lettered term most closely associated with the numbered word or phrase.

Questions 90 to 93
90. *Treponema pallidum*
91. Donovan body
92. Venereal wart
93. *Herpesvirus hominis*, Type II

    A. Granuloma inguinale
    B. Condyloma latum
    C. Condyloma acuminatum
    D. Herpes progenitalis   *(8:275-280)*

Questions 94 to 97
94. Tubal stenosis
95. *Hemophilus ducreyi*
96. Podophyllin
97. Frei's test

    A. Lymphogranuloma venereum
    B. Condyloma acuminatum
    C. Chancroid
    D. Gonorrhea   *(8:252-278)*

Questions 98 to 100
98. Hematogeneous dissemination to the fallopian tube

99. Dissemination through the veins and lymphatics of the broad ligament to the fallopian tube
100. Reaches the fallopian tube through the mucous membrane

    A. *Streptococcus*
    B. *Trichomonas*
    C. *Gonococcus*
    D. Tubercle bacillus
    E. *Candida albicans*   *(6:462, 484)*

Directions: The following clinical set problem consists of clinical information presented in the format of questions or incomplete statements followed by a group of the numbered options.

Indicate "T" if the option is true;
indicate "F" if the option is false.

A 24-year-old female computer programmer, complained of lower abdominal pain of 10-days duration. The pain was crampy, intermittent, and aggravated by intercourse. She has never been pregnant and has used an IUD for 2 years. She missed her menstrual period for 6 days and she was also annoyed by malodorous yellowish mucous vaginal discharge. You should now:
101. prescribe triple-sulfa vaginal cream
102. prescribe oral nystatin for 10 days
103. instruct the use of alkaline douches twice a day for 2 weeks
104. perform culdocentesis
105. order laparoscopy

A clinical diagnosis of PID has been established. If untreated, the likely complications include:
106. infertility
107. ectopic pregnancies
108. breast cancers
109. endometrial carcinomas

Appropriate managements include the following:
110. removal of IUD
111. total hysterectomy
112. chemotherapy of the sexual partners
                     (20:997-1003)

Answers and Explanations

1. **(E)** Patients with hydatidiform mole usually complain of vaginal bleeding without significant pelvic discomfort in the fourth or fifth month of pregnancy. The uterus is usually soft and of doughy consistency. The enlargement of the uterus is often out of proportion to the calculated duration of pregnancy.

2. **(E)** There is no ready answer to teenage contraception. The solution is determined by the individual problem, which needs to be clarified by exploration. Simply complying with the request or denying it usually is of little help to the girl who is really seeking help for the total problem. Contraceptive counseling is definitely needed.

3. **(C)** It is unlikely that a woman who has been having intercourse regularly (three pregnancies in the past two years) will stop simply because she is told it is wrong. Her problem is that she has already made the decision to have coitus and is in desperate need of contraception (her motivation is high if she has resorted to induced abortions three times). This patient is highly fertile and she possibly needs contractives with low pregnancy risk (i.e. IUD or oral contraceptives). Any patient undergoing induced abortion who does not want pregnancies in the near future should be on pills or have an IUD inserted. If this patient has difficulty following instructions to take pills daily, and IUD is an alternative. However, the decision has to be made by the patient.

4. **(E)** This is most probably a case of cervical polyp. Excision is in order and the tissue should be submitted for histological examination to be certain of its benign nature and to rule out cervical cancer in particular.

5. **(B)** Pregnant women with carcinoma in situ of the cervix should have invasive carcinoma ruled out (utilizing cold-knife cone biopsy, when necessary). The pregnancy may be allowed to continue and to terminate vaginally at term with subsequent postpartum re-evaluation (by conization biopsy). In invasive carcinoma, pregnancy should be terminated and radiation therapy instituted. With late pregnancy, if a viable infant can be delivered, cesarean section may be elected before instituting appropriate therapy.

6. **(B)** The cytologic report for Pap smears usually describes the specimen as I (normal, repeat in one year); II, III (abnormal, repeat immediately or in no more than three months); or IV, V (positive, take biopsy). The Class III or any abnormal Pap smear calls for immediate repeated smear, since *Trichomonas* infection may be the reason for abnormal cells. In no case is treatment justified until definite diagnosis has been established through biopsy studies. A repeated Class IV Pap smear with negative biopsies may pinpoint the possibility of ovarian or adnexal malignancies.

7. **(D)** Carcinoma of the cervix is diagnosed in about 1 in every 2000 pregnant women. Any suspicious cervical lesion requires a Pap smear or punch biopsies from obvious cervi-

73

cal lesions. However, unless microscopic study reveals anything but invasive cancer in women with abnormal cytology or suspicious cervical lesion, conization is necessary. Cone biopsy can usually be performed without disturbing the pregnancy.

8. **(A)** Trichomoniasis is characterized by pruritus and frothy, yellow-green, or clear discharge. Diagnosis is made by the presence of the flagellate in the wet smear.

9. **(C)** This appearance of the vagina is quite characteristic of *Trichomonas vaginalis*. The mucous membrane is reddened, and the posterior fornix often presents a granular or strawberry-like appearance, which is almost pathognomonic. Small petechial erosions may be seen on the cervix.

10. **(B)** Monilial vaginitis is characterized by the typical cheesy or curd-like, adherent discharge. Multiple brown-black colonies of 1-2 mm will grow on Nickerson's medium in 48 hours without incubation.

11. **(C)** Specific treatment of monilial vaginitis is the use of Mycostatin (nystatin) vaginal suppositories (100,000 units). One or two tablets are inserted high into the vagina every night before retiring for 10 to 14 days.

12. **(D)** The characteristic findings of a suburethral mass, which on compression produces purulent exudate from the urethral meatus, is diagnostic of a urethral diverticulum. Carcinoma of the female urethra may develop in urethral diverticulum but is not as localized and mostly occurs in older age groups. Gartner's duct cysts do not communicate with the urethra. Venereal urethritis is a diffuse process. Abscess of Skene's duct is extremely rare and generally occupies a position much closer to the external urinary meatus.

13. **(D)** In the presence of ascites, the lesion usually proves to be ovarian carcinoma with associated intra-abdominal metastases or ovarian fibroma with Meigs' syndrome.

14. **(D)** Meigs' syndrome is characterized by ovarian fibroma, hydrothorax, and ascites.

15. **(E)** Any patient presenting with amenor-

rhea is presumed to be pregnant until proved otherwise.

16. **(E)** Pseudomyxoma peritonei is an unusual condition characterized by the transformation of peritoneal mesothelium to mucus-secreting epithelium. Pseudomyxoma peritonei occurs in association with mucinous cystadenomas and appendiceal mucoceles. The rupture of malignant mucinous neoplasms also causes this condition. Huge amounts of mucinous material are secreted, and bowel obstruction and death can occur.

17. **(C)** The Stein-Leventhal syndrome is characterized by bilaterally enlarged polycystic ovaries, amenorrhea (or oligomenorrhea), infertility, obesity, and hirsutism. Grossly, the ovary is described as bilaterally enlarged and gray in color, with a firm, smooth cortex and a thickened fibrosed tunica. Beneath the surface are multiple cystic follicles and no evidence of corpora lutea.

18. **(C)** The most frequent complication of ovarian cyst is torsion or twisting of the pedicle, and the acute symptoms (pain and rigidity) thus precipitated are frequently the first indication of the presence of an ovarian tumor. This complication is more common in small or moderate-sized tumors than in large ones. When the cyst is on the right side, it often mimics acute appendicitis and often the diagnosis is made upon operation. The complication of torsion of an ovarian cyst is frequently peritonitis; treatment is immediate surgery.

19. **(B)** Submucous myomas comprise only 5% of all myomas, but are much more likely than other types of myomas to cause profuse bleeding and thus require hysterectomy, although their size is usually small.

20. **(B)** In the patient in her early forties who has completed her childbearing function, total hysterectomy is not looked on with disfavor. Preservation of the ovaries is desirable in premenopausal patients.

21. **(E)** Uncomplicated uterine retroversion is usually symptomless. Backache is one of the most common complaints in female patients and is usually an orthopedic backache. Back-

ache may be associated with retroversion of the uterus only in a severe case.

22. **(D)** Although patients with endometriosis may be asymptomatic, the classic symptomatology includes acquired dysmenorrhea, hypermenorrhea, polymenorrhea, cyclic bowel disturbances with painful defecation and rectal bleeding, and bladder irritability with hematuria. The physical finding is usually a hard, fixed, fibrotic nodule, usually noted as a beaded or "shotty" thickening in the uterosacral ligament, cul-de-sac, or posterior surface of the lower uterine wall or cervix. These patients are often unmarried or infertile.

23. **(C)** Two-thirds of endometrial carcinoma occurs in women beyond the menopause. Obesity, hypertension, diabetes, and sterility or poor fertility are associated with endometrial carcinoma. Any patients with postmenopausal bleeding should first be tested for cancer of the uterus, either of the cervix or of the body. Cervical cancer can usually be detected by careful inspection and office smears and biopsy. Once the vagina and cervix have been eliminated as sources of the bleeding, an intrauterine source may be safely assumed, and fractional dilatation and curettage should be in order.

24. **(C)** Uterine retrodisplacement is frequently associated with pregnancy, neoplasms (myoma uteri), trauma, adnexitis, and endometriosis. Endometriosis results in extensive scarring and contraction of the supporting tissue of the uterus, frequently causing fixation of the uterine fundus in the pelvis with retrodisplacement.

25. **(D)** Incision and drainage, sitz baths, and antibiotics are frequently useful adjuncts in management of an abscessed Bartholin's gland. Marsupialization is preferred, because it resolves the immediate problem and also prevents subsequent recurrence. In marsupialization, a linear incision is made over the medial border of the abscess in the region of the occluded duct opening. The gland lining is sutured to the vulvar skin and allowed to heal. If an incision of adequate length is made, the resultant opening will be widely patent and the Bartholin's cyst will usually not recur.

26. **(C)** Perforation of adnexal abscess causes pelvic or generalized peritonitis with severe abdominal pain (usually referred to the side of rupture), tachycardia, shock, and subnormal temperature that rises rapidly to 107-108°F. Pelvic examination may fail to demonstrate the previously palpable adnexal mass. Surgical exploration is immediately in order.

27. **(B)** Rupture of a tubo-ovarian abscess is an acute abdominal emergency that is rapidly fatal if not treated surgically. The treatment is total hysterectomy and bilateral salpingo-oophorectomy regardless of whether the abscess is bilateral or unilateral. Postoperatively, appropriate chemotherapy and supportive care for possible shock are indicated.

28. **(A)** Gonococcus is responsible for 65-75% of all pelvic inflammatory disease. Confirmation of the diagnosis is usually obtained by identifying the Gram-negative intracellular diplococci on a stained smear of the urethral, vaginal, or cervical discharge, of secretions milked from Skene's glands in the paraurethral area, or of material from rectal crypts obtained via anoscopy. A definite diagnosis is made by culture on Thayer-Martin medium.

29. **(D)** The irregular monophasic curve of BBT (basal body temperature) is characteristic of anovulatory cycle; biphasic temperature curve is indicative of ovulation and normal progesterone effect; and the sustained temperature elevation following ovulatory curve (biphasic) is the indication for pregnancy. Conception while the patient is maintaining a record of her basal body temperature curve occurs fairly frequently during the course of an infertility investigation.

30. **(E)** Although annual physicals of female patients are frequently directed towards the performance of Pap smears and sometimes are only limited to pelvic and abdominal organs, examination of the breasts and general survey of the entire physical make-up are musts as the basis of quality practice.

31. **(C)** Endometrial biopsy is the most accurate diagnostic technique of ovulation.

Phase	Day of menstrual cycle	Hormone
Proliferative (preovulation)	6-14	FSH, estrogen
Follicular secretory (ovulation)	15-28	FSH, estrogen, progesterone, and, LH
Luteal menstrual	1-5	FSH, estrogen, and progesterone (low titer)

32. **(A)** Ovulation usually occurs 14 days before the menstrual flow. However, in younger women, ovulation will possibly occur 10 days before the menstrual flow.

33. **(E)** The most common cause of congenital female pseudohermaphroditism is congenital adrenal hyperplasia. The defective adrenals are incapable of producing a normal amount of cortisol. The virilizing endogenous adrenal steroids produced cause virilization of patients who have normal female sex chromosome patterns.

34. **(B)** With an initial evaluation of normal pelvic findings, including normal vaginal estrogenic smear and normal arborization of cervical mucus, normal gonadotrophins (and 17-ketosteroids), and normal skull x-rays (normal visual field), a clinical test with IM injection of 100 mg progesterone (or 10 mg of medroxyprogesterone acetate daily for 10 days) can be employed after a negative pregnancy test. The withdrawal response to progestin administration indicates that the patient has a functional end-organ (uterine endometrium) and normal production of estrogen. A heavy dose of "tincture of time" will solve the problem.

35. **(D)** The combination pill (estrogen and progestin) with 50 μg of estrogen (such as orthonovum 1/50) is often used for young patients without contraindications (breast cancer, thromboembolism, stroke, estrogen-dependent neoplasia, and pregnancy). Hypomenorrhea or amenorrhea is due to estrogen deficiency and can be treated by increasing the estrogen content (80 or 100 μg).

36. **(B)** The absolute contraindications to using an intrauterine device (IUD) include pregnancy and active pelvic infections; the relative contraindications include recurrent pelvic infections, acute cervicitis, a history of ectopic pregnancy, valvular heart diseases (may lead to subacute bacterial endocarditis), and uterine abnormalities (cervical stenosis, a uterus smaller than 6 cm, endometriosis, endometrial polyps, bicornuate uterus, uterine myomata, endometrial hyperplasia, and severe dysmenorrhea and hypermenorrhea).

37. **(A)** After complete evacuation of the mole, the patient is instructed to avoid pregnancy; contraceptive pills should be prescribed. The persistent absence of an HCG (human chorionic gonadotrophin) titer for a year is reassuring, and the patient may be permitted to begin another pregnancy if she chooses. Quantitative HCG titers should be performed every one to two weeks until negative, and then monthly for the next year. Persistence of a titer or recurrence of a titer indicates persistent trophoblastic disease (a mole or malignant change of the mole—e.g., choriocarcinoma), and D and C is required to establish the diagnosis. A chest x-ray is mandatory to determine the presence of metastases. A persistent titer with negative D and C mandates chemotherapy with methotrexate. Actinomycin D is frequently used in combination with methotrexate.

38. **(A)** Chemotherapy is the primary therapy for chloriocarcinoma. Methotrexate (a folic acid antimetabolite that inhibits dihydrofolate reductase) is the drug most commonly used. Mercaptopurine (antimetabolite interfering with the biosynthesis of DNA) and actinomycin-D (an antibiotic binding DNA) are also used. Rifampin is an antibiotic inhibiting DNA-dependent RNA polymerase and is used for TB.

39. **(E)** Methotrexate is an extremely toxic drug which is used mainly for choriocarcinoma. Minor problems such as dermatitis, alopecia, and simple nausea and vomiting are common. Severe possibilities include bone marrow suppression, renal or hepatic complications, stomatitis, and GI ulcerations.

40. **(E)** Women with the complaint of pruritus vulvae are most likely to be patients who have monilial vaginitis during pregnancy, diabetics, or those who have received broad-spectrum antibiotics (tetracyclines) or are on oral contraceptives.

41. (E) Vesicovaginal fistulas are the most common type of urinary fistulas and usually result from surgical procedures. Vesicovaginal fistulas from radical hysterectomy are relatively rare.

42. (E) Urethrovaginal fistulas are less likely from obstetrical injury than postoperation or postirradiation. Lymphogranuloma venereum or inguinale may cause urethrovaginal fistulas. It is also frequently seen in the excision of a suburethral diverticulum.

43. (E) Rectovaginal fistula is the most common form of vaginal fecal fistula. The possible causes include birth injury, irradiation, vaginal surgery (vaginal puncture for pelvic abscess), hemorrhoidectomy, cancer, and lymphogranuloma inguinale. The treatment is observation and surgery.

44. (E) Diethylstilbestrol (stilbestrol) is a nonsteroid stilbene compound that has marked estrogenic properties. It has been effective for postcoital contraception, possibly by producing a premature fall in corpus luteum progesterone production and changes in the endometrium, which may provide an unacceptable implantation site for the fertilized ovum. lt is also often used in vaginal suppositories for atrophic vaginitis. Stilbestrol appears to be related to vaginal adenosis, cervical lesions, transverse vaginal septum, and clear-cell adenocarcinoma of the vagina in daughters whose mothers ingested stilbestrol during pregnancy.

45. (E) The ovary is one of the frequent sites of metastasis from almost any site. Cancers of all pelvic organs metastasize to the ovary, and the spread is usually bilateral. Five percent of endometrial carcinomas and 1% of cervical carcinomas metastasize to the ovary. The metastasis of vulvar and vaginal cancers to the ovary is usually in the late stage.

46. (C) Clomiphene citrate (Clomid), which is a nonsteroid compound, is an analogue of the estrogen chlorotrianisene (TACE). It is of greatest value in the treatment of anovulatory conditions in which there is some production of both gonadotrophins and estrogens but a complete loss of cyclicity. The drug acts at the estrogen receptor site in the hypothalamus and activates the negative feedback relationship between estrogens and gonadotrophins. Secretion of releasing factors and the ensuing increase in both FSH and LH induce follicle growth and ovulation by restoration of endocrine cyclicity. The patient with Stein-Leventhal's syndrome is the ideal candidate for Clomid therapy. Clomid is effective for some patients with Chiari Frommel's (amenorrhea-galactorrhea) syndrome but is ineffective in Turner's syndrome (ovarian dysgenesis) and Sheehan's syndrome (pituitary necrosis produced by postpartum hemorrhage or infection).

47. (B) In well-differentiated lesions, endometrial carcinoma is treated with hysterectomy and bilateral salpingo-oophorectomy. However, in moderately or poorly differentiated lesions, endometrial carcinoma is treated with preoperative radiation in the form of two radium insertions, followed in six weeks by total abdominal hysterectomy and bilateral salpingo-oophorectomy. For the moderately differentiated lesion, the surgery may be performed first, followed by irradiation.

48. (A) The triad of adenomyosis includes menorrhagia (heavier and longer menstrual flow), dysmenorrhea (pain during menstruation), and enlarged uterus (usually symmetrical, firm and globular, tender to palpation at the time of the menses). Frequently the uterus is nodular (nutmeg uterus). Dyspareunia, abdominal pain, and bowel irritability may also be present.

49. (A) The cervical cancer is frequently found to originate from the squamous-columnar junction. The histogenesis of cervical cancer postulates that the cancer cell is from the subcylindrical cell. Epidermoid carcinoma is believed to originate from the squamous epithelium of the portio vaginalis of the cervix. Adenocarcinoma of the cervix is less common and usually begins within the cervical canal with an atypical gland pattern. When cervical adenocarcinoma is found, it should be differentiated from secondary endometrial disease.

50. (A) A conservative approach to the treatment of endometriosis is first tried, since it is a nonneoplastic entity affecting women in the reproductive years. Pregnancy is desirable to treat endometriosis; however, frequently women with endometriosis are unable to conceive. Oral contraceptives and hormonal therapy (long-acting progesterone, Enovid) are frequently used with success. Primary surgical therapy is usually indicated only if there is significant enlargement of one or both ovaries, if the tubes are bound down in women who cannot conceive, if bowel obstruction is suspected, or if there is acute pain.

51. **(A)** Leukoplakia of the vulva, syphilis, lympnogranuloma inguinale, and lymphopathia venereum are associated with cancer of the vulva. They usually cause a syndrome of pruritus vulvae. Kraurosis of the vulva is a descriptive phrase connoting a shrunken, leathery vulva, the end stage of a variety of prior vulvar lesions, including simple atrophy; it rarely becomes cancer of the vulva.

52. **(E)** The imperforate hymen is rarely discovered before puberty. The frequent symptoms after menarche are cyclic abdominal pain, urinary retention with flank pain, and the accumulation of the blood in the vagina, uterus, and tubes (hematosalpinx).

53. **(B)** Venereal warts are more frequently found on both sexual partners. The virus is held to be the same as that of warts elsewhere but with different morphology because of local conditions. They have no relationship to lymphogranuloma venereum, but are frequently associated with vaginal discharges from trichomoniasis or moniliasis and have to be differentiated from secondary lues of condyloma latum (broad, flat, sessile growth), while condyloma acuminatum is a narrow-based pedunculated growth.

54. **(B)** In the first or second episode, conservative therapy with antibiotics and bed rest is recommended. The use of cortisone has been advocated in selected patients. Infertility is usually the case for PID patients, and surgical resection of uterus and ovaries is indicated in repeated flare-up cases.

55. **(E)** Side-effects of IUD (intrauterine device) use include breakthrough bleeding, leukorrhea, pelvic pain (dysmenorrhea), hypermenorrhea, psychiatric disturbances, PID (pelvic inflammatory disease), and chronic endometritis. Uterine perforation, ectopic IUD, peritonitis, and intestinal obstruction have been experienced.

56. **(D)** Vaginal bleeding is the most common complaint that prompts women to seek medical help. "Uterine apoplexy" is associated with hypertension. Physical examination should include a search for evidence of blood dyscrasia (e.g., ITP), such as petechiae or bleeding gums. It is unusual for vaginal bleeding to be due to serious systemic disease without other evidence of disease on physical examination. Dysfunctional uterine bleeding is due to a disruption of the normal hypothalamic-pituitary-ovarian interrelationship. Anovulatory cycle is often the cause and happens in menarche and menopause. If ovulation has occurred, a thorough study is needed.

57. **(C)** The most common etiology of abnormal vaginal bleeding is a pregnancy complication—usually a threatened or incomplete abortion. Postcoital bleeding is usually due to a cervical polyp or tumor in the vagina or cervix, and further investigation is needed. Until proved other wise, malignancy should be suspected as the cause of postmenopausal bleeding.

58. **(E)** Both an estrogen alone and progestin alone will prevent ovulation if large enough doses are given; the effect is apparently at the level of the hypothalamus or higher nerve centers. Small doses of progestins change endometrial metabolism and the type and amount of cervical mucus to prevent pregnancy. The oral pills seem certainly to increase the risk of thromboembolic disease. Oral pill users will have an increase in protein-bound plasma iodine and total thyroxine concentration in the blood due to the effect of estrogen on the binding capacity of globulin.

59. **(D)** Before prescribing oral contraceptives, patients with a positive family history of premature coronary heart diseases or hyperlipidemias, xanthomas, obesity, diabetes, or coronary or peripheral vascular diseases need studies on fasting serum triglycerides and cholesterol levels. D-thyroxine and cholestyramine are lipid-lowering drugs.

60. **(D)** Postmenopausal osteoporosis may be helped by estrogen therapy. However, the risk of endometrial carcinoma is increased in patients taking estrogen. A complete risk

factor analysis is required before instituting estrogen therapy. Endometrial carcinoma is associated with obesity, hypertension, diabetes mellitus, and nulliparity. The therapeutic benefit of estrogen (reduced frequency of fractures, lessened height loss, slowing of bone mineral loss) should be weighed against the increased risk of endometrial carcinoma and the possible side-reactions derived from estrogen use. When the decision is made to start estrogen therapy, cyclic therapy (20 of 30 days) should be instituted, and adequate follow-up visits (including pelvic examinations and Pap smears) should be performed.

61. **(E)** The acute subdural hematoma may be difficult to diagnose because of the associated cerebral injuries. This lesion is most commonly the result of high-speed impact, such as that occurring in automobile accidents. A rapid deterioration of the state of consciousness should arouse suspicion. Papillary dilatation and loss of extraocular movements, retinal hemorrhages, and papilledema may occur. Contralateral hemiparesis, Jacksonian convulsions, or generalized seizures may occur. Decerebrate rigidity and midbrain pontine signs are late manifestations.

62. **(D)** Malignancy, particularly breast cancer and multiple myeloma, frequently produces hypercalcemia by local bone reabsorption, prostaglandin synthesis, and production of parathormone-like substances. To prevent hypercalcemia, adequate hydration, active physical activity, and low calcium diet (avoidance of vitamin D) should be instituted. In acute hypercalcemia, stupor, delirium, psychosis, hyporeflexia, and coma may develop; adequate hydration, phosphate, glucocorticoids, and mithramycin can be instituted.

63. **(C)**

64. **(D)**

65. **(D)**

66. **(A)**

67. **(B)** Both IUDs and pills are used for fertilization prevention. IUDs probably prevent implantation however, the definite mechanism is not known. Contraceptive pills are ovulation-inhibiting agents which cause undesirable side-effects, including GI disturbances, breast fullness, and vaginal discharge (estrogen effect), and headache, dizziness, depression, apathy, fatigue, pelvic pain, and chloasma (progesterone effect). IUDs frequently cause breakthrough bleeding and infections. IUDs are almost as effective as pills in preventing pregnancy, although slightly more pregnancies may occur with IUD in situ. Contraceptive pills are effective only in highly motivated and relatively affluent consumers. IUDs are best suited for use in mass programs in developing societies where motivation is less and resources (economic and professional) are limited.

68. **(C)**

69. **(C)**

70. **(B)**

71. **(C)** Anovulatory cycle is seen in the first 1 to 2 years after menarche and in the climacterium. The bleeding is irregular in amount and duration in accordance with the prior stimulation and the withdrawal of estrogen. Climacterium is characterized by vasomotor disturbances (hot flashes), irritability, and musculoskeletal symptoms (osteoporosis). During anovulatory cycle, the basal body temperature (BBT) will show a monophasic curve which indicates the failure of ovulation.

72. **(A)**

73. **(C)**

74. **(A)** The growth of the duct system of the breast is stimulated by estrogen. Nipple erectility and pigmentation of the areola are also estrogen dependent. The development of acinar buds from the breast milk ducts and the formation of lobules and alveoli are stimulated by progesterone. Under the influence of estrogen, the endometrium proliferates, and under the effects of progesterone and estrogen, the secretory phase develops.

75. **(C)**

76. (B)

77. (C)

78. (B) In chronic pelvic inflammatory disease (PID), the menstrual rhythm is not disturbed and vaginal bleeding is in the form of menorrhagia. The pain in ectopic pregnancy is colicky, severe, and one-sided, frequently associated with nausea and attacks of faintness. The pain in PID is usually bilateral and of heavy bearing-down character. The culdocentesis will show turbid and serous character in PID and chocolate-colored blood in ectopic pregnancy (the blood usually does not clot). Vaginal bleeding in ectopic pregnancy is in the form of spotting.

79. (C)

80. (A)

81. (C) Endometrial polyp is frequently associated with bleeding (metrorrhagia) and offensive discharge. In postmenopausal women, endometrial polyp is often associated with malignancy and excision is recommended. Cervical polyp rarely becomes malignant. The bleeding is usually of the contact type (postcoital bleeding) and the treatment is excision.

82. (B)

83. (A)

84. (C) Ovarian granulosa cell tumors usually produce estrogen with symptoms of menorrhagia, pseudosexual precocity in children, vaginal bleeding, and breast enlargement in postmenopausal women. Granulosa cell tumors are low-grade malignancies. The ovarian arrhenoblastoma contains mixtures of Sertoli and Leydig cells and secretes androgen. The androgenic effect (virilism) is first manifested by defeminization (amenorrhea, breast atrophy, and loss of subcutaneous tissue) and is followed by masculinization (hirsutism, enlargement of clitoris, and deepening of the voice). Urinary 17-ketosteroids are usually increased slightly due to the production of a small amount of testosterone. (Urinary dehydroepiandrosterones are increased significantly.) Arrhenoblastomas are more malignant than granulosa cell tumors.

85. (B)

86. (A)

87. (B)

88. (A)

89. (C) Depression and amenorrhea occur more commonly with progestin-dominant pills, while gastric disturbance (nausea) and fluid retention occur more commonly with estrogen-dominant pills. Estrogen excess may cause acute weight gain (fluid retention) and progestogen excess may cause progressive (anabolic) weight gain. The preparation may be altered to counter the side-effects and still afford excellent birth control.

90. (B)

91. (A)

92. (C)

93. (D) Condyloma latum is secondary syphilis caused by *Treponema pallidum,* a spirochetal organism. Granuloma inguinale is caused by protozoan Donovan bodies. Condyloma acuminatum is multiple papillary proliferation on the vulva, vagina, or cervix and is of viral origin. Herpes progenitalis is caused by the Type II *Herpesvirus hominis.*

94. (D)

95. (C)

96. (B)

97. (A) Chronic gonorrheal pelvic inflammatory disease usually results in tubal stenosis with infertility. Chancroid (soft chancre) is caused by a small, Gram-negative, coccus-like bacillus, *Hemophilus ducreyi* (Ducrey's bacillus). Condyloma acuminatum is typically a narrow-based pedunculated growth (condyloma latum of syphilis is usually sessile, broad-based, and flat) which is treated with 25% podophyllin solution in tincture of benzoin. Frei's test is the skin test used for the diagnosis of lymphogranuloma venereum.

98. (D)

99. (A)

100. (C) The fallopian tubes constitute the initial seat of genital tuberculosis, which is usually secondary to extragenital tuberculosis (mostly pulmonary tuberculosis, although usually inactive) by hematogenous dissemination. Pyogenic acute salpingitis usually follows childbirth, abortion (septic or puerperal), or pelvic surgery (vaginal hysterectomy) when streptococci or staphylococci travel from a cervical or corporeal focus to the tube via veins and lymphatics of the broad ligament. Gonococci reach the tube via cervical focus by the mucous membrane, frequently with occlusion of the tubal lumen and subsequent sterility. Trichomonads are usually confined to vaginal mucosa to cause trichomonal vaginitis and are rare causes of salpingitis. *Candida albicans* causes monilial vaginitis in susceptible patients, including diabetics and patients on oral contraceptives or broad-spectrum antibiotics.

101. (F)

102. (F)

103. (F)

104. (F)

105. (F)

106. (T)

107. (T)

108. (F)

109. (F)

110. (T)

111. (F)

112. (T)

There are about half-million cases of PIDs (Pelvic Inflammatory Diseases) a year in the United States. Diagnosis is primarily on the clinical findings which include: abdominal tenderness, adnexal tenderness and cervical motion tenderness; fever (greater than 38°F), pelvic mass, positive onococcal culture, leukocytosis and pus on culdocentesis. Laparoscopic diagnosis is performed for differential diagnosis of ectopic pregnancy, appendicitis or ruptured abscess. Most common etiologic agents are gonococci (treated initially by penicillin G or ampicillin) and chlamydia trachomatis (treated initially by tetracyclines). Rarely it may be caused by turberculosis (mostly in postmenopausal women). Appropriate measures include the identification and treatment of the sexual contacts, antibiotic therapy, continuity of care and emotional supports. Health education of the sexually active women is urgently needed for preventive efforts.

Chapter 4

Obstetrics

1. A 35-year-old primigravida presents at term with the history of regular uterine contractions of increasing frequency for the past five hours. The interval between contractions is now five minutes. The abdominal examination reveals the following. The first maneuver reveals a hard, round, readily ballottable object occupying the fundus. The second maneuver identifies the back on the left side of the abdomen and the small parts on the right. The third maneuver identifies an irregular freely movable structure above the superior strait, and the fourth maneuver confirms absence of engagement of the presenting part. The fetal presentation is likely to be

   A. left occipito-transverse
   B. breech
   C. twin
   D. occipito-posterior
   E. right occipito-transverse   (*21:241*)

2. Lower leg edema during the last trimester of pregnancy is largely due to

   A. complete venous obstruction
   B. lymphatic stenosis
   C. intra-abdominal tumor
   D. increased venous pressure due to partial obstruction
   E. arterial obstruction in the pelvis   (*17:230*)

3. The plasma volume during normal pregnancy

   A. increases with the duration of the pregnancy
   B. decreases with the duration of the pregnancy
   C. reaches a peak at eighth month of gestation, then decreases
   D. remains constant throughout the pregnancy
   E. changes in no consistent pattern   (*17:230*)

4. At the end of 28 weeks of gestation (seven lunar months), the fetus weighs (in grams)

   A. 15
   B. 600
   C. 1000
   D. 1800
   E. 2500   (*16:65*)

5. The following laboratory tests are essential to good routine prenatal care for the multipara with a normal past history:

   A. glucose tolerance test
   B. chest x-ray
   C. x-ray pelvimetry
   D. protein-bound iodine
   E. none of the above   (*22:97*)

6. Presumptive signs of pregnancy include

   A. breast changes
   B. lassitude and somnolence

C. amenorrhea
D. nausea and vomiting
E. all of the above   (21:71-78)

7. Implantation of the fertilized ovum usually occurs

A. within 24 hours after ovulation
B. two to three days following ovulation
C. six to seven days following ovulation
D. ten to 12 days following ovulation
E. exactly 14 days following ovulation
                              (17:125)

8. Mastitis is commonly due to

A. breast carcinoma
B. lactation
C. traumatic infection
D. fibroadenoma of the breast
E. lipoma of the breast   (22:419)

9. Missed abortion means

A. the fetus was delivered prematurely
B. a dead fetus remained in the uterus for a period of time
C. inevitable abortion
D. the patient has recovered from the abortion
E. habitual abortion   (16:276)

10. The best evidence of progress in labor is gained by assessing

A. descent
B. dilatation
C. descent and dilatation
D. the degree of pain
E. the rapidity of the fetal heart beat
                              (17:390)

11. The most common fetal presentation and position at term is

A. right occipito-transverse (ROT)
B. left occipito-transverse (LOT)
C. right occipito-anterior (ROA)
D. left occipito-anterior (LOA)
E. left occipito-posterior (LOP)   (21:194)

12. Identical twins are usually

A. of the same sex
B. of the same body weight
C. of the same height
D. the result of several intercourses just before conception

E. of two chorions and two amnions
                              (22:213-215)

13. One minute after birth a pink infant is found to have a pulse of 98 with slow, irregular respirations; he sneezes when a catheter is placed in his nostril and demonstrates weak flexion of the extremities, which are blue in color. His one minute Apgar score is

A. 2
B. 3
C. 4
D. 6
E. 10   (17:454)

14. The umbilical cord in the neonate normally contains

A. two veins and one artery
B. two arteries and one vein
C. one vein and one artery
D. two arteries and two veins
E. none of the above   (22:27)

15. The largest diameter of the fetal head is the

A. occipitomental
B. occipitofrontal
C. biparietal
D. bitemporal
E. suboccipitobregmatic   (22:47-49)

16. All patients who develop acute infection of the kidneys during pregnancy should

A. have postpartum urinalysis
B. be treated with antibiotics for six months without urinalysis
C. not become pregnant again for a year
D. have surgery done in six months
E. have pyelograms done the day following delivery   (17:307)

17. A pregnant woman at term with a 4 cm dilated cervix is found to have marginal placenta previa with mild bleeding. The appropriate management is

A. cesarian section
B. rupture of the membrane
C. internal podalic version
D. use of an inflatable intrauterine rubber bag
E. use of Willett's scalp traction forceps
                              (22:264-265)

18. The most prominent sign of eclampsia is

A. headache
B. convulsion
C. edema
D. proteinuria
E. hypertension   *(21:169)*

19. A 43-year-old female, gravida 6, para 5, in her 32nd week of gestation, experienced the sudden onset of severe pelvic pains and dark, partly clotted blood (about half a bowl) discharging from her vagina. In the emergency room, a tube of blood without anticoagulant failed to clot, the abdomen was board-like, and the fetal heart tones were absent. The most likely diagnosis is

A. placenta previa
B. choriocarcinoma destruens
C. normal pregnancy
D. abruptio placentae
E. rupture of placental vessels   *(17:366)*

20. A 32-year-old female, gravida 3, para 2, presents in the emergency room with gushing bright red vaginal bleeding without abdominal pain in her ninth month of gestation. The blood clots well, and her blood pressure is 120/80 mmHg. The most probable diagnosis is

A. hydatidiform mole
B. abruptio placentae
C. marginal sinus bleeding
D. placenta previa
E. induced abortion   *(17:364)*

21. A multiparous pregnant woman is expected to deliver a full-term baby vaginally. At the 36th week of gestation during a normal prenatal vaginal examination, you find a complete placenta previa. You will deliver the baby by

A. rupture of the membrane
B. induction of labor
C. forceps delivery
D. the normal vaginal route
E. cesarean section   *(17:364)*

22. Which of the following complications is *not* more likely in diabetic then in nondiabetic gravidas?

A. pre-eclampsia
B. hydramnios
C. macrosomia
D. placenta previa
E. hyaline membrane disease   *(15:36-61)*

23. The important spectrophotometric peak of absorption for bilirubin pigments in amniotic fluid analysis for RH disease (in nm) is

A. 300
B. 350
C. 450
D. 600
E. 1000   *(17:431)*

24. Hydatidiform mole is most common in

A. the United States
B. the United Kingdom
C. Scandinavia
D. Eastern Europe
E. the Orient   *(17:217)*

25. The use of magnesium sulfate for severe pre-eclampsia is chiefly for its effect on

A. CNS
B. renal blood fiow
C. blood pressure
D. skeletal muscle
E. edema   *(17:348)*

26. The expected amount of amniotic fluid at term (in ml) is between

A. 1500 and 1800
B. 2000 and 2500
C. 200 and 500
D. 20 and 50
E. 800 and 1100   *(18:226-227)*

27. The L/S ratio in amniotic fluid helps in assessing

A. the kidney maturity of fetus
B. the skin maturity of fetus
C. the lung maturity of fetus
D. none of the above
E. all of the above   *(19:356)*

28. Alpha-fetoprotein levels in amniotic fluid are elevated in

A. congenital heart diseases
B. gastrointestinal anomalies
C. normal conditions
D. neural tube malformations
E. abnormal protein synthesis   *(14:186)*

29. A 23-year-old unmarried pregnant college girl (Gl PO) in her 18th week of gestation presents with a three day history of right calf aches. The physical examination reveals right calf swelling and tenderness. The use of Doppler has confirmed the diagnosis of a deep vein thrombophlebitis. The treatment of choice is

A. dextran
B. heparin
C. coumadin
D. indocin
E. high-dose salicylates   (20:331)

30. A 20-year-old known diabetic is found to be pregnant. This is her first pregnancy and she is currently at her eighth week of gestation. She is greatly overweight and on one dose of 35 units NPH and a weight-reduction, 1000 calorie diet. Records of the urine testings reveal persistent negative glucose, but off and on positive readings for ketones, especially during the early morning. The best course of action is to

A. split the NPH dose
B. increase the NPH dose to 54 units
C. start a 600 calorie diet
D. start an 1800 calorie diet
E. administer oral hypoglycemics   (16:359)

31. A 24-year-old pregnant woman with Grave's disease is best treated with

A. radioactive iodine
B. subtotal thyroidectomy
C. low-dose PTU
D. high-dose PTU
E. Inderal (propranolol)   (16:355)

32. A 25-year-old woman who delivered a normal full-term infant five days ago has fever, pleuritic pain, pelvic tenderness, and arterial hypoxemia. Management of this patient should consist of

A. immediate ligation of the inferior vena cava
B. administration of aspirin
C. administration of heparin
D. intermittent positive pressure breathing (IPPB)
E. antibiotics   (39:154)

Directions: For each of the incomplete statements below, ONE or MORE of the numbered completions is correct. In each case select:
A. if only 1, 2, and 3 are correct
B. if only 1 and 3 are correct
C. if only 2 and 4 are correct
D. if only 4 is correct
E. if all are correct

33. Maternal urinary estriols during pregnancy are of

1. fetal origin
2. paternal origin
3. maternal origin
4. fraternal origin   (18:159-160)

34. Common causes of shoulder presentations include

1. placenta previa
2. twins
3. hydramnios
4. contracted pelvis   (21:263)

35. Factors which may play a role in breech presentations are

1. prematurity
2. placenta previa
3. fetal malformation
4. abnormalities of the uterus   (21:238)

36. Frequent causes of uterine rupture during labor include

1. podalic version
2. classical cesarean scar
3. oxytocin administration
4. dysfunctional uterine labor   (17:551)

37. Acceptable indications for cesarean section in breech presentation include

1. cephalopelvic disproportion
2. fetal distress
3. elderly primigravidas
4. early delivery of a mother with diabetes   (17:517)

38. Urinary estriols are often low in

1. diabetic pregnancies
2. placental insufficiency
3. anencephaly
4. early fetal death   (22:112)

39. Indications for roentgen pelvimetry include

 1. dysfunctional labor
 2. normal cephalopelvic proportion
 3. abnormal presentation during labor at term
 4. routine procedures for every pregnant woman   (*17:486*)

40. The following conditions enter into the differential diagnosis of pregnancy:

 1. hematometra
 2. myoma
 3. ovarian cysts
 4. pseudocyesis   (*22:86-88*)

41. The following changes occur in the urinary system during normal pregnancy:

 1. increase in renal blood flow
 2. urinary frequency
 3. glycosuria
 4. dilatation of the urethra   (*17:240*)

42. Early in pregnancy the following laboratory test(s) are indicated:

 1. hemogloblin determination
 2. serology
 3. urinalysis
 4. blood typing   (*17:230*)

43. Predisposing causes for puerperal infection include

 1. prolonged labor
 2. excessive blood loss
 3. excessive numbers of vaginal examinations during labor
 4. premature rupture of membrane   (*17:585*)

44. A 25-year-old female who is ten weeks pregnant presents with fever, malaise, conjunctivitis, and postauricular lymphadenopathy. A maculopapular rash on her face, trunk, arms, and legs has been present for three days. You will recommend

 1. rest
 2. steroids
 3. hyperimmune gamma-globulin
 4. induced abortion   (*17:274*)

45. Excessive fetal development may be due to

 1. diabetes

2. multiparity
3. large size of the father
4. postmaturity   (*17:280*)

46. Kernicterus, a possible complication of severe hemolytic disease of the newborn, may cause the following:

 1. mental retardation
 2. opisthotonos
 3. muscle spasticity
 4. hypotonia   (*12:446*)

47. The infant born from a mother with hyperparathyroidism may be at increased risk for postpartum

 1. coma
 2. hyperglycemia
 3. hyaline membrane disease
 4. tetany   (*20:535*)

48. Rh immune globulin given to an Rh-negative mother immediately after delivery will

 1. prevent infusion of placenta blood into the mother's circulation
 2. prevent fetal blood from mixing with the maternal blood
 3. decrease the quantity of Rh-negative cells
 4. suppress Rh sensitization of the mother   (*16:203*)

49. Hydramnios is associated with

 1. maternal diabetes
 2. erythroblastosis
 3. fetal CNS anomalies
 4. renal agenesis   (*17:153*)

50. Fetal age is usually estimated by

 1. biparietal diameter via ultrasound
 2. the date of the last menses
 3. fundus height
 4. vaginal cytology for maturation index   (*16:194*)

51. A 42-year-old woman is accidentally pregnant. You would now

 1. help her to sort out her feelings about the pregnancy
 2. help her to reach the decision on the continuation of pregnancy

3. provide her with correct information on the risk of pregnancy

4. condemn her for not taking oral contraceptives faithfully   (39:1028)

52. Most diabetic patients are best delivered at

1. any time
2. before the 20th week of gestation
3. after the 40th week of gestation
4. at the 36th to 38th weeks of gestation   (16:360)

53. A woman with Class II (New York Heart Association Classification) cardiac disease is pregnant. Care should include

1. adequate bed rest
2. closer supervision of diet
3. vaginal delivery, if possible
4. treatment of congestive heart failure with no medications   (16:322)

Directions: Each group of numbered words or phrases is followed by a list of lettered statements. MATCH the lettered statement most closely associated with the numbered word or phrase.

Questions 54 to 57

54. A primigravida with a small normal pelvis and a membrane that has been ruptured for 24 hours is admitted. Her cervix is 6 cm dilated and the fetal heartbeat (FHB) is normal.

55. A multipara is found to have a ruptured membrane and a fully dilated cervix. The fetal heartbeat is 168 beats/minute.

56. In the third stage of labor, a nullipara is found to have one of the twins left in the uterus. There is prolapse of cord.

57. A nullipara is found to have prolapse of the cord down out of the vagina. The cord is pulsating and the cervix is 5 cm dilated.

A. External version
B. Internal version with forcep extraction
C. Forceps
D. Cesarean section
E. Cesarean section with hysterectomy   (22:447-466)

Questions 58 to 61

58. Placenta accreta
59. Placenta succenturiata
60. Placenta circumvallata
61. Placenta membranacea

A. May cause retention of the placenta
B. May fail to separate by hand
C. White fibrous ring
D. Thin membrane of the placenta   (22:277-278, 394-396)

Questions 62 to 67

62. Pituitary basophilic adenoma
63. Pituitary chromophobe adenoma
64. Pituitary acidophilic adenoma
65. Pituitary necrosis
66. Chiari-Frommel's syndrome
67. Frohlich's syndrome

A. Amenorrhea with hypertension
B. Amenorrhea and acromegaly
C. Amenorrhea with visual disturbance
D. Amenorrhea with hypometabolism
E. Amenorrhea and galactorrhea
F. Amenorrhea with obesity   (17:73-75)

Questions 68 to 70

68. Rupture of the membrane
69. Painless contraction, fourth month of pregnancy
70. Beginning of the second stage

A. Loss of vaginal acidity
B. Braxton-Hicks contraction
C. Bearing-down sensation   (22:79,169-174)

Questions 71 to 74

71. Average duration of labor in primigravidas
72. Average duration of labor in multigravidas
73. Median duration of the second stage of labor in primigravidas
74. Median duration of the second stage of labor in multigravidas

A. 13 hours
B. 50 minutes
C. 20 minutes
D. 8 hours   (22:154)

Questions 75 to 80

75. Twins
76. Alcoholism
77. Chronic smoker (greater than 1/2 pack a day)
78. Drug abuse

79. Weight gain of 25 lb
80. Polyhydramnios

   A. Fetal risk is increased
   B. Fetal risk is not increased   (16:86-102)

Questions 81 to 83
81. Elevated human placental lactogen level
82. Indication of oxytocin challenge test
83. Delta OD 450

   A. Pregnancy with hypertension
   B. Pregnancy with diabetes
   C. Both
   D. Neither   (108:137-176)

Directions: The following clinical set problem consists of clinical information presented in the format of questions or incomplete statements followed by a group of the numbered options.

Indicate "T" if the option is true;
indicate "F" if the option is false.

A 23-year-old unmarried female hypertensive patient (G1 P0) with 12-week gestation visited your office for the first time requesting prenatal care.

She has had essential hypertension for 2 years, controlled by thiazide diuretics and methyldopa (Aldomet). Physical examinations were essentially unremarkable. She indicates that she is interested in natural childbirth in the birthing room. You would now:

84. arrange for her therapeutic abortion to reduce risk of carrying through pregnancy with hypertension
85. tell her that you object strongly to natural childbirth and ask her to seek care elsewhere
86. explain to her that there may be time when natural childbirth is not in her best interest
87. discontinue thiazide diuretics and methyldopa during her pregnancy
88. refuse to see her because you do not like unmarried pregnant women

The possible complications of essential hypertension during pregnancy include:

89. preeclampsia
90. cerebral hemorrhage
91. macrosomia
92. erythroblastosis fetalis   (19:24-30)

Answers and Explanations

1. **(B)** Leopold's maneuvers will usually show the following in breech presentation: longitudinal lie, firm lower pole, limbs to one side, and hard head at fundus. Fetal heart is best heard above the umbilicus. Breech presentation is usually confirmed by pelvic examination.

2. **(D)** Venous pressure in the upper extremities remains fairly constant throughout pregnancy; in the lower extremities it rises progressively, beginning about the 12th week, and at term the pressure may reach a level as high as 10-20 cm of water above normal. The rise is due primarily to pressure of the gravid uterus on the adjacent pelvic veins, a factor that contributes to the development of ankle edema, varicose veins, and hemorrhoids.

3. **(C)** The plasma volume begins to increase during the first trimester, reaching a peak approximately 40% above normal at 32 to 34 weeks. From this time until term, there is a gradual reduction amounting to about 25% of the increase. During and immediately after the third stage of labor, there is a sharp temporary rise in plasma volume, followed by a rapid drop toward the normal nonpregnant range, although the original level is not actually reached until three or four weeks postpartum. The increase in plasma volume parallels the increase in cardiac output. Thus maximal risk for the patient with heart disease is reached early in pregnancy.

4. **(C)**

At the end of lunar month	Fetal weight (grams)
3	14
6	600
7	1000
8	1800
9	2500
10	3400

5. **(E)** Protein-bound iodine is frequently increased in pregnancy, and the glucose tolerance test is usually reserved for patients with diabetic tendency or patients with abnormal urine sugar and abnormal fasting blood sugar level. Chest x-ray and x-ray pelvimetry are reserved only for patients with definite indications (e.g., contracted pelvis, lung pathology) because unnecessary exposure to radiation should be avoided. Routine laboratory tests usually include urinalyses for protein, sugar, and sediments; blood examinations for syphilis, Rh factor, blood group, rubella antibody titer, hemoglobin or hematocrit value; and antibody screen, if indicated.

6. **(E)** Presumptive signs of pregnancy include cessation of menstruation, fatigue, nausea and vomiting, breast changes (tingling, enlargement, increased pigmentation, secondary areolae, veins, more prominent follicles of Montgomery, and striae), leukorrhea, abdominal striae, linea nigra (a line of pigmentation in the lower midline of the abdomen, ascending as pregnancy progresses), urinary fre-

quency, and discoloration of the vagina and cervix (Chadwick's sign—color changes in the vagina and cervix from pink to bluish, increasing to a deep purplish hue). Although these presumptive signs are not conclusive, they do offer presumptive evidence of pregnancy. They are valuable evidence, but never proof.

7. **(C)** Fertilization occurs probably within 24 hours after ovulation, and implantation occurs at the blastocyst stage six or seven days after ovulation.

8. **(B)** Mastitis is fairly common in the puerperium on the lactating breast. Mastitis seldom occurs prior to the end of the first week after delivery and often is seen for the first time three or four weeks postpartum. The usual symptoms are mild chills, fever, and breast soreness. Soon erythema and local heat develop over the infected and indurated segment of the breast. Tender, ipsilateral, axillary adenopathy is common. The infection is usually staphylococcal in origin and can be treated with antibiotics. If breast abscess develops, incision and drainage are frequently performed.

9. **(B)** Missed abortion is the failure of the uterus to expel its contents within eight weeks after the death of the embryo or fetus. The dead fetus may be retained for months or years. Disseminated intravascular coagulation, with resultant incoagulability of the blood, may occur after lengthy retention of a dead fetus in the uterus, particularly after the fourth month of gestation. Therapeutic abortion is often needed.

10. **(C)** The progress of labor is the result of the tendency for each uterine contraction to push the fetus downward through the pelvis and of the resistance of the soft tissue and the bony pelvis to its descent. This progress is best appreciated by assessing cervical dilatation, descent, and position and recording on a labor graph to detect obvious deviations from the normal course. The degree of descent is gauged by the station of the presenting part, which is its relationship to the plane of the ischial spines. If the presenting part is at the level of the spines, it is at Station 0; if it is 1 cm above the spines, it is at Station −1. If the lowest level of the presenting part is above Station −3, it is said to be floating. If the presenting part is 1 cm below the plane of the spines, it is at Station +1. When the presenting part reaches Station +3, it usually is resting on the pelvic floor. A sigmoid curve can be plotted for the relationship of passage of time of labor to the cervical dilatation. The curve shows latent and active phase (starting from 2 and 4 cm dilatation); deceleration sets in toward the end of the first stage (full dilatation of the cervix—10 cm).

11. **(B)** The most common presentation and position is left occipito-transverse (LOT); 95% of presentations are by head and 40% of these are LOT. Therefore, 38% of all births are LOT to start. The presenting part is the vertex, the area bounded by the bregma, the parietal eminences, and the posterior fontanelle. The denominator is the occiput.

12. **(A)** Twinning may result from the simultaneous fertilization of two ova (fraternal or dizygotic twins) or from the abnormal development of a single ovum (identical or monozygotic twins). Identical twins are always of the same sex; fraternal twins may be of the same or of different sexes. Identical twins usually have two amnions, one chorion, and one placenta. Fraternal twins have two amnions, two chorions, and two placentas. A twin infant is about 700 g lighter than a singleton infant at birth. Congenital malformations, prematurity, and stillbirths are more common in twins. Twinning is associated with toxemia, hydramnios, abnormal presentation, maternal anemia, and maternal circulatory and respiratory disturbances.

13. (D)

Sign	Apgar Score		
	0	1	2
Heart rate	Absent	Below 100	Over 100
Respiratory effort	Absent	Slow, irregular	Good crying
Response to catheter in nostril	None	Grimace	Cough or sneeze
Muscle tone	Limp	Some flexion of extremities	Active motion
Color	Blue, pale	Body pink, extremities blue	Completely pink

The highest possible score, 10, indicates an optimal condition; most normal infants are scored between 7 and 10. Those who are moderately depressed will usually have scores between 4 and 7 (as with the above infant); they will usually respond to stimuli and can be resuscitated without difficulty. Those with scores below 4 are severely depressed and require immediate treatment.

14. (B) The umbilical cord (funis) extends from the navel of the fetus to the placenta. It transmits fetal venous blood from the fetus through two arteries to the placenta, returning arterial blood by one vein from the placenta. Its diameter ranges from 1 to 2.5 cm and its length from 30 to 100 cm. The right umbilical vein usually disappears early, leaving only the original left vein. A common vascular anomaly is the absence of one umbilical artery, a condition often associated with other severe fetal anomalies, such as esophageal atresia and imperforate anus. The absence of one umbilical artery has been noted in 1% of the cords of singletons and in 5% of the cords of at least one twin.

15. (A) The occipitomental (OM) is the largest diameter (13.5 cm), extending from the most prominent portion of the occiput to the chin. This is the anteroposterior diameter presented to the maternal pelvis with brow presentations. The diameter of the bitemporal (BT—8 cm), the smallest diameter of the fetal head, is the greatest distance between the two temporal sutures. Biparietal (BP—9.25 cm) is the greatest transverse diameter of the head from one parietal bone to the other. This is customarily the greatest transverse diameter that must traverse the maternal pelvis. Suboccipitobregmatic (SOB—9.5 cm) extends from the middle of the large fontanel to the undersurface of the occipital bone, just where it joins the neck. This is the anteroposterior diameter presented to the maternal pelvis with occipital presentations and is the one most commonly seen. With the biparietal diameter, it forms a nearly circular plane and presents the smallest possible circumference, 29 cm. Occipitofrontal (OF—11.5 cm) extends from the most prominent portion of the occipital bone to the root of the nose, seen in syncipital presentations.

16. (A) The urine should be examined for the presence of infection during the early puerperium and again after involution in all women who have had acute pyelonephritis during pregnancy. If the infection has been recurrent or if bacteriuria persists, pyelograms should be made two or three months after delivery in an attempt to demonstrate a lesion that could have caused the attacks or any damage that may have been produced by the infection.

17. (B) When the placenta is lateral or only slightly over the os (marginal placenta previa) and the cervix has dilated enough to admit one or two fingers, rupture of the membranes may permit the head to press the placenta against the uterine wall and stop the bleeding. When the child is not viable, the Braxton Hicks version (internal podalic version), the inflatable intrauterine rubber bag, and Willett's scalp traction forceps may be used.

18. (B) Pre-eclampsia is characterized by hypertension, proteinuria, and edema, while eclampsia is mainly characterized by convulsion and coma (rarely coma alone).

19. **(D)** Abruptio placentae is the early separation of the placenta from its normal implantation site in the upper segment of the uterus before the birth of the baby. It frequently occurs in women of high parity (more than five children) and it recurs in about 10% of patients who had abruptio placentae in previous pregnancies. A clotting defect (fibrinogenopenia, intravascular coagulation) frequently develops with complete placental separation. Some patients may develop acute tubular necrosis or bilateral renal cortical necrosis to cause anuria. The principle of treatment is to control bleeding, to replace the blood loss, and to empty the uterus.

20. **(D)** The cause of placenta previa is unknown and it occurs more frequently in multiparas, increasing with the degree of parity. The differential diagnosis of abruptio placentae and placenta previa is summarized as follows.

Placenta previa	Abruptio placentae
The bleeding is painless	Bleeding accompanied by pain
Bright red blood	Blood is usually dark
Shock comparable with bleeding	Profound shock
Slight bleeding at onset, usually recurs	Profuse initial bleeding
Soft, nontender, contracting uterus	Firm, tender, tetanically contracted uterus
Easily felt fetus; FHB present	Difficult to feel fetus; FHB irregular or absent
Placenta may be felt	Placenta cannot be felt
No evidence of toxemia	May be associated with toxemia; BP low due to bleeding
Normal urine	Proteinuria or anuria
Blood clots normally	Clotting defect present

21. **(E)** In almost every instance, even though the baby is dead, the patient with complete placenta previa should be delivered by cesarean section. It is seldom necessary to delay termination if the pregnancy is of at least 36 weeks' duration. Cesarean section is the best method for terminating pregnancy with incomplete placenta previa. If the fetus is dead, the cervix is soft and patulous, and only the edge of the placenta can be felt; if bleeding is minimal, vaginal delivery is possible. Vaginal delivery usually increases the hazard for the infant because compression of the placenta by the presenting part obstructs fetal vessels, leading to severe anoxia. If a large enough area of fetal circulation is eliminated, the infant will die of anoxia.

22. **(D)** The course of pregnancy in the diabetic is characterized by an increased incidence of a variety of complications affecting both mother and fetus. Maternal mortality is negligible for diabetic gravidas, while fertility and spontaneous abortion rates among diabetics and among healthy subjects are the same. The most important problem is fetal mortality, which, despite improvements and increased experience in obstetrics and medical care, continues at rates of 10-20%, or three to six times the rate observed in the general population. Fetal mortality includes stillbirths, hyaline membrane disease, and congenital anomalies. Fetal morbidity includes macrosomia, hypoglycemia, respiratory distress syndrome, hyperbilirubinemia, hypocalcemia, and congenital anomalies. Maternal morbidity includes hydramnios and pre-eclampsia.

23. **(C)** The spectrophotometric analysis of amniotic fluid is a useful evaluation of fetal erythroblastosis. The bilirubin in the amniotic fluid of babies affected by erythroblastosis alters the optical density and produces a deviation at about 450 nm. The exact peak of this deviation from linearity is expressed as the difference between expected and actual optical density at 450 nm as measured from a tangent line drawn between 365 and 550 nm using semilogarithmic graph paper. Those in the lower zone (normal curve or a slight rise) need no special treatment. Those in the middle zone (a higher peak) should be delivered early or require exchange transfusions. Those in the upper zone (even higher peak) require intrauterine transfusion or treatment by immediate delivery.

24. **(E)** Hydatidiform mole is a neoplastic proliferation of the trophoblast in which the terminal villi are transformed into vesicles filled with clear, viscid material. Although it is usually benign, it has malignant potentialities and precedes the development of choriocarci-

noma. It is uncommon in the U.S.A., occurring once in 2500 pregnancies. In the Orient, it was estimated to occur once in 200 pregnancies in the Philippines and once in 100 (82–120) pregnancies in Taiwan.

25. **(A)** Sedation is the mainstay of the treatment of severe or progressive pre-eclampsia. The cerebral depressive action of magnesium sulfate produces general sedation; thus its ability to decrease vascular tone and its depression of the myoneural junction tend to lower blood pressure, promote excretion of urine, and help to prevent convulsions by decreasing hyperactive reflexes. Magnesium sulfate not only lowers blood pressure, but also relieves cerebral vasospasm, increases cerebral blood flow, and increases oxygen utilization by brain tissue. All these tend to reverse the changes of pre-eclampsia-eclampsia.

26. **(E)** The amniotic fluid increases rapidly to an average volume of 50 ml at 12 weeks' gestation and 400 ml at midpregnancy; it reaches a maximum of about a liter at 36 and 38 weeks of gestation. The volume decreases to 600 ml by 43 weeks.

27. **(C)** The ratio of dipalmityl lecithin to sphingomyelin (L/S ratio) in amniotic fluid can be used to assess pulmonary maturity, and, more specifically, to predict the probability of hyaline membrane disease. The ratio is low in cases of hyaline membrane disease and tends to be higher in prematures than in their gestational peers.

28. **(D)** Elevated alpha-fetoprotein levels in amniotic fluid have been shown to be associated with various neural tube malformations, including anencephaly and spina bifida.

29. **(B)** Untreated patients with deep vein thrombophlebitis in pregnancy may be at increased risk of developing pulmonary embolism. Heparin does not cross the placenta and is the drug of choice, whether used in a continuous intravenous infusion or in q 4h bolus doses. Coumadin agents cross the placenta and have been associated with teratogenic effects (similar to chondrodysplasia punctata with nasal bone hypoplasia and bone stippling). Low-dose subcutaneous heparin is used primarily for prophylaxis with prior phlebitis. Dextran has

little beneficial effect. Indocin has been shown to be associated with premature closure of the ductus arteriosus. Salicylate may cause fetal hemorrhage, and prolonged use of high-dose salicylate (as in patients with rheumatoid arthritis) may cause a postmaturity state.

30. **(D)** A well balanced diet of at least 1800 calories (with needed folic acid and iron supplementation) is needed during pregnancy to achieve an acceptable weight gain of 25 to 27 pounds in meeting nutritional requirements of the pregnant woman and her baby. Strict weight reduction is to be avoided during pregnancy, as it will lead to starvation ketosis, which may be harmful to the fetus. Following the administration of an 1800 calorie diet, blood and urine testing are indicated to assess the adequacy of the NPH insulin dose.

31. **(C)** Surgical procedure may cause recurrent laryngeal nerve paralysis, parathyroid removal, and anesthesic effects on the fetus. Radioactive iodine is contraindicated during pregnancy due to the fetal radiation exposure. PTU (propylthiouracil) crosses the placenta, and high-dose (or regular-dose) PTU may cause a hypothyroid infant (goitrous cretin). The patient should be controlled with low-dose PTU and the mother maintained in mild hyperthyroidism to minimize the effects of PTU on the fetus. Inderal may induce labor and may cause fetal bradycardia.

32. **(C)** The treatment of pulmonary embolism is anticoagulation using heparin or coumadin. Urokinase and streptokinase may be used.

33. **(B)** A marked increase in urinary output occurs during pregnancy. The bulk of the steroid hormones elaborated during pregnancy are synthesized in a cooperative effort—partly by the fetus and partly by the placenta, although the fetal adrenals are the essential source. Between 80% and 90% of the estrogen excreted during pregnancy is in the form of the 16-alpha-hydroxylated compound, estriol. Since the enzyme responsible for 16-alpha-hydroxylation exists only in the fetus, urinary estriol is used as a measure of fetal viability.

34. **(E)** Shoulder presentation is more common in multiparas than in primiparas and in prema-

ture than in mature labors. Twins, hydramnios, placenta previa, contracted pelvis, undue mobility or unusual shape of the fetus, or abnormal shape of the uterus (e.g., subseptate uterus) will frequently cause shoulder presentation.

35. **(E)** The breech is the presenting part in 25% of cases before 30 weeks; therefore, prematurity is an important factor. Multiple pregnancies, fetal malformation, hydrocephalus, hydramnios, lax uterus and pendulous abdomen, abnormal shape of pelvic brim or uterus (partial uterine septa), and placenta previa are all associated with breech presentations.

36. **(A)** The most common cause of uterine rupture is the separation of a scar from previous cesarean section. Spontaneous rupture occurs frequently in patients of high parity whose labor has been obstructed by malpresentation or disproportion. Administration of oxytocin in large doses or to patients in whom stimulation is contraindicated (obstructed labor, abnormal presentation) often causes uterine rupture. Operative deliveries (podalic version) often result in uterine rupture, particularly in prolonged labor, which overstretches the lower segment.

37. **(E)** Outcome for infants will be improved by performing cesarean section for any breech presentation in which easy, uncomplicated delivery cannot be anticipated. Frequent indications for cesarean section include pelvic contraction, a large fetus, a primigravida over 35 years of age, fetal distress (abnormal fetal heart rate), and dysfunctional labor. Cesarean section should also be used for women requiring an early delivery because of medical problems—e.g., diabetes and hypertension.

38. **(E)** The estriol level fails to rise in molar pregnancy, anencephaly, placental sulfatase deficiency, placental insufficiency, toxemia, diabetes, and prematurity. In late pregnancy, the level falls slowly or abruptly with fetal death.

39. **(B)** Indications for roentgen pelvimetry include: (1) dysfunctional labor, particularly when considering using oxytocin; (2) contracted pelvis with no progress in labor; (3) breech or other abnormal presentation during labor; (4) evidence of disproportion; (5) abnormal clinical measurements of the pelvis before conception.

40. **(E)** In myoma, menses are not absent, the uterine size usually does not increase steadily, and the pregnancy test is usually negative. In ovarian cysts, no presumptive or positive signs of pregnancy can be determined and the pregnancy test is usually negative. In pseudocyesis (spurious pregnancy), subjective signs of pregnancy may develop with abdominal size increased by fat, tympanites, or ascites, but the pregnancy test is usually negative.

41. **(E)** During normal pregnancy, renal blood flow increases 25% during the first and second trimesters and glomerular filtration increases 50% until the last two or three weeks of gestation. Urethral dilatation is common, especially on the right side. Dilatation of the kidney pelvis favors a diagnosis of pyelonephritis. Urinary frequency is common early in pregnancy because of bladder compression by the enlarging uterus and again in late pregnancy if the fetal head enters the pelvic cavity. Urinary frequency is also due to hyperemia of the bladder mucosa associated with pelvic venous congestion. Glycosuria is common because of increased glomerular filtration.

42. **(E)** Essential laboratory studies in the normal pregnant woman include determination of the hemoglobin or hematocrit, blood type, Rh factor, serological test for syphilis, urine tests for protein and sugar, and a screening cytological examination of cervical secretions.

43. **(E)** Puerperal infection is more common in women who are exhausted and dehydrated from prolonged labor; who bleed excessively without replacement and who are already anemic; who have experienced traumatic deliveries; whose placental fragments are retained; who received excessive vaginal examinations and unsterile intrauterine manipulation during labor, who are nulliparous; who are under 20 years of age; and whose membranes ruptured prematurely.

44. **(D)** Therapeutic abortion is justifiable whenever unquestioned rubella is contracted during the first 20 weeks after the onset of the

last menstrual period, unless the woman and her husband are willing to accept the risk of the infant's being affected. If the maternal infection occurred during the first four months of pregnancy, 75% of infants will develop congenital malformation (congenital heart lesions, cataracts, and glaucoma). Abortion should also be considered for women who acquire infection after the 20th week of pregnancy because the infant is more likely to suffer psychomotor disturbances or have a small head or congenital anomalies. The definite diagnosis of rubella should be established by hemagglutination-inhibition (HI) antibody studies before performing an abortion.

45. **(A)** The birth weight often increases progressively in each pregnancy. Babies whose parents are large generally weigh more than those born to smaller individuals. Giant babies are often associated with maternal diabetes. Postmaturity has little to do with the development of large infants; the typical postmature baby is thin and undernourished because of placental insufficiency.

46. **(E)** Erythroblastotic babies are very rarely jaundiced at birth, since the placenta and maternal liver metabolize and excrete most of the bilirubin. Soon after the birth, however, clinical jaundice may develop as a result of hemolysis and decreased liver function. If the indirect bilirubin of the infant exceeds critical levels for gestation age (20 mg/100 ml), kernicterus may develop, resulting in mental retardation, lethargy, hypotonia, muscle spasticity, opisthotonos, or even death.

47. **(D)** During intrauterine life, the infant of a hyperparathyroid mother is exposed to high serum calcium levels which may result in tetany when no longer present after birth. Tetany in newborns may be the first indication of maternal hyperparathyroidism. However, the majority of these infants are normal.

48. **(D)** Rh immune globulin will suppress Rh sensitization if given intramuscularly to an unsensitized Rh-negative woman within 72 hours after delivery of an Rh-positive infant. The major transfer of fetal Rh-positive blood to the maternal system occurs during labor, particularly at the time of placental separation. Fetal Rh-positive cells are eliminated from the circulation by the antigen-antibody reaction before they can stimulate an innate and permanent maternal antibody response.

49. **(A)** The accumulation of amniotic fluid in excess of 2000 ml is termed hydramnios. It is frequently associated with maternal diabetes, erythroblastosis, and fetal anomalies, including anencephaly, spina bifida, duodenal atresia, or tracheoesophageal fistula. Marked deficiency or absence of amniotic fluid (oligohydramnios) is exceedingly rare and is usually associated with fetal urinary tract anomalies, particularly fetal renal agenesis.

50. **(A)** Laboratory tests for assessing fetal age/maturity are as follows
    1. X-ray of the fetal skeleton
    2. Biparietal diameter by ultrasound
    3. Biochemical tests on the amniotic fluid
        a. Creatinine
        b. Lecithin/sphingomyelin ratio
        c. Shake or foam test
        d. Other tests
            1. Amylase
            2. Bilirubin and/or AOD 450 nm
            3. Protein
            4. Osmolarity
            5. Triglycerides
            6. Lipid-staining cells

The estimation of fetal skeletal age by x-ray is decreasing in popularity due to radiation exposure to the fetus. The presence of the distal femoral and proximal tibial epiphysial centers suggest a gestation of 36 to 38 weeks, respectively.

51. **(A)** When a woman accidentally becomes pregnant, she is usually already distressed; condemning her for not faithfully taking oral contraceptives prescribed by you may increase her guilty feelings. The risk of occurrence of Trisomy 21 Down's syndrome is directly correlated with the increased maternal age. The risk of Down's syndrome is 1:2000 live births at maternal age 20; it increases to 1:300 at maternal age 35; to 1:100 at age 40; and to 1:40 at age 45. The increased maternal age is also associated with the increased frequency of Trisomy 13 and 18. These risks should be fully explained to the patient, and the patient should undergo amniocentesis at 12 to 16 weeks of gestation if she decides to continue the pregnancy. The family physician will assist the patient (and possibly the husband or

significant others) in thinking through the problem of pregnancy so that the patient can reach the decision about the continuation of pregnancy. Whatever the patient's decision, the family physician should support the patient and provide needed care.

52. **(D)** The risk of hyaline membrane disease is quite high before the 36th week of gestation. Most pregnant diabetic patients are delivered at 38 weeks' gestation with pulmonary maturity. The method of delivery may be induction of labor or cesarean section, depending on the size and well-being of the baby and the status of labor readiness. Many diabetics are delivered by the vaginal route.

53. **(A)** Patients with Class I or II cardiac disease should have little trouble with pregnancy, although those with Class II disease require additional rest and closer supervision of diet to prevent the development of congestive heart failure, which would call for digitalization, diuretics, and oxygen therapy.

54. **(D)**

55. **(C)**

56. **(B)**

57. **(D)** External version is done to change a breech or transverse to a vertex presentation before labor starts. Internal version and forcep extraction are often needed for the second twin when prolapse or nonengagement occurs. Forceps are indicated when fetal circulation is embarrassed (FHB more than 160 or less than 100) with ruptured membrane and fully dilated cervix (without cephalopelvic disproportion). C-section is indicated for contracted pelvis with uterine inertia, prolapse with distress, maternal diabetes, fulminating preeclampsia, and malpresentation.

58. **(B)**

59. **(A)**

60. **(C)**

61. **(D)** Placenta accreta is the condition in which villi erode directly into the muscularis and manual separation is dangerous, causing hemorrhage; thus hysterectomy may be required on occasion. In placenta succenturiata, one or more small lobes (accessory lobes) are often found in the membranes, unconnected with the main placental mass except by vessels. They may be retained in the uterus, causing postpartum bleeding; manual removal is indicated. In placenta membranacea, a membrane surrounds the entire ovum and is difficult to separate during the third stage of labor. Manual separation is required. In placenta circumvallata, an elevated fibrous ring has formed at or near the margin of the fetal surface of the placenta, which may cause intermittent bleeding.

62. **(A)**

63. **(C)**

64. **(B)**

65. **(D)**

66. **(E)**

67. **(F)** Basophilic adenoma (Cushing's syndrome) consists of amenorrhea, obesity, hirsutism, abdominal striae, hypertension, and osteoporosis. Chromophobe adenoma is the most common type of pituitary adenoma and is characterized by amenorrhea, sterility, headache, progressive optic atrophy, and enlargement of sella turcica visible on x-ray. In acidophilic adenoma, there is gigantism or acromegaly with amenorrhea in late stages. Pituitary necrosis (Sheehan's syndrome) consists of postpartum hemorrhage or puerperal infection, no lactation, atrophic genital organs, amenorrhea, loss of pubic and axillary hair, and hypometabolism. The Chiari-Frommel's syndrome consists of amenorrhea and galactorrhea, Frohlich's syndrome is amenorrhea, obesity, and facial hirsutism, with adipose tissue deposited mainly about the hips, shoulders, breasts, and abdomen.

68. **(A)**

69. **(B)**

70. **(C)** Braxton Hicks contractions are characterized by intermittent, painless contrations that begin almost as soon as implantation occurs and continue at irregular intervals throughout gestation. They may be felt by manual

examination, but they are not infallible signs of pregnancy, since they may be caused by an irritation (myoma or hematometra). Normal vaginal secretions are acid but amniotic fluid is alkaline. Thus rupture of the membrane will increase the pH of the vagina. Rupture of the membranes often marks the beginning of the second stage of labor (full dilatation of the cervix). After a short lull, the contractions are renewed with increasing vigor and decreasing intervals. The patient soon feels like bearing down. These voluntary efforts grow increasingly irresistible and involuntary.

71. **(A)**

72. **(D)**

73. **(B)**

74. **(C)** The median duration of labor in primigravidas is 11 hours, with mode as seven hours. The median duration in multipara is six hours, with mode as four hours. Labors lasting over 30 hours usually are classified as "prolonged."

75. **(A)**

76. **(A)**

77. **(A)**

78. **(A)**

79. **(B)**

80. **(A)** Alcoholism may cause fetal alcohol syndrome, and the mother should not drink during pregnancy. A mother who is a chronic smoker of more than a half pack of ciagrettes a day may cause fetal intrauterine growth retardation, and the mother should abstain from cigarette smoking during pregnancy. Mothers who are drug abusers may produce drug-dependent infants who may develop withdrawal syndromes. The mother is required to stop drugs during pregnancy. Twins may cause preterm delivery, abnormal presentation, intrauterine fetal growth retardation, and twin-twin transfusion. Polyhydramnios may increase the risk of fetal abnormalities, including anencephaly and gastrointestinal obstructions. A weight gain of 25 lb is normal and there is no associated fetal risk.

81. **(B)**

82. **(C)**

83. **(D)** Patients with high-risk pregnancy (either with hypertension or with diabetes) require frequent clinical evaluation to assess fetal well-being. Before 34 weeks, serial ultrasonographic examinations are generally performed to estimate fetal age through biparietal diameter; at the 32nd week, serial estriol measurements are made to watch for signs of falling; at the 34th week, the oxytocin challenge test is performed to assess placental function; amniocentesis is performed to estimate L/S (lecithin/sphingomyelin) ratio for assessing fetal lung maturity, which determines the optimal time for delivery. In pregnant diabetics, the human placental lactogen level is generally elevated; in placental insufficiency, the level may be reduced, but it is not sensitive. In hypertension and toxemia during pregnancy, the human placental lactogen level is generally reduced; a nonstress test followed by an oxytocin challenge test should be performed to assess placental condition. The L/S ratio is estimated to decide the timing of delivery (when the fetus is mature and eclampsia is superimposed). A high Delta OD 450 of the amniotic fluid may indicate the need for fetal transfusion in erythroblastosis fetalis.

84. **(F)**

85. **(F)**

86. **(T)**

87. **(F)**

88. **(F)**

89. **(T)**

90. **(T)**

91. **(F)**

92. **(F)**

Traditional family structure is changing, a family physician may see more unmarried females determined to start a single parent family. These females are badly in need of comprehensive and continuous total health care from their family physicians. The patients with essential hypertension during pregnancy are at a higher risk to develop preeclampsia and eclampsia, left ventricular failure, cerebral hemorrhage, malignant encephalopathy, ablatio placentae and a baby of small birth weight. These patients require frequent prenatal care and the patients should be informed of occasional needs of surgical intervention rather than natural childbirth. During pregnancy antihypertensive medical regimens are continued and outcomes are usually excellent. Most patients are treated with thiazide diuretics and central adrenergic blockers (e.g., methyldopa and clonidine). Some clinicians may withdraw diuretics to avoid hypokalemia which may cause fetal arrhythmia. Diuretics may rarely cause jaundice or thrombocytopenia in the fetus. Arteriolar dilators such as hydralazine are used when pre-eclampsia supervenes.

Chapter 5

Dermatology, Ophthalmology, Orthopedics, Urology, and Otorhinolaryngology

Directions: Each of the questions or incomplete statements below is followed by five suggested answers or completions. Select the BEST answer in each case.

1. A 25-year-old female comes to your office because of malaise for four weeks, fever for two weeks, generalized pain in her joints, and swelling of her vulva. Physical examination reveals a mass in the right inguinal region discharging pus and associated with very marked engorgement of the vulva. Laboratory data showed: hemoglobin 12 g/100 ml, white blood count 12,000 with 55% segmented neutrophils, 45% lymphocytes; total protein 7.4 g/100 ml with albumin 3.4 g/100 ml and globulin 4.0 g/100 ml. The most likely diagnosis is

   A. chancroid
   B. syphilis
   C. lymphogranuloma venereum
   D. tuberculous lymphadenitis
   E. granuloma inguinale   (25:45)

2. A teenager came to you last month for acne. He has 24 palpable papules on his face plus innumerable red marks from former lesions. You prescribed dietary restrictions and tetracycline 250 mg twice a day. Today he returns complaining that his acne is no better, even though he has taken the medication and stuck to the diet faithfully. There are still plenty of red marks, but only eight palpable papules. What do you do?

   A. continue the same treatment
   B. give him a strong peeling lotion
   C. send him to a dermatologist

   D. double the dose of tetracycline
   E. tell him to forget the diet   (25:86-87)

3. A teenager consults you about profuse comedos of his face. You tell him to apply retinoic acid (e.g., Retin A cream) to his face every night. One week later he returns with a face that is redder and scalier than any you've seen before. Which of the following do you do?

   A. tell him to stop using the medicine and never use it again
   B. tell him to keep up the good work and continue treatment every night, just as he has been doing
   C. tell him to stop treatment for the present and use the medication less frequently once the irritation has subsided
   D. tell him to apply retinoic acid three times a day, then everything will be alright
   E. tell him to expose his face to strong sunlight after applying the medication   (25:86-87)

4. An eight-year-old girl has had a scaly, itching rash on the dorsal aspect of her toes each winter for the past three years. Her father has athlete's foot, her mother has hay fever, and one maiden aunt has psoriasis. The most likely diagnosis is

   A. dermatophytosis
   B. atopic eczema
   C. psoriasis
   D. candidiasis
   E. contact dermatitis from shoes   (25:121)

5. You have a middle-aged female patient who has had dry skin on the soles of her feet for many years and whose toenails are undermined with crumbly material. During the past few summers she has had circumscribed, itchy, and scaly patches of dermatitis about her ankles. Steroid creams aggravate rather than help, but the rash disappears in the winter. What is your diagnosis?

A. psoriasis
B. atopic dermatitis
C. *T. rubrum* infection
D. lichen planus
E. pityriasis rosea   (50:928)

6. A strawberry mole on a one-year-old child's neck which has grown to the size of a half dollar since its first appearance at about one month of age is best treated by

A. surgical excision
B. subintensive roentgen therapy
C. freezing
D. radium implantation
E. reassurance   (11:691)

7. The following statements are true of Leiner's disease (erythroderma desquamativum) *except* that

A. it occurs most frequently in breast-fed infants
B. its onset is between one and three months of age
C. a virus has been identified as the etiological agent
D. fresh plasma is one modality of treatment
E. it is characterized by the seborrhea of the scalp, intertrigo of the groins and axillae, and diffuse redness and scaling   (12:1688)

8. A 23-year-old female complains of nasal discharge, nasal obstruction, and pain in the face. The pain is throbbing in nature and is referred to the supraorbital area. The pain is worsened by head movements, walking, or stooping. On examination, tenderness is elicited over the antrum, which fails to transilluminate clearly. The most likely diagnosis is

A. frontal sinusitis
B. dental infection
C. chronic tonsillitis
D. maxillary sinusitis
E. chronic hypertrophic rhinitis   (36:113-115)

9. An insidious, indolent, inflammatory disease of a salivary gland with sinus tract formation would suggest

A. Mikulicz's disease
B. syphilis
C. tuberculosis
D. actinomycosis
E. sarcoidosis   (34:39)

10. Unilateral nasal discharge in children suggests

A. papilloma
B. vasomotor rhinitis
C. foreign bodies
D. juvenile angiofibroma
E. nasal polyps   (34:234)

11. Cerebrospinal rhinorrhea is frequently due to

A. fracture of the frontal bone
B. fracture of the occipital bone
C. fracture of the ethmoid bone
D. tumor of the parietal lobe
E. pituitary tumor   (34:235)

12. The most common cause of epistaxis is

A. trauma
B. hypertension
C. purpura
D. leukemia
E. avitaminosis C   (34:199)

13. A 30-year-old housewife complains of long-standing nasal obstruction; profuse clear, watery nasal discharge; conjunctival infection, and annoying sneezing. Physical findings of the lungs and heart are essentially negative. The nasal mucosa appears to be thickened and edematous with bluish-tinged inferior turbinates. The microscopic examination of the nasal secretion may reveal

A. neutrophilia
B. numerous staphylococci
C. numerous *E. coli*
D. eosinophilia
E. numerous spirochetes   (34:228-229)

14. A 20-year-old male has had tonsillitis for 10 days with some improvement. Two days ago he noted that the right side of the throat was becoming increasingly painful, and he was having trouble swallowing; he also noted that his voice was becoming muffled and he

had an earache. His temperature is now 102° F. On examination, trismus is present and the buccal mucosa is dirty. The right tonsil is pushed downward and medially. The uvula resembles a white grape. This clinical picture is most commonly caused by

A. *Staphylococcus*
B. Vincent's organism
C. *Streptococcus*
D. herpes simplex
E. actinomycosis   *(34:61)*

15. A 75-year-old male who has been smoking for 45 years has developed an ulcerative lesion of the tongue which did not heal with conservative treatment. The most likely diagnosis is

A. carcinoma of the tongue
B. tuberculosis of the tongue
C. gonorrhea of the tongue
D. hemangioma of the tongue
E. leukoplakia of the tongue   *(34:43-44)*

16. A patient suddenly feels the need to tilt his head toward his left shoulder in order to see "comfortably." He possibly has a lesion involving the following cranial nerve:

A. II
B. III
C. IV
D. V
E. VI   *(26:218)*

17. A patient with a sudden ptosis notes that his eye is turned outwards. You examine the eye and find the pupil reacts normally. The most likely diagnosis is

A. carotid aneurysm
B. diabetic neuropathy
C. hypertension
D. trauma
E. strabismus   *(26:245)*

18. In spontaneous, extensive subconjunctival hemorrhage, the treatment should consist of the following:

A. internal corticosteroid
B. topical corticosteroid
C. internal antibiotics
D. topical antibiotics
E. reassurance   *(26:83)*

19. A 72-year-old lady complains that her "trav-

eling rheumatism" has now affected her head. She has had pain on chewing and anorexia for two months. She has a tender area on her right temple. The most probable diagnosis is

A. temporal arteritis
B. tension headache
C. migraine headache
D. acute rheumatic fever
E. climacteric syndrome   *(26:265)*

20. A patient with bilateral cataracts appearing at age 30 who has signs of premature aging and diabetes most likely has

A. Thomson's syndrome
B. Werner's syndrome
C. Waardenburg's syndrome
D. Cogan's syndrome
E. Naphthalene poisoning   *(26:265)*

21. Proliferative retinopathy may be seen in all of the following *except*

A. methemoglobinemia
B. macroglobulinemia
C. diabetes
D. central retinal vein occlusion
E. hemorrhage from hypertension   *(26:141)*

22. Which of the following is most likely to lead to secondary (hemorrhagic, thrombotic) glaucoma?

A. central retinal artery occlusion
B. branch artery occlusion
C. branch retinal vein occlusion
D. internal carotid artery occlusion
E. central retinal vein occlusion   *(26:235)*

23. A 49-year-old man calls you to say that he has just had three episodes of blindness in his right eye. These episodes all occurred within two days of one another, lasted six to seven minutes, and then cleared—first in the inferior field of vision and then in the superior field of vision. Retinal findings in the involved eye show yellow flecks at two bifurcations of the inferior temporal arteriole. The most likely pathology is

A. atheromatous occlusion of the right internal carotid artery
B. sclerosis of the retinal vessels
C. embolization of the retinal vessels of calcific particles from a diseased aortic valve

D. cholesterol emboli that probably originated from the right carotid siphon

E. an ulcerating atheroma in the wall of the right carotid bifurcation   *(26:27)*

24. One of your strabismus patients with accommodative esotropia is being treated with echothiophate iodide drops. You discover an incarcerated inguinal hernia which requires immediate care. What is your advice to the surgeon and anesthesiologist?

A. increase the preoperative dose of atropine over the usual amount

B. use Fluothane (halothane) as a general anesthetic and not ether

C. avoid succinylcholine for abdominal wall relaxation

D. monitor the temperature closely for suspected malignant hyperpyrexia

E. use an intravenous fluid such as Ringer's lactate because of increased acidosis
    (26:373)

25. A patient with a perforating wound involving the uveal tract in one eye developed uveitis in the other eye two weeks later. This phenomenon is possibly due to

A. secondary glaucoma

B. direct bacterial invasion

C. virus infection in the other eye

D. autoimmune hypersensitivity to uveal pigment

E. infected embolism   *(26:116)*

26. A 10-year-old boy with itching eruptions over the nasolabial angles on the face was found to have progressive protrusion of the right eye and headache. The most likely diagnosis is

A. orbital cellulitis

B. cavernous sinus thrombosis

C. acute conjunctivitis

D. hordeolum

E. Horner's syndrome   *(26:200)*

27. A 45-year-old male suddenly develops headache, blurred vision, and excruciating eye pain; he vomits frequently. The most likely diagnosis is

A. acute conjunctivitis

B. acute glaucoma

C. corneal ulcer

D. acute iritis

E. episcleritis   *(26:158)*

28. A two-year-old child comes in for a routine physical and strabismus is noted. The parents should know the following *except* that

A. a large number of children with strabismus have some degree of amblyopia

B. amblyopia should be prevented rather than treated

C. in children with pure alternating strabismus, orthoptic treatment is usually unrewarding

D. practically all deviating eyes can be straightened by treatment

E. the surgery should be carried out after age ten   *(12:1578-1962)*

29. Acute purulent conjunctivitis in the first 10 days of life is least likely to be associated with

A. *Neisseria gonorrheae*

B. chemical irritation due to silver nitrate

C. dacryostenosis

D. other bacterial (e.g., *Staphylococcus, Pneumococcus, Streptococcus viridans, Escherichia coli*) infections

E. inclusion blennorrhea   *(12:408-409)*

30. Combined ulnar and median nerve injury at the level of the wrist is usually manifested by the following *except*

A. ape hand

B. claw hand

C. the inability to approximate the small finger to the thumb

D. the inability to spread the fingers apart

E. wrist drop   *(80:92)*

31. Sciatica is most commonly due to one of the following clinical conditions in a young man:

A. osteoarthritis

B. disk herniation

C. spinal cord tumor

D. abnormal posture

E. psychoneurosis   *(80:97)*

32. Hyperlateralization of the knee joint most likely will cause

A. rupture of the anterior cruciate ligaments

B. rupture of the medial meniscus

C. rupture of the lateral meniscus

D. rupture of the posterior cruciate ligament

E. rupture of the lateral collateral ligament
    (82:1224)

33. A 48-year-old woman has suffered from rheumatoid arthritis for 20 years. Recently she developed mild hypertension, general edema, proteinuria, and splenomegaly. Hyaline casts and a few RBCs were found in the urine. The most likely diagnosis is

A. gout
B. secondary amyloidosis
C. nephrotic syndrome
D. liver cirrhosis
E. acute glomerulonephritis   (82:1119)

34. An 18-year-old athlete complained of swelling and pain in his left thigh for three weeks. The pain prevented him from participating in athletic activities. The x-ray showed faint calcification. The most likely diagnosis is

A. myositis ossificans
B. osteoarthritis
C. rheumatoid arthritis
D. sprain
E. normal physical   (50:566)

35. Thickening of frontal and temporal bones is seen in the skull x-ray. The patient is probably suffering from

A. gargoylism
B. hydrocephalus
C. pituitary tumor
D. no disorder
E. hyperthyroidism   (73:1146)

36. A 60-year-old man falls down with his hand stretched. His problem is possibly

A. fracture of the clavicle
B. supracondylar fracture of the humerus
C. fracture of the shoulder
D. Colles' fracture
E. fracture of the shaft of the humerus   (32:223)

37. A 20-year-old male has been suffering from chronic backache with stiffness. On examination, the lumbar curve is flattened, with limited back motion. X-ray of the spine shows erosion and sclerosis of the sacroiliac joints. The most likely diagnosis is

A. ankylosing spondylitis
B. rheumatoid arthritis
C. osteoporosis
D. acute lumbosacral sprain
E. psoriatic arthritis   (73:1919)

38. The most common complaint of patients with Sjögren's syndrome is dry eyes manifested by symptoms of chronic conjunctival irritation. The diagnosis is established most definitely by

A. the finding of salivary gland enlargement
B. the finding of a dry tongue and a dry mouth with much dental decay
C. the demonstration of hypergammaglobulinemia and a reactive latex fixation test for rheumatoid factor
D. a biopsy of the inner surface of the lip
E. sialography   (76:1985)

39. A seven-year-old boy stopped riding his bicycle because of pain in his left knee. During the next four weeks he was observed to limp with any activity and continued to complain of pain in his left knee. There was no history of trauma to the knee and no obvious lesion on inspection. The most likely diagnosis is

A. a dislocated internal meniscus of the left knee
B. osteoid osteoma of the femur
C. early osteomyelitis
D. leukemia
E. osteochondrosis of the femoral head   (11:547)

40. Your elderly patient develops within six weeks a bulky tumor on his face the size of the end of your thumb. It has rounded, bulging sides and a central core filled with keratin. The most likely diagnosis is

A. squamous cell carcinoma
B. basal cell carcinoma
C. keratoacanthoma
D. common wart
E. seborrheic keratosis   (73:2297)

41. Nephrocalcinosis is seen in all of the following conditions except

A. primary nephrocalcinosis
B. breast cancer with bone metastasis
C. milk-alkali syndrome
D. sarcoidosis
E. hypoparathyroidism   (39:572)

42. A 40-year-old male has developed flank pain, albuminuria, and hematuria. On physical examination, there are smooth masses palpable in both flanks, with tenderness. Blood pressure is 160/100 mmHg. The most likely diagnosis is

A. nephrosclerosis
B. hydronephrosis
C. glomerulonephritis
D. essential hypertension
E. polycystic kidneys   *(38:413-416)*

43. A 30-year-old male patient has vomited out everything he has ingested for four days. The urine specific gravity is 1.014. He possibly has

A. poor renal function
B. good renal function
C. diabetes insipidus
D. normal renal function
E. diabetes mellitus   *(38:48)*

44. A patient received a severe blow over the left flank region. Two hours later, he developed gross hematuria. The first procedure you would order is

A. surgical exploration
B. cystogram
C. infusion urography
D. renal angiogram
E. EKG   *(38:248)*

45. The first diagnostic procedure to be done in a patient suffering from hematuria following pelvic injury is

A. renal angiography
B. cystogram
C. IVC
D. chest x-ray
E. EKG   *(38:252-253)*

46. A young man complains of fever, chills, burning, and micturition urgency. There is no hematuria. Rectal examination reveals an exquisitely tender, enlarged mass. The most likely diagnosis is

A. acute urethritis
B. acute prostatitis
C. internal hemorrhoids
D. acute pyelonephritis
E. acute glomerulonephritis   *(38:177)*

47. Vesicocolic fistula most commonly occurs as a complication of

A. pelvic surgery
B. carcinoma of the bladder
C. carcinoma of the sigmoid or rectum
D. diverticulitis of the sigmoid
E. pelvic irradiation   *(38:479)*

48. Which of the following symptoms is usually lacking in the early stage of renal cancer?

A. hematuria
B. palpable flank mass
C. pain
D. loss of weight
E. anemia   *(38:276)*

49. The administration of aminoglycosides and cephalosporins to a 75-year-old female who is currently on furosemide may increase the risk of developing

A. necrotizing enteropathy
B. acute renal failure
C. hypocalcemic tetany
D. pulmonary fibrosis
E. thrombocytopenic purpura   *(39:962)*

50. A merchant marine sailor whose route was mainly the Pacific and Indian Oceans came to the office complaining of progressive weakness of his left hand accompanied by wasting and anesthesia. On examination, his left ulnar nerve was grossly thickened. There was a red-brown indolent pigmented swelling of his right ear. Other parts of the physical examinations are essentially normal. CBC, urinalysis, and tuberculin test results are all negative. The most likely diagnosis is

A. syphilis
B. leprosy
C. tuberculosis
D. rheumatoid arthritis
E. multiple sclerosis   *(73:1634-1639)*

51. A 16-year-old girl has had two years of winter nasal congestion and rhinorrhea without sneezing. She has used antihistamine-decongestants, which have helped some. Skin tests are negative with common environmental allergens and some nasal eosinophils are present. The most likely diagnosis is

A. perennial nonallergic rhinitis
B. perennial allergic rhinitis
C. common cold
D. atrophic rhinitis
E. seasonal allergic rhinitis   *(34:231)*

52. In a one-day-old infant, mucoid ocular discharge, conjunctival hyperemia, and swollen eyelids are most frequently due to

A. gonococcal infection

B. infection due to *Hemophilus influenzae*
C. inclusion conjunctivitis
D. congenital toxoplasmosis
E. instillation of silver nitrate   *(12:408)*

53. A 45-year-old man has developed chronic, pruritic, red-brown and red-blue, well defined plaques in the chest wall. You would now

A. order chest x-rays
B. perform skin biopsy
C. perform bone marrow aspiration
D. order serum electrophoresis
E. perform wood light examination

(25:555-558)

54. A 45-year-old woman presents with recent onset of inflammatory arthritis involving both hands. Which is the *least* likely diagnosis?

A. rheumatoid arthritis
B. osteoarthritis
C. scleroderma
D. Reiter's syndrome
E. systemic lupus erythematosus

(73:1920-1921)

55. A 70-year-old man has developed acute renal failure after having an intravenous pyelogram. The *least* likely cause is

A. multiple myeloma
B. prostatic hypertrophy
C. volume depletion
D. diabetes mellitus
E. prior renal insufficiency   *(73:488)*

56. A 19-year-old sexually active female presents with hemorrhagic crusting of her lips with oral erosions, fever, malaise, and a generalized skin eruption consisting of round, raised plaques with tense blisters. The most likely diagnosis is

A. secondary syphilis
B. gonococcemia
C. herpes simplex
D. lymphogranuloma venereum
E. venereal warts   *(73:1714-1717)*

57. A 10-year-old girl complains of oliguria. Her blood pressure is 80/40 mmHg, urinalysis is normal, BUN is 60, and creatinine is 1.0. The most likely diagnosis is

A. acute poststreptococcal glomerulonephritis

B. volume depletion
C. urolithiasis
D. chronic glomerulonephritis
E. hemolytic uremic syndrome   *(73:1920-1921)*

58. A 60-year-old female has had a hearing impairment in her left ear for almost 15 years. Intermittently, there was severe pain on the left side of her face. During the office visit for her upper respiratory infection, you noticed a swelling coming out from the external ear. Following manipulation, profuse bleeding has developed. The most likely diagnosis is

A. acoustic neuroma
B. pyogenic abscess
C. glomus jugulare tumor
D. cholesteatoma
E. foreign body in the left ear canal

(34:365-366)

59. Uveitis is commonly associated with all of the following conditions *except*

A. diabetes mellitus
B. hypertension
C. rheumatoid arthritis
D. tuberculosis
E. sarcoidosis   *(26:114-118)*

60. A 6-year-old boy complains of right earache following swimming in a pool. Now you would

A. prescribe oral decongestants
B. prescribe oral polymyxin B
C. prescribe oral corticosteroids
D. prescribe polymyxin B eardrops
E. examine both ear canals   *(34:334-335)*

61. A 55-year-old patient was well on retiring after heavy alcohol intake but was unable to walk on arising. His right great toe was red and swollen, with exquisite tenderness. Among the following, the most specific test for the diagnosis is

A. polarizing light microscopy of the synovial fluid
B. erythrocyte sedimentation rate
C. white blood cell count
D. serum uric acid level
E. serum urea level   *(78:1175-1176)*

62. A 27-year-old female bank teller complains of an irritated red left eye. On physical examination, there is a moderate injection of

the larger conjunctival vessels, watery discharge, and a palpable preauricular lymph node. The most likely diagnosis is

A. retinal detachment
B. subconjunctival hemorrhage
C. chronic simple glaucoma
D. acute viral conjunctivitis
E. acute iritis   (26:69)

63. A young patient suddenly develops weakness of the left side of his face accompanied by severe pain inside the left external ear. The otoscopic examination reveals vesicular eruption on the left ear drum. The most likely diagnosis is

A. herpes simplex
B. otomycosis
C. pemphigus vulgaris
D. pemphigoid
E. Ramsay Hunt's syndrome   (34:438)

64. Pain and swelling of the submandibular region due to eating are most likely caused by

A. mixed tumor
B. thyroid nodule
C. trigeminal neuralgia
D. salivary calculi
E. paranasal sinusitis   (34:452-453)

65. Shortwave diathermy is indicated for all of the following conditions *except*

A. cardial pacemakers
B. osteoarthritis
C. tenosynovitis
D. cervical spondylitis
E. frozen shoulder   (82:709)

Directions: For each of the incomplete statements below, ONE or MORE of the numbered completions is correct. In each case select:
   A. if only 1, 2, and 3 are correct
   B. if only 1 and 3 are correct
   C. if only 2 and 4 are correct
   D. if only 4 is correct
   E. if all are correct

66. A housewife complains that she has been losing three of her fingernails during the past four weeks. You note that the affected nails are partially undermined from their distal aspects, but show no subungual debris. There is tender red swelling of the paronychial tissue at the bases of the affected nails. Which of the following measures do you suggest?

1. thorough scrubbing with soap and water
2. strict avoidance of soap, water, and detergents
3. griseofulvin orally
4. 4% thymol in chloroform applied q.i.d.
                                    (50:1110)

67. Tuberous sclerosis is characterized by

1. mental deterioration
2. adenoma sebaceum
3. convulsions
4. retinal phacoma   (12:1763-1764)

68. A patient with herpes zoster infection

1. has characteristic skin lesions which tend to follow dermatomes
2. has the primary lesion in the anterior horn cells of the spinal cord
3. will develop antibodies which cross-react with herpes zoster and varicella viruses
4. is almost always under 10 years of age
                                (76:1121-1124)

69. A 23-year-old female college student complains of a generalized rash all over the trunk. She also complains of headache, sore throat, and lacrimation. On inspection, there are maculopapular lesions on the palms and soles. Moist papules are also found in the anogenital region. The following procedures will confirm the diagnosis:

1. antinuclear antibody
2. STS
3. blood cultures × 3
4. darkfield examination of a skin lesion
                                (25:258-261)

70. Mènière's syndrome in a middle-aged woman usually includes the following clinical features:

1. vertigo
2. nausea and vomiting
3. deafness
4. tinnitus   (36:74-75)

71. Adenoid hypertrophy may cause

1. nasal obstruction
2. serous otitis media
3. adenoid facies
4. fluctuating hearing loss   (*34:71*)

72. A patient complains of a mild right-sided sore throat which progresses in severity. He also complains of intermittent right earache and a bad taste in the mouth. The possible etiological agents are

1. viruses
2. spirochetes
3. psyche
4. fusiform bacilli   (*34:54*)

73. The most frequent causes of paralysis of any of the three cranial nerves (III, IV, and VI) are

1. aneurysm
2. trauma
3. diabetes
4. hyperthyroidism   (*26:218*)

74. Fibrositis syndrome is characterized by

1. pain and stiffness
2. trigger points
3. sleep disturbance
4. highly elevated ESR   (*82:1083-1090*)

75. Fracture of the navicular without displacement is usually treated by

1. immobilization
2. applying a walking heel and permitting weight bearing
3. exercising the toes actively
4. open reduction   (*81:1684*)

76. The following may be true for the management of fracture of the neck of the femur:

1. closed reduction is usually sufficient
2. replacement of the head on the neck may cause aseptic necrosis
3. the blood supply of the femoral head after internal fixation will rapidly return to normal
4. arthroplasty is a useful method of management   (*81:1186*)

77. Nonunion of fractures is frequently associated with

1. inadequate immobilization

2. inappropriate reduction
3. severe fracture
4. extensive soft tissue damage   (*32:256*)

78. Septic arthritis is best treated by

1. open drainage of the joint
2. parenteral antibiotics
3. intra-articular antibiotics
4. irradiation   (*32:244*)

79. The following statements are correct concerning fractures in children:

1. they are simpler to treat than fractures in adults
2. anatomical reduction is generally not necessary
3. correct application of the cast is important
4. open reduction is always indicated
                                       (*32:251*)

80. Meniscus and ligament diseases of the knee joint are usually diagnosed by

1. evaluation of the history
2. x-ray alone
3. clinical findings
4. ESR   (*50:735*)

81. Volkmann's contracture is commonly seen in

1. humeral supracondylar fracture
2. forearm fracture-dislocation
3. cast of the humeral supracondylar fracture
4. cast of forearm fracture-dislocation
                                       (*32:260*)

82. A 55-year-old executive complains of persistent pain in the neck, at the shoulder girdle, in the right arm, and in the right hand for a year. X-rays of his cervical spines may show the following changes:

1. narrow intervertebral disk and lipping of the bodies
2. osteoarthritic changes
3. sclerosis
4. destruction of C3-C4 vertebrae   (*50:587*)

83. A 30-year-old white male complains of fleeting arthralgia for six months, which has been followed in the last month by bilateral knee swelling with heat and tenderness. Rheumatoid factor in a titer of 1:640 is present. Which of the following statements are correct?

1. the presence of a low synovial fluid complement is caused by deposition of immune complexes in synovium
2. rheumatoid factor is an isoantibody that can be safely transferred to another individual
3. there is a family of rheumatoid factors which are of 19S or 7-11S species
4. chronic antigenic stimulation can lead to the development of rheumatoid factor
(73:1913)

84. The following features are true for progressive systemic sclerosis (PSS):

1. a positive latex fixation test for rheumatoid factor
2. a positive ANA
3. elevated ESR
4. agammaglobulinemia   (76:2002-2006)

85. Fractured clavicle has the following signs in newborns:

1. Moro's reflex is absent on the affected side
2. crepitus may be elicited
3. the arm on the affected side not moving freely
4. rarely fractured by delivery   (12:361)

86. Vocal nodules are often associated with

1. constant screaming in children
2. singing above one's normal range
3. abuse of the voice in laryngitis
4. mutism   (34:104)

87. An eight-year-old girl has been suffering from vague abdominal pain with diarrhea and low-grade fever for a week. Her mother has noted that she has hesitancy in initiating the urinary stream and an intermittent stream. Renal tenderness is elicited on examination. Otherwise the physical examination is within normal limits. Pyuria and bacteriuria are found on urinalysis. The plain film of the abdomen reveals spina bifida. The following procedures are helpful to establish the diagnosis:

1. excretory urogram
2. simple cystogram
3. voiding cystourethrography
4. delayed cystography   (38:145-148)

88. Diabetic nephropathy may include the following clinical pictures:

1. intercapillary glomerulosclerosis
2. nephrotic syndrome
3. renal insufficiency
4. Wilm's tumor   (73:1339)

89. Tabes dorsalis may cause

1. incontinence
2. bladder distention
3. Charcot's joint
4. Argyll Robertson's pupils   (73:1656)

90. The complications of benign prostatic hypertrophy (BPH) include

1. epididymitis
2. bladder stones
3. hydronephrosis
4. uremia   (38:301)

91. Tuberculosis of the genital tract is characterized by the following clinical features:

1. painless swelling is usually presented in tuberculous epididymitis
2. often associated with extragenital tuberculosis
3. may often cause persistent "sterile" pyuria
4. IVP may show a "moth-eaten" appearance of the involved ulcerated calyces
(38:201-204)

92. Nephrotic syndrome is often associated with the following diseases:

1. glomerulonephritis
2. systemic lupus erythematosus (SLE)
3. amyloidosis
4. diabetic nephropathy   (38:439)

93. Bartter's syndrome is an uncommon form of secondary hyperaldosteronism. It is characterized by

1. edema
2. hypokalemia
3. hypertension
4. alkalosis   (76:1345)

94. Diuretics have been used extensively for the treatment of patients with edema and with hypertension. They may be useful in the treatment of patients with which of the following nonedematous conditions?

1. diabetes insipidus
2. idiopathic hypercalciuria
3. bromism

4. hypercalcemia   (76:1360-1362)

95. Hypocalcemia is frequently associated with

1. acute pancreatitis
2. anticonvulsants
3. hypovitaminosis D
4. hypoalbuminemia   (79:300-306)

96. Hyperuricosuria may be caused by

1. ulcerative colitis
2. leukemia
3. gout
4. allopurinol usage   (78:157)

97. Cotton wool spots are commonly seen in

1. hypertension
2. cataract
3. vascular insufficiency syndrome
4. toxoplasmosis   (26:244)

98. Central retinal vein occlusion is associated with

1. hypertension
2. anemias
3. hyperviscosity syndrome
4. lipemia retinalis   (26:235)

99. The following factors may increase the risk of perpetuating urinary tract infection:

1. vesicoureteral reflux
2. vesical residual urine
3. renal calculi
4. vaginal colonization by pathogenic bacteria
                                (73:622-623)

100. A 50-year-old farmer has had three episodes of blurring and pain in his right eye which lasted about two hours and were relieved by sleep. A few hours ago the symptom recurred. The examination showed that there were no conjunctival injection or exudates. His visual acuity was 20/200 OD. Now you would

1. reassure the patient
2. start corticosteroid eyedrops
3. prescribe a hypnotic flurazepam (Dalmane)
4. measure intraocular pressure   (26:160)

101. A 26-year-old black female has developed fever, arthralgia, and red-hot, painful, deep-seated nodules on the lower anterior legs. You would now

1. order chest x-rays
2. order a blood culture
3. perform skin biopsy
4. order bone scans for both lower legs
                                (73:2266)

102. A 55-year-old obese female has had chronic backache which has become increasingly unbearable. The x-ray of the lumbar spine revealed a narrowed joint space with osteophyte formation. You would now

1. prescribe oral steroids
2. start megadose fluorides
3. give cyclic estrogen therapy
4. institute a weight reduction program
                                (73:1951-1954)

103. Rheumatoid arthritis is frequently associated with

1. pericarditis
2. Baker's cyst
3. pulmonary fibrosis
4. glomerulonephritis   (73:1911-1912)

104. A seven-year-old girl has developed itchy rashes in the antecubital areas, wrists, popliteal areas, and neck. The skin covering the involved areas is thickened. The patient's history shows seasonal sneezing and nasal discharges. Now you would

1. start immunotherapy
2. prescribe oral antihistamines
3. administer BCG
4. initiate topical steroids   (73:2249)

105. Kyphosis may be associated with

1. neurofibromatosis
2. poliomyelitis
3. syringomyelia
4. Frederick's ataxia   (73:2187)

106. A 27-year-old engineer complains of moderate discomfort and redness in his right eye after working in his garden over the weekend. Visual acuity is normal (20/20 o.u.) and the right eye has mild hyperemia of the conjunctival vessels with a little mucoid discharge. The right cornea appears clean to penlight examination. You would now

1. advise the use of dexamethasone eye drops for three days
2. perform allergy skin tests

3. start systemic amphoterecin B
4. perform fluorescein staining of the cornea
(26:63)

107. The dietary regimen for patients with recurrent calcium oxalate stones should stress

1. alkaline-ash diet
2. daily megavitamin C
3. strict avoidance of meat
4. high fluid intake   (38:229)

108. Chronic urethritis is characterized by

1. urethral stenosis
2. urethral discomfort
3. burning on urination
4. normal urinalysis   (38:500)

109. Corneal annulus

1. is the first sign of a cataract
2. is always associated with hypercholesteremia
3. is caused by herpes simplex type II
4. is frequently seen in the elderly   (26:101)

110. Exophthalmos can be associated with

1. high myopia
2. macrophthalmos
3. rhabdomyosarcoma
4. fibroma   (26:198)

111. Necrotizing papillitis may be associated with

1. diabetes mellitus
2. sickle cell traits
3. vesicoureteral reflux
4. chronic use of analgesics   (38:167)

112. A 19-year-old complains of nasal obstruction for three months. Physical examination reveals a fiery red nasal mucosa; otherwise the examination is essentially normal. You would now

1. give him nose drops
2. prescribe oral antibiotics
3. perform bronchoscopy
4. ask about his medication history   (34:233)

Directions: Each group of numbered words or phrases is followed by a list of lettered statements. MATCH the lettered statement most closely associated with the numbered word or phrase.

Questions 113 to 117
113. Tight, shiny, indurated skin; face mask-like
114. Chronic irregular red plaques, may be butterfly type
115. Papules to nodules forming raised peripheral rings and central clearing
116. Flat-topped, polygonal, shiny to scaly violaceous papules
117. Blisters

A. Lichen planus
B. Pemphigus
C. Granuloma annulare
D. Scleroderma
E. Lupus erythematosus   (50:924-937)

Questions 118 to 121
118. Acanthosis nigricans   (25:420)
119. Lichen planus   (25:355)
120. Pellagra   (25:420)
121. Mongolian spot   (25:528)

A. Color plaque at the buttock
B. Psychosis and photosensitivity
C. Adenocarcinoma of the stomach
D. Violaceous flat pruritic papules in an emotionally tense individual

Questions 122 to 124
122. Dermatomyositis   (25:157)
123. Hirradenitis suppurativa   (25:91)
124. Hodgkin's disease   (25:555)

A. Staphylococcus
B. Bronchogenic carcinoma
C. Pruritus

Questions 125 to 127
125. Tinea versicolor   (25:279)
126. Erythema nodosum   (25:219)
127. Stevens-Johnson's syndrome   (25:215)

A. Subepidermal vesiculation seen histologically
B. Coccidioidomycosis
C. Pale areas on tanned skin

Questions 128 to 131
128. Sarcoidosis   (25:489)
129. Vitiligo   (25:422)
130. Lupus erythematosus   (25:149)
131. Pemphigus   (25:134)

A. Abnormality of intercellular mucopolysaccharide protein complex

B. Apresoline
C. Kveim test
D. Depigmentation in neck

Questions 132 to 135
132. Xanthelasma
133. Xanthoma tuberosum
134. Elevated serum triglycerides
135. Plane xanthomas

    A. Type II hyperlipoproteinemia
    B. Type III hyperlipoproteinemia
    C. Both
    D. Neither   *(25:378-386)*

Questions 136 to 141
136. Still's disease
137. Rheumatoid arthritis
138. Aortic insufficiency
139. Hypertriglyceridemia
140. Sickle cell anemia
141. Severe anemia

    A. Pale, whitish retinal vessels
    B. Pulsating retinal arterioles
    C. Uveitis
    D. Bluish spots on the sclera in an elderly woman
    E. Retinal detachment
    F. Blotchy hemorrhage and cotton wool exudates   *(26:115)*

Questions 142 to 146
142. Toxoplasmosis
143. Marfan's syndrome
144. Trichinosis
145. Sarcoidosis
146. Avitaminosis A

    A. Nodular uveitis
    B. Chorioretinitis
    C. Eyelid edema
    D. Keratomalacia
    E. Subluxation of the lens   *(26:112)*

Questions 147 to 149
147. Rosacea
148. Hypertension
149. Sturge-Weber's syndrome

    A. Hemangioma of choroid
    B. Blepharoconjunctivitis
    C. A-V nicking, absorbent cotton   *(26:112)*

Questions 150 to 154
150. Chiasma lesion
151. Complete lesion of the right optic nerve
152. Lesion of the left optic tract
153. Occipital lesion
154. Lesion in optic radiation

    A. Total blindness, right eye
    B. Right homonymous hemianopsia
    C. Bitemporal hemianopsia
    D. Homonymous hemianopsia with macular sparing
    E. Congruous homonymous hemianopsia without macular sparing   *(26:206)*

Questions 155 to 158
155. Paget's disease
156. Hyperparathyroidism
157. Rickets
158. Osteoporosis

	Serum-Ca	Serum-P	NPN	Alk-ptase
A.	High	low	normal	increased
B.	Normal	normal	normal	increased
C.	Normal	normal	normal	normal
D.	Normal (or low)	low	normal	increased
E.	Low	low	high	decreased

    (82:1306)

Questions 159 to 161
159. Osgood-Schlatter's disease
160. Legg-Perthes' disease
161. Köhler's disease

    A. Capital femoral epiphysis
    B. Tibial tuberosity
    C. Tarsal navicular   *(32:245)*

Questions 162 to 165
162. Osteogenic sarcoma
163. Ewing's sarcoma
164. Giant cell tumor
165. Osteoid osteoma

    A. "Onion peel" appearance
    B. Sunburst pattern in the humeral shaft
    C. Dense sclerotic lesion with radiolucent center
    D. Osteolytic lesion with irregular margin, bone cyst   *(39:536-537)*

Questions 166 to 170
166. Tennis elbow   *(32:226)*
167. Frozen shoulder   *(50:727)*
168. Thoracic outlet syndrome   *(32:224)*
169. Trigger finger   *(32:228)*
170. Carpal tunnel syndrome   *(32:228-229)*

    A. Hyperabduction of the arm may decrease
       the radial pulse
    B. Tenderness over the lateral epicondyle
    C. Calcific bursitis
    D. First trimester of pregnancy
    E. Pain along the radial styloid

Questions 171 to 174
171. Polyarteritis nodosa
172. Wegener's granulomatosis
173. Gout
174. Dermatomyositis

    A. Sinusitis
    B. Cholecystitis
    C. Chondrocalcinosis
    D. Bronchogenic carcinoma
              (76:352, 935, 1888, 2055)

Questions 175 to 177
175. Peyronie's disease   *(38:491)*
176. Reiter's syndrome   *(38:182)*
177. Goodpasture's syndrome   *(38:438)*

    A. Conjunctivitis and arthritis
    B. Plastic induration of the penis
    C. Pulmonary hemorrhage

Questions 178 to 181
178. Acute glomerulonephritis   *(38:436)*
179. Pyelonephritis   *(38:157)*
180. Kidney TB   *(38:199)*
181. Urinary stone   *(38:223)*

    A. The urine is usually cloudy, shows a little
       protein, and contains large amounts of
       pus and bacteria
    B. Persistent pyuria; bacteria smear stained
       with methylene blue is negative
    C. Coffee-colored or grossly bloody urine
    D. Gross hematuria with calcium phosphate
       casts

Questions 182 to 185
182. Pain
183. Pyuria

184. Parotitis
185. Before puberty

    A. Torsion of the testicle
    B. Acute epididymitis
    C. Both
    D. Neither   *(38:511)*

Questions 186 to 189
186. Intense itching
187. HLA B8
188. Malabsorption
189. Sun exposure

    A. Dermatitis herpetiformis
    B. Transient acantholytic dermatosis
    C. Both
    D. Neither   *(105:326-330, 976)*

Questions 190 to 193
190. 4000 Hz notch
191. Carhart's notch
192. No air-bone gap
193. Loss of low tones

    A. Mènière's disease
    B. Noise exposure
    C. Both
    D. Neither   *(34:372)*

Questions 194 and 195
194. Diabetes mellitus
195. Steroid therapy

    A. Glaucoma
    B. Cataract
    C. Both
    D. Neither   *(26:132, 166-179)*

Questions 196 and 197
196. Cytoid bodies
197. Cherry red spot with pallor of retina

    A. Herpes simplex
    B. Retinal artery embolism
    C. Lead poisoning
    D. Systemic lupus erythematosus
    E. Vertiligo   *(26:274)*

Questions 198 and 199
198. Sjögren's syndrome
199. Ankylosing spondylitis

A. HLA B5
B. HLA B17
C. HLA B27
D. HLA DW$_2$
E. HLA DW$_3$ (73:1919-1936)

Questions 200 to 202
200. Roth spots
201. Xanthopsia
202. Pigmentary retinopathy

A. Hypervitaminosis D
B. Use of phenothiazines
C. Use of chlorothiazide (Diuril)
D. Use of diazepam (Valium)
E. Subacute bacterial endocarditis

(26:233-257)

Questions 203 to 207
203. RBC cast
204. WBC and bacteria
205. WBC cast, fever, CVA tenderness
206. Refractile fat body in a polarized light
207. Hexagonal cystine crystal

A. Nephrotic syndrome
B. Cystine stone
C. Acute glomerulonephritis
D. Cystitis
E. Pyelonephritis   (38:45)

Questions 208 to 210
208. Depressed bone and air conduction curves
209. A bone conduction curve at or near the zero decibel level and a lower air conduction curve
210. A sharp dip at high frequencies

A. Presbycusis
B. Otitis media
C. Congenital rubella syndrome
D. Normal
E. Petit mal epilepsy   (35:25)

Questions 211 and 212
211. Internal hordeolum
212. Meibomian gland

A. Chalazion
B. Sty
C. Both
D. Neither   (26:44-46)

Questions 213 to 217
213. Myasthenia gravis
214. Gargoylism
215. Diabetes mellitus
216. Premature baby under high oxygen therapy
217. Osteogenesis imperfecta

A. Corneal opacity
B. Ptosis
C. Rubeosis iridis
D. Retrolental fibroplasia
E. Blue sclera   (26:151, 244, 258, 278, 279)

Questions 218 to 220
218. Acetylcholine
219. Distal oncholysis
220. Liquid nitrogen

A. Senile lentigines
B. Pustular psoriasis
C. Secondary syphilis
D. Heat urticaria
E. Gonorrhea dermatitis syndrome
(105:241, 649, 924)

Questions 221 to 223
221. Propranolol
222. Pyridoxine
223. Halothane

A. Gardner's syndrome
B. Malignant hyperthermia
C. Homocystinuria
D. Hemochromatosis
E. Marfan's syndrome   (78:435)

Questions 224 to 226
224. Ring scotoma
225. Central scotoma
226. Arcuate scotoma

A. Early glaucoma
B. Optic neuritis
C. Temporal lobe lesion
D. Retinitis pigmentosa
E. Parietal lobe lesion   (26:162-163)

Questions 227 to 229
227. Reduced complement level in synovial fluid
228. Calcium pyrophosphate crystals in synovial fluid
229. Phagocytosis of leukocytes by macrophages

A. Gout
B. Rheumatoid arthritis
C. Pseudogout
D. Traumatic arthritis
E. Reiter's syndrome   (78:1134)

Directions: The following clinical set problem consists of clinical information presented in the format of questions or incomplete statements followed by a group of the numbered options.
Indicate "T" if the option is true;
indicate "F" if the option is false.

A female nurse caught you at the hospital cafeteria; she asked you to help her nine-month-old girl who was irritable with a fever of 100.2°F. She was anorexic and vomited twice this morning. You would now:

230. prescribe Prochlor-Perazine (campazine) 5 mg/teaspoonful q.i.d.
231. instruct her to use trimethobenzamide (Tigan) suppository ½ tablet
232. tell her that you are fully occupied and run away from her
233. instruct her to try ice chips

The detailed history revealed that the baby also has had slight cough, and the mother noticed that the baby has been pulling at the ears. The examination of both of the girl's eardrums revealed patchy bright red spots on the tympanic membranes which were not bulged. The throat was injected; the tonsils were enlarged, not red; lungs were clear to percussion and auscultation. The remaining parts of the examination were unremarkable. You would now:

234. perform myringotomy
235. order a culture of the aspirate from tympanocentesis

236. perform a culture from nasopharyngeal secretions
237. perform an audiogram
238. order x-rays of both ears

A diagnosis of acute otitis media is considered. You would now prescribe which of the following antibiotics?

239. Ampicillin p.o. 75 mg/kg/day for ten days
240. INH p.o. 10 mg/kg/day for ten days
241. Amoxicillin p.o. 75 mg/kg/day for ten days
242. Amphotericin B p.o. 1.0 mg/kg/day for 14 days

Complications of acute otitis media include

243. meningitis
244. recurrent infections
245. brain abscess
246. serous otitis media
247. facial nerve paralysis   (12:1025-1029)

A twenty-three-year-old female was married four days ago; she developed dysuria for 3 days. You will now:

248. prescribe nitrofurantoin 100 mg 1 tablet q.i.d. for 10 days
249. give her 3 g oral amoxicillin stat
250. prescribe phenazopyridine (Pyridium) 200 mg 1 tablet t.i.d. for 3 days

A diagnosis of urinary tract infection is entertained; the high risk groups of urinary tract infection include:

251. patients taking cyclophosphamide
252. patients with diabetes mellitus
253. patients with pulmonary tuberculosis
254. patients receiving indwelling catheters
255. male with prostatic hypertrophy
                    (66, 67, 68, 69, 76:892-895)

Answers and Explanations

1. **(C)** The most important test in routine diagnosis of lymphogranuloma venereum is by the intradermal Frei's test. A serious complication is rectal stricture; the effective mode of antibiotic therapy is tetracycline.

2. **(A)** The reduction of palpable papules from 24 to 8 in a month is highly significant, and you can continue therapy with confidence that improvement will continue. The patient has been misled by the persistent red marks. You must counsel him that these do not count in evaluating the initial response to therapy, since it may take quite a few months for them to disappear. In another month, if improvement continues, the acne will probably be sufficiently under control to permit experimentation with foods.

3. **(C)** Note that it is usually wiser to start treatment with retinoic acid applications every third night, then gradually work up to every night, if tolerated. Many patients will find that they cannot use the medication even once; others will become intolerant after six months to a year. Always warn patients using retinoic acid to avoid sun light—they burn very easily. The medication should be discontinued during the summer, or a sunscreen should be prescribed.

4. **(B)** Always be reluctant to diagnose pedal dermatophytosis in prepubertal children. Contact dermatitis from shoes seems unlikely, since her feet have been growing and she has probably worn different shoes each year. Psoriasis is unusual at this age, and candidiasis of the toes is a rarity.

5. **(C)** *T. rubrum* infection (tinea pedis) is treated with griseofulvin.

6. **(E)** Most capillary hemangiomas will disappear by the age of six without any treatment and with excellent cosmetic results. Parental counseling and reassurance are required. Unless complications occur or the mass is in such a location as to interfere with function, no treatment is advisable.

7. **(C)** The cause is unknown, although in a familial type of Leiner's disease there is a deficiency of the opsonic activity of the C5 component of complement. Administration of fresh plasma to infants with C5 dysfunction may be lifesaving.

8. **(D)** X-ray of the maxillary sinus will show opacity and sometimes a fluid level. If there is swelling of the cheek, either dental infection or antral tumor should be considered. The complications include spread to other sinuses (e.g., frontal sinusitis), otitis media, laryngitis, pneumonia, or chronic paranasal sinusitis.

9. **(D)** In actinomycosis, the pathognomonic "sulfur granules" are found in the pus. Treatment is with penicillin or clindamycin.

10. **(C)** Children often put foreign bodies in their noses. Paper wads, peas, pebbles, rub-

117

ber erasers, and beans are the most common objects. The cardinal symptom is unilateral purulent nasal discharge.

11. **(C)** Sparkling clear unilateral discharge which contains sugar is highly suspicious of cerebrospinal rhinorrhea, which frequently results from head injury (mostly of the ethmoid bone), tumor (nasopharyngeal carcinoma), crushing otolaryngeal operation, congenital defect (encephalocele), or primary spontaneous CSF rhinorrhea.

12. **(A)** The most common cause of nosebleed is trauma. Nose picking is commonly the etiology of epistaxis in children. Nosebleed may be precipitated by trauma in patients with hypertension (the patients are usually older and the nosebleed may recur), rheumatic fever, purpura, and leukemia. A patient who is not bleeding from any other part of the body rarely has nosebleed due to a hematological disorder.

13. **(D)** Allergic rhinitis (hay fever) is best treated by eliminating the allergens or desensitization. Microscopically, the nasal secretions may reveal eosinophilia. Antihistamines are often used and environmental control is needed.

14. **(C)** Quinsy is a collection of pus arising outside the capsule of the tonsil in close relationship to its upper pole. It is most frequently caused by *Streptococcus* as a complication of acute tonsillitis. Tonsillectomy is often indicated because peritonsillar infection (or abscess) tends to recur.

15. **(A)** Metastasis of tongue cancer occurs early with bilateral metastases. Hemiglossectomy with radical neck dissection is often done.

16. **(C)** When the fourth cranial nerve is affected, a gross deviation is not often observed. The affected superior oblique muscle, however, will fail to intort the eye and diplopia will result unless the patient tilts his head to the shoulder opposite the affected eye. This eliminates the need for intorsion, and fusion may be maintained.

17. **(B)** The most common causes of oculomotor paralysis (third cranial nerve) include trauma, carotid aneurysm, and diabetes. In diabetes, the pupillary reponses are usually intact; in carotid aneurysm, they almost never are spared.

18. **(E)** In the common and benign form of subconjunctival hemorrhage, it should be noted that the gross hemorrhages that appear without cause are usually not related to hypertension or arteriosclerosis. However, when such hemorrhage is associated with extensive ecchymosis in the lids, one should consider an orbital neoplasm or a hemorrhagic dyscrasia. There is no treatment and the hemorrhage is usually reabsorbed in about two to three weeks. The best treatment is reassurance.

19. **(A)** A symptom complex of headache, pain on chewing, malaise, or polymyalgia rheumatica in an elderly female with a high sedimentation rate may establish the diagnosis of temporal arteritis. One should look temporal to the eyes to find nodular, tortuous, or tender temporal arteries. Prompt treatment with high-dosage steroids appears to significantly prevent the irreversible blindness which occurs in 50% of cases.

20. **(B)** Werner's syndrome is a rare hereditary disorder characterized ocularly by juvenile cataracts, glaucoma, and corneal opacities. It is probably transmitted as a recessive trait. The onset is usually between ages 20 and 30, with graying and thinning of the hair of the scalp, genital region, and axillas. Atrophic skin changes may also occur.

21. **(A)** The proliferative retinopathy (often referred to as retinitis proliferans) consists of the growth of retinal vessels into the vitreous, usually at the disk. They proliferate in a network pattern, may bleed and cause massive hemorrhage into the vitreous, or contract in scar formation that will detach the retina. It is now felt that patients with any significant degree of retinopathy should be evaluated by fluorescein angiography.

22. **(E)** About one-third of patients with central retinal vein occlusion have open-angle glaucoma in both eyes. This is considered to be a predisposing factor.

23. **(E)** Episodes of amaurosis fugax frequently occur as a result of atherosclerotic lesions of the ipsilateral internal carotid artery.

OTEN® TABLETS
opril Tablets
CRIPTION

OTEN (captopril) is the first of a new class of antihypertensive agents, a specific competitive itor of angiotensin I-converting enzyme (ACE), the enzyme responsible for the conversion of otensin I to angiotensin II. Captopril is also effective in the management of heart failure.

POTEN (captopril) is designated chemically as 1-[(2S)-3-mercapto-2-methylpropionyl]-L-proline 217.29].

ptopril is a white to off-white crystalline powder that may have a slight sulfurous odor; it is le in water (approx. 160 mg/mL), methanol, and ethanol and sparingly soluble in chloroform thyl acetate.

POTEN (captopril) is available in potencies of 12.5 mg, 25 mg, 50 mg, and 100 mg as scored ts for oral administration. Inactive ingredients: cellulose, corn starch, lactose, and stearic acid.

ICAL PHARMACOLOGY

hanism of Action

nechanism of action of CAPOTEN (captopril) has not yet been fully elucidated. Its beneficial ts in hypertension and heart failure appear to result primarily from suppression of the renin-otensin-aldosterone system. However, there is no consistent correlation between renin levels response to the drug. Renin, an enzyme synthesized by the kidneys, is released into the lation where it acts on a plasma globulin substrate to produce angiotensin I, a relatively inactive peptide. Angiotensin I is then converted by angiotensin converting enzyme (ACE) to angiotensin potent endogenous vasoconstrictor substance. Angiotensin II also stimulates aldosterone etion from the adrenal cortex, thereby contributing to sodium and fluid retention.

POTEN (captopril) prevents the conversion of angiotensin I to angiotensin II by inhibition of a peptidyldipeptide carboxy hydrolase. This inhibition has been demonstrated in both healthy an subjects and in animals by showing that the elevation of blood pressure caused by enously administered angiotensin I was attenuated or abolished by captopril. In animal es, captopril did not alter the pressor responses to a number of other agents, including otensin II and norepinephrine, indicating specificity of action.

E is identical to "bradykininase," and CAPOTEN (captopril) may also interfere with the degra-n of the vasodepressor peptide, bradykinin. Increased concentrations of bradykinin or aglandin E_2 may also have a role in the therapeutic effect of CAPOTEN.

ibition of ACE results in decreased plasma angiotensin II and increased plasma renin activity), the latter resulting from loss of negative feedback on renin release caused by reduction in otensin II. The reduction of angiotensin II leads to decreased aldosterone secretion, and, as a t, small increases in serum potassium may occur along with sodium and fluid loss.

e antihypertensive effects persist for a longer period of time than does demonstrable inhibition culating ACE. It is not known whether the ACE present in vascular endothelium is inhibited er than the ACE in circulating blood.

macokinetics

oral administration of therapeutic doses of CAPOTEN (captopril), rapid absorption occurs with blood levels at about one hour. The presence of food in the gastrointestinal tract reduces rption by about 30 to 40 percent; captopril therefore should be given one hour before meals. d on carbon-14 labeling, average minimal absorption is approximately 75 percent. In a 24-hour d, over 95 percent of the absorbed dose is eliminated in the urine; 40 to 50 percent is anged drug; most of the remainder is the disulfide dimer of captopril and captopril-cys-disulfide.

proximately 25 to 30 percent of the circulating drug is bound to plasma proteins. The apparent nation half-life for total radioactivity in blood is probably less than 3 hours. An accurate mination of half-life of unchanged captopril is not, at present, possible, but it is probably less 2 hours. In patients with renal impairment, however, retention of captopril occurs (see DOSAGE ADMINISTRATION).

macodynamics

inistration of CAPOTEN (captopril) results in a reduction of peripheral arterial resistance in rtensive patients with either no change, or an increase, in cardiac output. There is an increase nal blood flow following administration of CAPOTEN (captopril) and glomerular filtration rate is lly unchanged.

ductions of blood pressure are usually maximal 60 to 90 minutes after oral administration of an idual dose of CAPOTEN (captopril). The duration of effect is dose related. The reduction in d pressure may be progressive, so to achieve maximal therapeutic effects, several weeks of apy may be required. The blood pressure lowering effects of captopril and thiazide-type tics are additive. In contrast, captopril and beta-blockers have a less than additive effect.

ood pressure is lowered to about the same extent in both standing and supine positions. ostatic effects and tachycardia are infrequent but may occur in volume-depleted patients. pt withdrawal of CAPOTEN has not been associated with a rapid increase in blood pressure.

patients with heart failure, significantly decreased peripheral (systemic vascular) resistance blood pressure (afterload), reduced pulmonary capillary wedge pressure (preload) and pul-ary vascular resistance, increased cardiac output, and increased exercise tolerance time (ETT) been demonstrated. These hemodynamic and clinical effects occur after the first dose and ar to persist for the duration of therapy. Placebo controlled studies of 12 weeks duration show olerance to beneficial effects on ETT; open studies, with exposure up to 18 months in some s, also indicate that ETT benefit is maintained. Clinical improvement has been observed in e patients where acute hemodynamic effects were minimal.

udies in rats and cats indicate that CAPOTEN (captopril) does not cross the blood-brain barrier y significant extent.

CATIONS AND USAGE

ertension: CAPOTEN (captopril) is indicated for the treatment of hypertension.

using CAPOTEN, consideration should be given to the risk of neutropenia/agranulocytosis (see NINGS).

APOTEN may be used as initial therapy for patients with normal renal function, in whom the risk atively low. In patients with impaired renal function, particularly those with collagen vascular ase, captopril should be reserved for hypertensives who have either developed unacceptable effects on other drugs, or have failed to respond satisfactorily to drug combinations.

APOTEN is effective alone and in combination with other antihypertensive agents, especially ide-type diuretics. The blood pressure lowering effects of captopril and thiazides are approxi-ly additive.

eart Failure: CAPOTEN (captopril) is indicated in patients with heart failure who have not onded adequately to or cannot be controlled by conventional diuretic and digitalis therapy. OTEN is to be used with diuretics and digitalis.

NINGS

tropenia/Agranulocytosis

ropenia (<1000/mm³) with myeloid hypoplasia has resulted from use of captopril. About half of neutropenic patients developed systemic or oral cavity infections or other features of the drome of agranulocytosis.

e risk of neutropenia is dependent on the clinical status of the patient:

In clinical trials in patients with hypertension who have normal renal function (serum creatinine less than 1.6 mg/dL and no collagen vascular disease), neutropenia has been seen in one patient out of over 8,600 exposed.

In patients with some degree of renal failure (serum creatinine at least 1.6 mg/dL) but no collagen vascular disease, the risk of neutropenia in clinical trials was about 1 per 500, a frequency over 15 times that for uncomplicated hypertension. Daily doses of captopril were relatively high in these patients, particularly in view of their diminished renal function. In foreign marketing experience in patients with renal failure, use of allopurinol concomitantly with captopril has been associated with neutropenia but this association has not appeared in U.S. reports.

In patients with collagen vascular diseases (e.g., systemic lupus erythematosus, scleroderma) and impaired renal function, neutropenia occurred in 3.7 percent of patients in clinical trials.

While none of the over 750 patients in formal clinical trials of heart failure developed neutropenia, it has occurred during the subsequent clinical experience. About half of the reported cases had serum creatinine $\geq$ 1.6 mg/dL and more than 75 percent were in patients also receiving procainamide. In heart failure, it appears that the same risk factors for neutropenia are present.

The neutropenia has usually been detected within three months after captopril was started. Bone marrow examinations in patients with neutropenia consistently showed myeloid hypoplasia, frequently accompanied by erythroid hypoplasia and decreased numbers of megakaryocytes (e.g., hypoplastic bone marrow and pancytopenia); anemia and thrombocytopenia were sometimes seen.

In general, neutrophils returned to normal in about two weeks after captopril was discontinued, and serious infections were limited to clinically complex patients. About 13 percent of the cases of neutropenia have ended fatally, but almost all fatalities were in patients with serious illness, having collagen vascular disease, renal failure, heart failure or immunosuppressant therapy, or a combination of these complicating factors.

Evaluation of the hypertensive or heart failure patient should always include assessment of renal function.

If captopril is used in patients with impaired renal function, white blood cell and differential counts should be evaluated prior to starting treatment and at approximately two-week intervals for about three months, then periodically.

In patients with collagen vascular disease or who are exposed to other drugs known to affect the white cells or immune response, particularly when there is impaired renal function, captopril should be used only after an assessment of benefit and risk, and then with caution.

All patients treated with captopril should be told to report any signs of infection (e.g., sore throat, fever). If infection is suspected, white cell counts should be performed without delay.

Since discontinuation of captopril and other drugs has generally led to prompt return of the white count to normal, upon confirmation of neutropenia (neutrophil count <1000/mm³) the physician should withdraw captopril and closely follow the patient's course.

Proteinuria

Total urinary proteins greater than 1 g per day were seen in about 0.7 percent of patients receiving captopril. About 90 percent of affected patients had evidence of prior renal disease or received relatively high doses of captopril (in excess of 150 mg/day), or both. The nephrotic syndrome occurred in about one-fifth of proteinuric patients. In most cases, proteinuria subsided or cleared within six months whether or not captopril was continued. Parameters of renal function, such as BUN and creatinine, were seldom altered in the patients with proteinuria.

Since most cases of proteinuria occurred by the eighth month of therapy with captopril, patients with prior renal disease or those receiving captopril at doses greater than 150 mg per day, should have urinary protein estimations (dip-stick on first morning urine) prior to treatment, and periodically thereafter.

Hypotension

Excessive hypotension was rarely seen in hypertensive patients but is a possible consequence of captopril use in severely salt/volume depleted persons such as those treated vigorously with diuretics, for example, patients with severe congestive heart failure (see PRECAUTIONS [Drug Interactions]).

In heart failure, where the blood pressure was either normal or low, transient decreases in mean blood pressure greater than 20 percent were recorded in about half of the patients. This transient hypotension may occur after any of the first several doses and is usually well tolerated, producing either no symptoms or brief mild lightheadedness, although in rare instances it has been associated with arrhythmia or conduction defects. Hypotension was the reason for discontinuation of drug in 3.6 percent of patients with heart failure.

BECAUSE OF THE POTENTIAL FALL IN BLOOD PRESSURE IN THESE PATIENTS, THERAPY SHOULD BE STARTED UNDER VERY CLOSE MEDICAL SUPERVISION. A starting dose of 6.25 or 12.5 mg tid may minimize the hypotensive effect. Patients should be followed closely for the first two weeks of treatment and whenever the dose of captopril and/or diuretic is increased.

Hypotension is not *per se* a reason to discontinue captopril. Some decrease of systemic blood pressure is a common and desirable observation upon initiation of CAPOTEN (captopril) treatment in heart failure. The magnitude of the decrease is greatest early in the course of treatment; this effect stabilizes within a week or two, and generally returns to pretreatment levels, without a decrease in therapeutic efficacy, within two months.

PRECAUTIONS

General

Impaired Renal Function

Hypertension—Some patients with renal disease, particularly those with severe renal artery stenosis, have developed increases in BUN and serum creatinine after reduction of blood pressure with captopril. Captopril dosage reduction and/or discontinuation of diuretic may be required. For some of these patients, it may not be possible to normalize blood pressure and maintain adequate renal perfusion.

Heart Failure—About 20 percent of patients develop stable elevations of BUN and serum creatinine greater than 20 percent above normal or baseline upon long-term treatment with captopril. Less than 5 percent of patients, generally those with severe preexisting renal disease, required discontinuation of treatment due to progressively increasing creatinine; subsequent improvement probably depends upon the severity of the underlying renal disease.

See CLINICAL PHARMACOLOGY, DOSAGE AND ADMINISTRATION, ADVERSE REACTIONS [Altered Laboratory Findings].

Valvular Stenosis: There is concern, on theoretical grounds, that patients with aortic stenosis might be at particular risk of decreased coronary perfusion when treated with vasodilators because they do not develop as much afterload reduction as others.

Surgery/Anesthesia: In patients undergoing major surgery or during anesthesia with agents that produce hypotension, captopril will block angiotensin II formation secondary to compensatory renin release. If hypotension occurs and is considered to be due to this mechanism, it can be corrected by volume expansion.

Information for Patients

Patients should be told to report promptly any indication of infection (e.g., sore throat, fever), which may be a sign of neutropenia, or of progressive edema which might be related to proteinuria and nephrotic syndrome.

All patients should be cautioned that excessive perspiration and dehydration may lead to an excessive fall in blood pressure because of reduction in fluid volume. Other causes of volume depletion such as vomiting or diarrhea may also lead to a fall in blood pressure; patients should be advised to consult with the physician.

Patients should be warned against interruption or discontinuation of medication unless instructed by the physician.

Heart failure patients on captopril therapy should be cautioned against rapid increases in physical activity.

Patients should be informed that CAPOTEN (captopril) should be taken one hour before meals (see DOSAGE AND ADMINISTRATION).

(continued on last page)

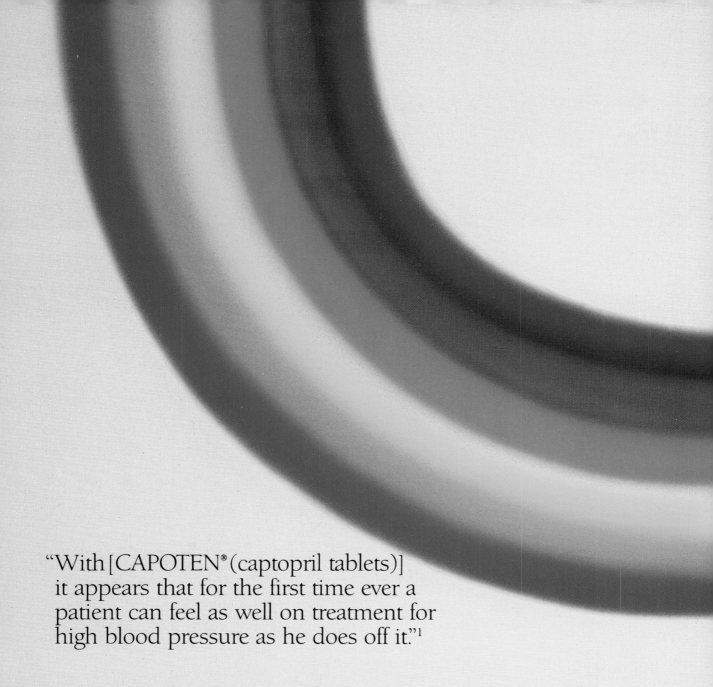

"With [CAPOTEN® (captopril tablets)] it appears that for the first time ever a patient can feel as well on treatment for high blood pressure as he does off it."[1]

*Angiotensin Converting Enzyme

†CAPOTEN may be used as initial therapy only for patients with normal renal function in whom the risk of neutropenia/agranulocytosis is relatively low (1 out of over 8,600 in clinical trials). Use special precautions in patients with impaired renal function, collagen vascular disorders, or those exposed to other drugs known to affect the white cells or immune response. Evaluation of hypertensives should always include assessment of renal function. See INDICATIONS AND USAGE, WARNINGS, and ADVERSE REACTIONS in the full prescribing information on the adjacent pages.

‡The most frequently occurring adverse reactions are skin rash and taste alteration; both effects are generally mild, reversible, or self-limited.

Reference:
1. Stumpe KO, Overlack A, Kolloch R, et al: Long-term efficacy of angiotensin-converting-enzyme inhibition with captopril in mild-to-moderate essential hypertension. Br J Clin Pharmacol 14(suppl 2):121S-126S, 1982.

Expanded Prescribing Freedom–
Mild-to-Moderate Hypertension

Capoten for Initial Therapy of Hypertension†

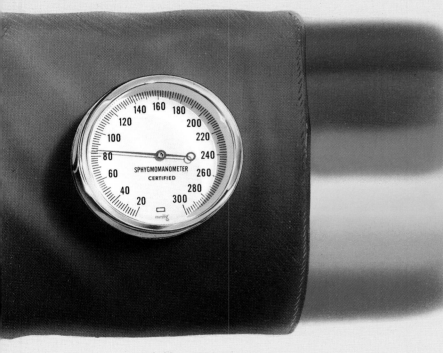

☐ Fatigue, loss of libido, impotence, and mental impairment <u>almost never</u> occur‡

☐ Effective <u>alone</u> or in combination with diuretics

☐ <u>Convenient</u> bid dosage

ACE*INHIBITOR

CAPOTEN®
captopril tablets

FIRST-LINE THERAPY THAT PUTS QUALITY OF LIFE FIRST

Drug Interactions

Hypotension—Patients on Diuretic Therapy: Patients on diuretics and especially those in whom diuretic therapy was recently instituted, as well as those on severe dietary salt restriction or dialysis, may occasionally experience a precipitous reduction of blood pressure usually within the first hour after receiving the initial dose of captopril.

The possibility of hypotensive effects with captopril can be minimized by either discontinuing the diuretic or increasing the salt intake approximately one week prior to initiation of treatment with CAPOTEN (captopril) or initiating therapy with small doses (6.25 or 12.5 mg). Alternatively, provide medical supervision for at least one hour after the initial dose. If hypotension occurs, the patient should be placed in a supine position and, if necessary, receive an intravenous infusion of normal saline. This transient hypotensive response is not a contraindication to further doses which can be given without difficulty once the blood pressure has increased after volume expansion.

Agents Having Vasodilator Activity: Data on the effect of concomitant use of other vasodilators in patients receiving CAPOTEN (captopril) for heart failure are not available; therefore, nitroglycerin or other nitrates (as used for management of angina) or other drugs having vasodilator activity should, if possible, be discontinued before starting CAPOTEN. If resumed during CAPOTEN therapy, such agents should be administered cautiously, and perhaps at lower dosage.

Agents Causing Renin Release: Captopril's effect will be augmented by antihypertensive agents that cause renin release. For example, diuretics (e.g., thiazides) may activate the renin-angiotensin-aldosterone system.

Agents Affecting Sympathetic Activity: The sympathetic nervous system may be especially important in supporting blood pressure in patients receiving captopril alone or with diuretics. Therefore, agents affecting sympathetic activity (e.g., ganglionic blocking agents or adrenergic neuron blocking agents) should be used with caution. Beta-adrenergic blocking drugs add some further antihypertensive effect to captopril, but the overall response is less than additive.

Agents Increasing Serum Potassium: Since captopril decreases aldosterone production, elevation of serum potassium may occur. Potassium-sparing diuretics such as spironolactone, triamterene, or amiloride, or potassium supplements should be given only for documented hypokalemia, and then with caution, since they may lead to a significant increase of serum potassium. Salt substitutes containing potassium should also be used with caution.

Inhibitors Of Endogenous Prostaglandin Synthesis: It has been reported that indomethacin may reduce the antihypertensive effect of captopril, especially in cases of low renin hypertension. Other nonsteroidal anti-inflammatory agents (e.g., aspirin) may also have this effect.

Drug/Laboratory Test Interaction

Captopril may cause a false-positive urine test for acetone.

Carcinogenesis, Mutagenesis and Impairment of Fertility

Two-year studies with doses of 50 to 1350 mg/kg/day in mice and rats failed to show any evidence of carcinogenic potential.

Studies in rats have revealed no impairment of fertility.

Animal Toxicology

Chronic oral toxicity studies were conducted in rats (2 years), dogs (47 weeks; 1 year), mice (2 years), and monkeys (1 year). Significant drug related toxicity included effects on hematopoiesis, renal toxicity, erosion/ulceration of the stomach, and variation of retinal blood vessels.

Reductions in hemoglobin and/or hematocrit values were seen in mice, rats, and monkeys at doses 50 to 150 times the maximum recommended human dose (MRHD). Anemia, leukopenia, thrombocytopenia, and bone marrow suppression occurred in dogs at doses 8 to 30 times MRHD. The reductions in hemoglobin and hematocrit values in rats and mice were only significant at 1 year and returned to normal with continued dosing by the end of the study. Marked anemia was seen at all dose levels (8 to 30 times MRHD) in dogs, whereas moderate to marked leukopenia was noted only at 15 and 30 times MRHD and thrombocytopenia at 30 times MRHD. The anemia could be reversed upon discontinuation of dosing. Bone marrow suppression occurred to a varying degree, being associated only with dogs that died or were sacrificed in a moribund condition in the 1 year study. However, in the 47-week study at a dose 30 times MRHD, bone marrow suppression was found to be reversible upon continued drug administration.

Captopril caused hyperplasia of the juxtaglomerular apparatus of the kidneys at doses 7 to 200 times the MRHD in rats and mice, at 20 to 60 times MRHD in monkeys, and at 30 times the MRHD in dogs.

Gastric erosions/ulcerations were increased in incidence at 20 and 200 times MRHD in male rats and at 30 and 65 times MRHD in dogs and monkeys, respectively. Rabbits developed gastric and intestinal ulcers when given oral doses approximately 30 times MRHD for only 5 to 7 days.

In the two-year rat study, irreversible and progressive variations in the caliber of retinal vessels (focal sacculations and constrictions) occurred at all dose levels (7 to 200 times MRHD) in a dose-related fashion. The effect was first observed in the 88th week of dosing, with a progressively increased incidence thereafter, even after cessation of dosing.

Pregnancy: Category C

Captopril was embryocidal in rabbits when given in doses about 2 to 70 times (on a mg/kg basis) the maximum recommended human dose, and low incidences of craniofacial malformations were seen. These effects in rabbits were most probably due to the particularly marked decrease in blood pressure caused by the drug in this species.

Captopril given to pregnant rats at 400 times the recommended human dose continuously during gestation and lactation caused a reduction in neonatal survival.

No teratogenic effects (malformations) have been observed after large doses of captopril in hamsters and rats.

Captopril crosses the human placenta.

There are no adequate and well-controlled studies in pregnant women. Captopril should be used during pregnancy or for patients likely to become pregnant, only if the potential benefit justifies a potential risk to the fetus.

Nursing Mothers

Concentrations of captopril in human milk are approximately one percent of those in maternal blood. The effect of low levels of captopril on the nursing infant has not been determined. Caution should be exercised when captopril is administered to a nursing woman, and, in general, nursing should be interrupted.

Pediatric Use

Safety and effectiveness in children have not been established although there is limited experience with the use of captopril in children from 2 months to 15 years of age with secondary hypertension and varying degrees of renal insufficiency. Dosage, on a weight basis, was comparable to that used in adults. CAPOTEN (captopril) should be used in children only if other measures for controlling blood pressure have not been effective.

ADVERSE REACTIONS

Reported incidences are based on clinical trials involving approximately 7000 patients.

Renal—About one of 100 patients developed proteinuria (see WARNINGS).

Each of the following has been reported in approximately 1 to 2 of 1000 patients and are of uncertain relationship to drug use: renal insufficiency, renal failure, polyuria, oliguria, and urinary frequency.

Hematologic—Neutropenia/agranulocytosis has occurred (see WARNINGS). Cases of anemia, thrombocytopenia, and pancytopenia have been reported.

Dermatologic—Rash, often with pruritus, and sometimes with fever, arthralgia, and eosinophilia, occurred in about 4 to 7 (depending on renal status and dose) of 100 patients, usually during the first four weeks of therapy. It is usually maculopapular, and rarely urticarial. The rash is usually mild and disappears within a few days of dosage reduction, short-term treatment with an antihistaminic agent, and/or discontinuing therapy; remission may occur even if captopril is continued. Pruritus, without rash, occurs in about 2 of 100 patients. Between 7 and 10 percent of patients with skin rash have shown an eosinophilia and/or positive ANA titers. A reversible associated pemphigoid-lik lesion, and photosensitivity, have also been reported.

Angioedema of the face, mucous membranes of the mouth, or of the extremities has bee observed in approximately 1 of 1000 patients and is reversible on discontinuance of captopr therapy. One case of laryngeal edema has been reported.

Flushing or pallor has been reported in 2 to 5 of 1000 patients.

Cardiovascular—Hypotension may occur; see WARNINGS and PRECAUTIONS [Drug Interactions for discussion of hypotension on initiation of captopril therapy.

Tachycardia, chest pain, and palpitations have each been observed in approximately 1 c 100 patients.

Angina pectoris, myocardial infarction, Raynaud's syndrome, and congestive heart failure hav each occurred in 2 to 3 of 1000 patients.

Dysgeusia—Approximately 2 to 4 (depending on renal status and dose) of 100 patients develope a diminution or loss of taste perception. Taste impairment is reversible and usually self-limited (2 to months) even with continued drug administration. Weight loss may be associated with the loss of tast

The following have been reported in about 0.5 to 2 percent of patients but did not appear a increased frequency compared to placebo or other treatments used in controlled trials: gastri irritation, abdominal pain, nausea, vomiting, diarrhea, anorexia, constipation, aphthous ulcer peptic ulcer, dizziness, headache, malaise, fatigue, insomnia, dry mouth, dyspnea, cough, alope cia, paresthesias.

Altered Laboratory Findings

Elevations of liver enzymes have been noted in a few patients but no causal relationship to captop use has been established. Rare cases of cholestatic jaundice, and of hepatocellular injury with c without secondary cholestasis, have been reported in association with captopril administration.

A transient elevation of BUN and serum creatinine may occur, especially in patients who ar volume-depleted or who have renovascular hypertension. In instances of rapid reduction of long standing or severely elevated blood pressure, the glomerular filtration rate may decrease transientl also resulting in transient rises in serum creatinine and BUN.

Small increases in the serum potassium concentration frequently occur, especially in patien with renal impairment (see PRECAUTIONS).

OVERDOSAGE

Correction of hypotension would be of primary concern. Volume expansion with an intravenou infusion of normal saline is the treatment of choice for restoration of blood pressure.

Captopril may be removed from the general circulation by hemodialysis.

DOSAGE AND ADMINISTRATION

CAPOTEN (captopril) should be taken one hour before meals. Dosage must be individualized.

Hypertension—Initiation of therapy requires consideration of recent antihypertensive drug trea ment, the extent of blood pressure elevation, salt restriction, and other clinical circumstances. possible, discontinue the patient's previous antihypertensive drug regimen for one week befo starting CAPOTEN.

The initial dose of CAPOTEN (captopril) is 25 mg bid or tid. If satisfactory reduction of bloo pressure has not been achieved after one or two weeks, the dose may be increased to 50 mg bid c tid. Concomitant sodium restriction may be beneficial when CAPOTEN is used alone.

The dose of CAPOTEN in hypertension usually does not exceed 50 mg tid. Therefore, if the bloo pressure has not been satisfactorily controlled after one to two weeks at this dose (and the patient not already receiving a diuretic), a modest dose of a thiazide-type diuretic (e.g., hydrochlorothiazid 25 mg daily), should be added. The diuretic dose may be increased at one- to two-week interva until its highest usual antihypertensive dose is reached.

If CAPOTEN (captopril) is being started in a patient already receiving a diuretic, CAPOTEN therap should be initiated under close medical supervision (see WARNINGS and PRECAUTIONS [Dru Interactions] regarding hypotension), with dosage and titration of CAPOTEN as noted above.

If further blood pressure reduction is required, the dose of CAPOTEN may be increased to 100 m bid or tid and then, if necessary, to 150 mg bid or tid (while continuing the diuretic). The usual dos range is 25 to 150 mg bid or tid. A maximum daily dose of 450 mg CAPOTEN should n be exceeded.

For patients with severe hypertension (e.g., accelerated or malignant hypertension), when tempo rary discontinuation of current antihypertensive therapy is not practical or desirable, or whe prompt titration to more normotensive blood pressure levels is indicated, diuretic should b continued but other current antihypertensive medication stopped and CAPOTEN dosage prompt initiated at 25 mg bid or tid, under close medical supervision.

When necessitated by the patient's clinical condition, the daily dose of CAPOTEN may b increased every 24 hours or less under continuous medical supervision until a satisfactory bloo pressure response is obtained or the maximum dose of CAPOTEN (captopril) is reached. In th regimen, addition of a more potent diuretic, e.g., furosemide, may also be indicated.

Beta-blockers may also be used in conjunction with CAPOTEN therapy (see PRECAUTION [Drug Interactions]), but the effects of the two drugs are less than additive.

Heart Failure—Initiation of therapy requires consideration of recent diuretic therapy and th possibility of severe salt/volume depletion. In patients with either normal or low blood pressure, wh have been vigorously treated with diuretics and who may be hyponatremic and/or hypovolemic, starting dose of 6.25 or 12.5 mg tid may minimize the magnitude or duration of the hypotensive effe (see WARNINGS, [Hypotension]); for these patients, titration to the usual daily dosage can the occur within the next several days.

For most patients the usual initial daily dosage is 25 mg tid. After a dose of 50 mg tid is reache further increases in dosage should be delayed, where possible, for at least two weeks to determir if a satisfactory response occurs. Most patients studied have had a satisfactory clinical improve ment at 50 or 100 mg tid. A maximum daily dose of 450 mg of CAPOTEN (captopril) should n be exceeded.

CAPOTEN is to be used in conjunction with a diuretic and digitalis. CAPOTEN therapy must b initiated under very close medical supervision.

Dosage Adjustment in Renal Impairment—Because CAPOTEN (captopril) is excreted primari by the kidneys, excretion rates are reduced in patients with impaired renal function. These patien will take longer to reach steady-state captopril levels and will reach higher steady-state levels for given daily dose than patients with normal renal function. Therefore, these patients may respond smaller or less frequent doses.

Accordingly, for patients with significant renal impairment, initial daily dosage of CAPOTE (captopril) should be reduced, and smaller increments utilized for titration, which should be qui slow (one- to two-week intervals). After the desired therapeutic effect has been achieved, the dos should be slowly back-titrated to determine the minimal effective dose. When concomitant diuret therapy is required, a loop diuretic (e.g., furosemide), rather than a thiazide diuretic, is preferred patients with severe renal impairment.

HOW SUPPLIED

12.5 mg tablets in bottles of 100, **25 mg tablets** in bottles of 100 and 1000, **50 mg tablets** in bottles 100, and **100 mg tablets** in bottles of 100. Bottles contain a desiccant-charcoal canister.

Unimatic® unit-dose packs containing 100 tablets are also available for each potency: **12.5 m 25 mg, 50 mg.** and **100 mg.**

The **12.5 mg tablet** is a flat oval with a partial bisect bar; the **25 mg tablet** is a biconvex rounde square with a quadrisect bar; the **50 and 100 mg tablets** are biconvex ovals with a bisect bar.

All captopril tablets are white and may exhibit a slight sulfurous odor. Tablet identificatic numbers: 12.5 mg, **450**; 25 mg, **452**; 50 mg, **482**; and 100 mg, **485**.

Storage

Do not store above 86° F. Keep bottles tightly closed (protect from moisture). (J3-658D

24. **(C)** Echothiophate iodide is an indirect-acting, irreversible anticholinesterase drug; thus, succinylcholine use should be avoided. Echothiophate iodide (phospholine iodide) is also believed to be cataractogenic in some patients.

25. **(D)** Sympathetic ophthalmia is probably due to hypersensitivity to uveal pigment. It very rarely occurs following uncomplicated surgery for cataract or glaucoma.

26. **(B)** Thrombosis of the cavernous sinus is usually due to infection spreading along the venous channels which drain the orbit, central face, throat, and nasal cavities.

27. **(B)** Acute glaucoma is an ophthalmological emergency. The intraocular pressure is markedly increased, vision is severely decreased, the pupil is fixed and moderately dilated, and the cornea is edematous.

28. **(E)** Parents should know that practically all deviating eyes can be straightened by corrective lenses, miotic therapy, orthoptics, surgery, or some combination thereof, and that the straightening should be accomplished at the earliest possible time.

29. **(C)** Dacryocystitis usually results from obstruction (dacryostenosis) of long standing.

30. **(E)**

Peripheral nerve	Involvement
Median	Thumb and thenar eminence
Ulnar	Little finger and hypothenar eminence
Radial	Wrist drop
Femoral	Absent knee jerk
Peroneal	Foot drop
Sciatic	Pain down lateral thigh, absent ankle jerk

31. **(B)** Sciatica is a sensory disturbance beginning in the buttock and moving down the lateral aspect of the thigh caused by irritation of the nerve root from L4 to S3. The most common cause is lumbar disk protrusion (pain may be precipitated by coughing or sneezing), often with absent ankle jerk.

Straight leg raising aggravates the back pain.

32. **(B)** The medial meniscus is much more prone to laceration than the lateral. The typical cause of injury is a blow against the lateral aspect of the knee while it is flexed and the foot is fixed on the ground in an outwardly twisted position; thus it is frequently incurred by young athletes and the elderly.

33. **(B)** The renal lesion of amyloidosis is usually not reversible and in time leads to progressive azotemia. The diagnosis is accurately made by renal biopsy.

34. **(A)** Treatment consists of resting the part and allowing the disorder to take its course.

35. **(A)** Hurler's syndrome (gargoylism) is characterized by the excessive accumulation of intracellular mucopolysaccharides. X-ray often shows an enlarged skull with frontal and occipital hyperostosis; hypertelorism; a long, shallow sella turcica with anterior pocketing; and deformities of the facial bones.

36. **(D)** Colles' fracture of the wrist occurs in the elderly very frequently, due to osteoporosis. Although the bones are weak, they heal well. The median nerve is frequently injured.

37. **(A)** Ankylosing spondylitis (Marie-Strumpell's disease) is frequently seen in a young white man with chronic backache who develops progressive limitation of back motion, transient peripheral arthritis, uveitis, and aortic insufficiency. The late radiographic sign is "bamboo spine." Psoriatic arthritis may also cause backache and spondylitis but is a late manifestation, although it may occur as a primary disease. It is often associated with Reiter's syndrome, psoriatic arthritis, and ulcerative arthritis.

38. **(D)** Sjögren's syndrome consists of dry eyes (keratoconjunctivitis sicca), dry mouth (xerostomia), and a chronic arthritis. Lip biopsy specimens show infiltrates of plasma cells and lymphocytes in the minor salivary glands.

39. **(E)** Osteochondrosis of the femoral capital epiphysis (Legg-Calve-Perthes' disease) is

most often unilateral. It is usually found in boys of four to nine years and is characterized by hip joint irritation (protective limp and pain on forced motion) and referred knee joint pain.

40. **(C)** This is a classical history and description. Keratoacanthomas almost always respond to simple conservative surgical removal, but on rare occasions can be aggressive and even lethal.

41. **(E)** Chronic hypercalciuria and hyperphosphaturia may result in precipitation of calcium salts in the renal parenchyma. The most common causes are hyperparathyroidism, hypervitaminosis D, high intake of calcium and alkali, osteoporosis following immobilization, sarcoidosis, De Toni-Fanconi's syndrome, destruction of bone by metastatic carcinoma, and chronic pyelonephritis.

42. **(E)** Wine glass sign is usually seen in the calyces (spider crescent deformity). Sonography may reveal the association with polycystic liver. The treatment is usually symptomatic and supportive. In adults, the condition is transmitted by autosomal dominance, while in children, at least in some families, it is transmitted by autosomal recessive traits. Aneurysms of the arteries of the circle of Willis are frequently found. A normal hematocrit and renal failure may coexist.

43. **(A)** A normal young person can concentrate urine to 1.040. The urine specific gravity increases as excessive water is lost. However, if the patient previously was unable to concentrate urine normally, the specific gravity may not rise even if severe water loss is present.

44. **(C)** Injury to the kidney usually can be revealed by a plain x-ray film. However, infusion urography should be done as soon as is practical. Retrograde urograms delineate the degree of injury quite clearly, but they are seldom needed. Infusion urography shows normal function and configuration if injury is minimal, delayed visualization if injury is present, and deformed renal pelvis or calyces if lacerations have occurred.

45. **(B)** Vesical injury can be revealed by a plain film x-ray and excretory urograms. However, a cystogram is the most dependable test for vesical injury.

46. **(B)** Prostatic secretion should be subjected to culture and sensitivity tests, though the cultures are usually negative. Only three antimicrobials are active in prostatic tissue: erythromycin, oleandomycin, and trimethoprim. Since the bacteria are usually Gram-negative rods, a combination of a sulfonamide and trimethoprim may be administered.

47. **(D)** Diverticulitis accounts for 50-60% of the vesical fistulas, followed by colonic cancer and Crohn's disease.

48. **(C)** Adenocarcinoma of the kidney frequently causes painless gross hematuria. Early metastases (to lungs, liver, and long bones) with enlarged palpable kidneys may be found. Fever and infection may also be present. Pain is rarely the initial symptom and is usually a late manifestation.

49. **(B)** In the elderly with dehydration or pre-existing renal insufficiency, or who are using furosemide, the administration of aminoglycosides (gentamycin) and cephalosporins may cause acute renal failure (tubulointerstitial injury). The kidney's ability to concentrate urine may decrease, the glomerular filtration rate may decrease, proteinuria may develop, and blood urea nitrogen (BUN) and creatinine may be increased. Urine sediments may show eosinophils.

50. **(B)** Nerve thickening and erythematous anesthetic lesion are characteristic of leprosy. Biopsy of the skin or nerve lesion usually confirms diagnosis. Dapsone (DDS) and rifampin in combination are quite effective; however, they may cause "Lepra reaction" (fever, anemia, leukopenia, gastrointestinal symptoms, allergic dermatitis, hepatitis, mental disturbances), which can be treated with steroids.

51. **(A)** The characteristic findings of allergic rhinitis, perennial nonallergic rhinitis, and vasomotor rhinitis are as follows.

Characteristics	Alergic rhinitis	Perennial nonallergic rhinitis	Vasomotor rhinitis
Onset	Childhood	Adult	Adult
Nasal congestion	+	+ +	+
Sneezing	+ +	+	−
Nasal Secretion	Watery	Mucoid	Watery
Cells	Eosinophils	Eosinophils	Neutrophils
Nasal polyps	+ −	+	−
Allergy skin tests	+	−	−
Antihistamines	+ +	+	−
Decongestants	+	+	−
Steroids	+ + +	+ + +	−
Cromolyn	+ + +	−	−
Desensitization	+ + +	−	−

52. **(E)** Acute conjunctivitis, characterized by redness, chemosis, and mucopurulent discharge, is common in children, particularly in newborn infants. Instillation into the eyes of prophylactic silver nitrate (for gonorrhea prophylaxis) frequently produces in the newborn a chemical irritation with a purulent discharge lasting 24 to 48 hours.

53. **(B)** The patient is very likely suffering from mycosis fungoides, which is lymphoma originating in the skin, and biopsy is required for diagnosis.

54. **(D)** Reiter's syndrome is characterized by nonspecific urethritis, conjunctivitis, keratoderma blennorrhagica, and arthritis. It is commonly seen in young men, and the arthritis is commonly asymmetric, with involvement of knees, ankles, and sacroiliac joints. The HLA B27 test is frequently positive. The other four types of arthritis all may involve both hands in a middle-age woman with inflammatory reactions.

55. **(B)** Acute renal failure may occur after exposure to x-ray contrast media with good prognosis. Risk factors include old age (beyond 60 years), prior renal insufficiency (cre-

atinine greater than 1.6), diabetes mellitus, volume depletion, and multiple myeloma. Prostatic hypertrophy may cause acute renal failure by obstruction, but it usually does not increase the risk to the contrast media.

56. **(C)** In secondary syphilis, the skin lesions are often bright red vesicles with scaling. In gonococcemia, a few peripheral raised hemorrhagic necrotic pustules may be seen with arthralgias. In lymphogranuloma venereum, ulcers and papules are centered in the genitalia with fluctuant inguinal lymphadenopathy. In venereal warts, the lesions are commonly seen in the vulvar or perianal areas with pointed edges.

57. **(B)** Acute renal failure can be classified into prerenal causes, renal causes (proliferative glomerulopathies, contrast media, aminoglycosides, acute tubular necrosis, disseminated intravascular coagulation) and postrenal causes (obstructive uropathies). Prerenal causes are very common in the elderly and in children due to volume depletion. In volume depletion, urinalysis is normal (no proteinuria, no hematuria, no RBC casts, no eosinophils in the sediments), blood pressure is at normotension, and the ratio of BUN to creatinine is greater than 15.

58. **(C)** The glomus jugulare tumor arises from the glomus bodies located in the adventia of the dome of the jugular bulb. It may cause tinnitus; hearing loss; throbbing, pulsating discomfort; and multiple cranial nerve paralyses (particularly nerve VII); profuse bleeding may follow manipulation. Surgical excision or irradiation is indicated.

59. **(B)** Uveitis is characterized by acute painful red eye with photophobia and blurred vision. It is often associated with diabetes mellitus, rheumatoid arthritis, gout, ankylosing spondylitis (HLA B27), Behcet's disease (relapsing iritis, aphthous and genital ulceration, HLA B5), Crohn's disease, ulcerative colitis, Reiter's disease (urethritis, conjunctivitis, arthritis, HLA B27), tuberculosis, sarcoidosis, toxoplasmosis, sympathetic ophthalmia, histoplasmosis, and nematode endophthalmitis; hypertension mainly causes retinopathy.

60. **(E)** Acute otitis externa is often associated with swimming ("swimmer's ear"), seborrheic dermatitis, or diabetes. It is characterized by pain, itching, and discharges. The ear canal shows crusting, scaling, erythema, and swelling. Topical antibiotics such as polymyxin B or neomycin can be used; corticosteroid ear drops are useful for underlying dermatitis.

61. **(A)** The diagnosis of gout is strongly suggested in a male by acute arthritis in the great toe following heavy alcohol ingestion. The presence of urate crystal in the synovial fluid is diagnostic. However, in clinical practice, the diagnosis of gouty arthritis is usually made through a detailed history and characteristic physicals with minimal laboratory tests findings, including leukocytosis, elevated ESR, hyperuricemia, and dramatic therapeutic response to colchicine. However, in equivocal cases, synovial analysis and biopsy of a soft tissue mass or synovial membrane are required.

62. **(D)** In viral conjunctivitis, the discharge is serous, the conjunctiva is injected, and the periauricular adenopathy is present. Usually a history of precedent upper respiratory infection with pharyngitis (sore throat) can be elicited. Itching is usually not present in viral conjunctivitis but is a prominent symptom of allergic conjunctivitis. In iritis, a small pupil and keratic precipitates are present; blurred vision with vomiting is present in glaucoma. In viral conjunctivitis, lymphocytes are found in scrapings from the infected eye. There is no specific treatment available. Antibiotics and corticosteroids are not indicated. The disease is contagious and the patient should be advised to remain at home.

63. **(E)** Ramsay Hunt's syndrome is herpes zoster oticus, characterized by facial paralysis, otalgia, and vesicles in the external auditory canal. Treatment includes topical anesthetic (dibucaine), systemic steroids, and vitamin B12.

64. **(D)** Calculi of the salivary glands are most commonly found in the submaxillary glands, followed by the parotid glands and the sublingual glands. The presence of a stone in the submaxillary gland can be determined by bimanual palpation of the floor of the mouth, probing of the duct, and x-ray examination.

65. **(A)** Ice packs and cold compresses are useful for an acute localized problem, while diathermy is used for chronic focal conditions. Diathermy should not be used in patients with pacemakers or metal implants. In addition to shortwave, diathermy can utilize microwave and ultrasound.

66. **(C)** The description is classical for candidal onychia and paronychia. It is normally associated with excessive moisture and detergents, so that these should be avoided as much as possible. Thymol in chloroform should be applied. Neither griseofulvin nor tolnaftate is effective against *Candida albicans*.

67. **(E)** The characteristic cerebral lesions are sclerotic patches (tubers) scattered throughout the cortical gray matter. Convulsions, mental defect, rhabdomyoma of the heart, and renal tumors are often associated. Adenoma sebaceum is the most characteristic skin lesion. It consists of small bright red or brownish nodules in a butterfly configuration on the nose and cheeks. Hypopigmented skin macules on the arms, legs, and trunk are usually present from birth.

68. **(B)** The agent of herpes zoster is the V-Z virus, the same virus that causes varicella. The skin lesions are unilateral and are distributed along the course of a nerve. The disease is self-limited, usually lasting several weeks.

69. **(C)** Primary syphilis is usually characterized by a moist ulceration of the chancre, frequently seen in the penis, anus, lip, or tongue (the site of first contact with the spirochete). It may be symptomless in the female. Secondary syphilis usually commences approximately six to eight weeks after the onset of the primary chancre. The complaints of headache, loss of weight, arthralgia, and sore throat are common in secondary syphilis. Occasionally, there is iritis with photophobia, lacrimation, and ocular redness. Physical examination may reveal mucous patches involving the pharynx and oral cavity; generalized maculopapular lesios, including the palms and soles; generalized nontender, palpable adenopathy; patchy hair loss with a "moth-eaten" appearance; paronychia and onychia; hepatitis; periostitis; meningeal irritation; and transient nephrotic syndrome. Diagnosis is by positive serologic test for syphilis (STS), positive darkfield examination, and positive fluorescent treponemal antibody absorption test (FTA-ABS). The treatment is penicillin. Bicillin 2.4 million units IM in each buttock is usually administered.

70. **(E)** Vertigo is intermittent, the attacks lasting between several minutes and several hours and taking the form of a definite feeling of rotation. It is preceded by pressure in the ear and is followed by malaise for several days. Deafness is perceptive and is more marked before and during an attack. The audiogram shows a perceptive deafness. The curve is fairly flat (the losses for high tones and low tones are similar). A calorigram may show a pattern of canal paresis.

71. **(E)** Adenoid hypertrophy may cause nasal obstruction, leading to mouth breathing, poor rest at night, and a slight nasality of the voice. Chronic mouth breathing during

the age when facial bones are changing toward the adult configuration often produces a high arch to the hard palate, pinching in of the nose, shortening of the upper lip, malocclusion of the teeth, and a dull facial expression (adenoid facies). Partial blocking of the eustachian tube may cause recurrent suppurative otitis media, serous otitis media, tinnitus, and fluctuating hearing loss.

72. **(C)** A deep, circumscribed ulcer of the right tonsil may be found. Vincent's angina can be diagnosed by the smear examination. Treatment is usually local cautery with phenol.

73. **(A)** The three ocular motor nerves—III (oculomotor), IV (trochlear), and VI (abducens)—may be affected by many intracranial disorders, but the three major causes of paralysis are aneurysms, diabetes, and trauma.

74. **(A)** Of the adults screened by the U.S. Public Health Survey, 22% of men and 32% of women reported morning stiffness and 13% reported joint pain and tenderness. Fibrositis syndrome is usually seen in young or middle-aged patients who experience emotional distress, chronic fatigue, poor sleep, and morning stiffness. SGOT, rheumatoid factor test, ANF, muscle enzymes, ESR, and sacroiliac films are all normal.

75. **(A)** Fractures of the navicular are usually due to forcible dorsiflexion of the foot. No reduction is usually needed. To avoid the development of avascular necrosis, immobilization by cast is indicated.

76. **(C)** The lesion cannot be reduced by closed methods; open operation is necessary because of the difficulty in controlling the head. Replacement of the head on the neck and internal fixation cause aseptic necrosis due to the disrupted blood supply to the head. Management is usually by arthroplasty, arthrodesis, or replacement of the head by prosthesis.

77. **(E)** In nonunion, the fracture is not united and will remain so indefinitely. The actual causes for this are not clear. Radiologically, there is a definite gap at the fracture site, the ends of the bone are sclerotic and smooth, and occasionally one end of the fragment has a cupped appearance.

78. **(A)** Septic arthritis is common in children under two years of age. Staphylococci, streptococci, pneumococci, and *Hemophilus influenzae* are the most common causative organisms. Treatment is removal of the septic effusion to decrease joint distention and to eliminate the proteolytic enzymes of the septic effusion.

79. **(A)** Children heal faster than adults. It is usually sufficient to bring the broken ends of the bone in proximity to one another; an anatomical or open reduction is seldom necessary. Children are excellent patients, and should the child show signs of distress despite a good reduction, the reason can usually be found in the cast, which is either too tight or has been improperly applied.

80. **(B)** X-rays fail to disclose abnormalities in most cases unless one of the ligaments has avulsed a small flake of bone with it. This would be diagnostic.

81. **(E)** Volkmann's ischemia is a paralysis and contracture of the forearm muscles supplied by the brachial artery. Median nerve palsy may develop secondary to a traction injury. In adolescents, ulnar nerve palsy may develop through the abnormal bone growth subsequent to the injury. Late ulnar palsy in children frequently follows supracondylar humeral fracture-dislocation. The most important early sign of Volkmann's contracture is pain.

82. **(B)** Chronic neck sprain (spondylosis) is a common cause of headache. It is likewise the most common cause of pain over the upper and midthoracic areas of the back. The chronic degenerative change may be exacerbated by injury (such as auto accident) which disrupts the relationship of the nerve roots in the cervical area and causes acute symptoms.

83. **(E)** Rheumatoid arthritis (RA) is frequently seen in women. Painful swollen small joints with morning stiffness are frequently experienced. Rheumatoid nodules in the lung may cavitate to resemble malignant lesions roentgenographically. Synovial fluid analysis may show inflammatory reactions with lymphocytosis. Aspirin remains the best drug for RA. The dosage for anti-inflammatory effects is higher than that for analgesic effect, and the doses tolerated by individuals tend to vary inversely with their ages. Gold salt therapy is useful but often must be discontinued due to unwanted side-effects, which include the involvement of oral mucosa, bone marrow, kidney and skin.

84. **(A)** PSS is often seen with Raynaud's phenomenon; firm, tight, waxy skin; pulmonary fibrosis; intestinal malabsorption; peptic esophagitis; polyarthritis; and hypergammaglobulinemia (elevated IgG).

85. **(A)** The clavicle is fractured more frequently than any other bone during labor and is particularly vulnerable in difficult delivery of the shoulder in vertex presentations and of the extended arms in breech deliveries. Treatment consists of immobilization of the arm and the shoulder on the affected side.

86. **(A)** Vocal nodules (singer's nodes) are frequently caused by misuse of the voice.

87. **(E)** Vesicoureteral reflux is more common in girls. The diagnosis is usually confirmed by cystoscopy and x-ray findings.

88. **(A)** Diabetic nephropathy may cause renal artery arteriosclerosis, glomerulonephritis, and pyelonephritis. The patient frequently develops a full-blown nephrotic syndrome with hypoalbuminemia, edema, proteinuria, and increased circulating beta-lipoproteins.

89. **(E)** Tabes dorsalis is a type of neurosyphilis which causes progressive degeneration of the parenchyma of the posterior columns of the spinal cord and of the posterior sensory ganglia and nerve roots. Signs of neurogenic bladder (painful bladder spasm, distention of bladder, and incontinence) may develop. Crises are common, including abdominal pain and dyspnea. Argyll Robertson pupils are poorly reactive to light but well reactive to accommodation. Charcot's joint is joint damage as a result of lack of sensory innervation.

90. **(E)** The symptoms of BPH include hesitancy and straining to initiate micturition, reduced force and caliber of the urinary stream, and

nocturia. The complications are due to obstructions (infections, calculi, and uremia). Uremia may often lead to death in untreated BPH.

91. **(E)** Tuberculosis of the prostate and seminal vesicles usually causes no symptoms. The first clue is tuberculous epididymitis characterized by painless swelling and chronic draining scrotal sinus. Diagnosis is by chest x-ray showing pulmonary tuberculosis and observation of tuberculous bacilli in urine.

92. **(E)** Children with nephrotic syndrome usually run a fairly benign course. Adults with nephrosis fare less well, particularly when disease is associated with glomerulonephritis, SLE, amyloidosis, renal vein thrombosis, or diabetic nephropathy.

93. **(C)** Bartter's syndrome is characterized by the signs of severe hyperaldosteronism (hypokalemic alkalosis), with moderate to marked increase in renin activity but normal blood pressure and absence of edema.

94. **(E)** Both chlorothiazide and hydrochlorothiazide have been shown to increase free-water reabsorption in diabetes insipidus. However, the diuretics will only decrease urine flow by 30-50% and patients require vasopressin therapy. The thiazides are very useful in treating polyuria in nephrogenic diabetes insipidus. Bromism resulting from chronic use of "nerve tonics" (Bromo-Seltzer) may be treated with sodium chloride and mercurial or thiazide diuretics, which promote bromide diuresis. Hypercalcemia and hypercalciuria are often helped by the saline/furosemide regimen. Furosemide is a potent natriuretic agent. The loop diuretic ethacrynic acid is also effective for hypercalcemia. In fact, long-term therapy with chlorothiazide may produce hypocalcemia. Thiazide diuretics may also cause hypokalemia; however, spironolactone (Aldactone) may cause hyperkalemic acidosis.

95. **(E)** Long-term phenytoin and phenobarbital therapy may cause hypocalcemia and osteomalacia. Starvation, a diet deficient in total calories, calcium, phosphorus, and vitamin D (as in chronic alcoholism), may

produce hypocalcemia with slow, progressive osteomalacia. Malabsorption syndrome with defective absorption of vitamin D and calcium may lead to rickets in children and osteomalacia in adults. Low serum calcium is a constant feature in hypoparathyroidism. Low serum magnesium may also cause tetany, which is a chief clinical feature of severe hypocalcemia.

96. **(A)** Hyperuricosuriais is caused by hyperuricemia with normal renal excretion. Secondary hyperuricemia may be caused by polycythemia, hyperparathyroidism, sarcoidosis, renal tubular acidosis, chronic hemolytic anemia, distal bowel diseases, chemotherapy of malignancies (excessive breakdown of tumor cells), administration of low dosage salicylate (less than 2 g in 24 hours), and chronic use of drugs, including thiazide diuretics, acetazolamide, pyrazinamide, and ethambutal. Acute alcohol ingestion may also cause hyperuricemia, which may result in acute gouty attacks.

97. **(B)** The cotton wool spots are soft exudates due to superficial retinal hemorrhages and may be caused by hypertension, vascular insufficiency syndrome, diabetes mellitus, and collagen diseases (such as systemic lupus erythematosus). Toxoplasmosis may cause chorioretinitis and intracranial calcified foci. A cataract is a lens opacity.

98. **(B)** Central retinal vein occlusion is associated with hypertension, diabetes mellitus, collagen vascular diseases, hyperviscosity syndrome (Waldenstrom's macroglobulinemia, angioimmunoblastic lymphadenopathy, polycythemia, leukemia), blood dyscrasias, inflammatory disorders (tuberculosis, syphilis), and sarcoidosis.

99. **(E)** Urinary tract infections are often associated with urinary tract anomalies, urinary stasis and obstruction or stenosis of the urinary tract, instrumentations, diabetes mellitus, pregnancy, renal calculi, initial sexual activities ("Honeymoon cystitis"), and neurogenic bladders. Chronic urinary tract infections can be suppressed by daily ingestion of trimethoprim-sulfamethoxazole (Bactrim) for 6 to 12 months.

100. (D)

Acute conjunctivitis	Acute iritis	Acute glaucoma
Mild discomfort, itching	Moderate pain	Severe pain
Watery or purulent discharges	No discharges	No discharges
	Photophobia	Nausea and vomiting
Conjunctival injection	Perilimbal injection	Perilimbal injection
Normal vision	Impaired vision	Blurred vision
Clear cornea	Clear cornea	Cloudy cornea
Normal pupil	Small and irregular pupil	Dilated and fixed pupil

101. (B) The skin lesion is likely to be erythema nodosum, which is commonly associated with sarcoidosis, tuberculosis, chronic inflammatory bowel diseases, ingestion of sulfonamides or progestogens, and streptococcal infections. With other systemic signs and symptoms present, the likelihood of sarcoidosis is very high and skin biopsy is recommended. Chest x-rays show hilar adenopathy and fibrous infiltrations.

102. (D) Osteoarthritis rarely occurs in young patients without trauma and is the most common form of arthritis in the elderly group. It is not associated with extra-articular symptoms, and the treatment is symptomatic. In obese patients, a weight reduction program may diminish stress on lumbar joints. Salicylates (600 g q.i.d.) are used to relieve pain. Local heat may be helpful. Overuse of the affected joints should be avoided, and bending and lifting should be minimized. Systemic steroids are not recommended; intra-auricular steroid injection can be tried in severe cases.

103. (A) Rheumatoid arthritis is often associated with vasculitis (digital gangrene), pleurisy, pericarditis with cardiac tamponade, Baker's popliteal cyst, pulmonary fibrosis (Kaplan's syndrome), splenomegaly (Felty's syndrome), cryoglobulinemia, temporal arteritis, and amyloidosis.

104. (C) Atopic dermatitis is characterized by pruritus and lichenification (thickening of skin) and is associated with asthma, hay fever, xerosis, cutaneous autonomic dysfunctions, emotional stress, histiocytosis X (seen after 9 months of age), Wiskatt-Aldrich's syndrome (eczema, thrombocytopenia, and infections), and phenylketonuria. Atopic dermatitis may be complicated by staphylococcal, herpes simplex, and *Trichophyton rubrum* infections, otitis externa, and cataracts. The IgE level is elevated and is correlated with the severity and extent of the disease. Treatments include wet dressings, oral antihistamines (to break the itch-scratch cycle), and topical steroids. Allergy desensitization treatment has no proven benefit.

105. (E) Most causes of kyphoscoliosis are unknown. The onset is usually insidious and is more common in girls than in boys. There appears to be a familial incidence. The condition may cause psychological problems, and empathetic support is necessary.

106. (D) Allergic conjunctivitis is a possibility, and the patient is likely to be allergic to pollen or grasses encountered in working in his garden. However, the absence of itching and the unilateral presentation makes it likely that the conjunctivitis is caused by herpes simplex. If there are any doubts about the diagnosis, a fluorescein staining of the cornea should be performed to be sure that the cornea is normal. The intraocular pressure should also be measured if vision is impaired to rule out glaucoma. Steroid eyedrops are to be avoided in herpes and fungal conjunctivitis. In herpes, conjunctival scrapings may show multinucleated giant epithelial cells, and in allergic conjunctivitis, eosinophils may be seen in the scrapings. Topical corticosteroids are to be used only when the diagnosis of allergic conjunctivitis is certain, because they may potentiate herpes simplex and fungal infections of the cornea.

107. (D) Patients with recurrent calcium oxalate stones need to reduce calcium and oxalate intake. The urinary calcium level can be lowered by a moderate restriction of milk and dairy products (cheese and ice cream) and by avoidance of excessive intake of vitamin D. Excessive ingestion of vitamin C (ascorbic acid) and fruit juices high in vitamin C (orange juice) will increase urinary oxalate excretion and should be avoided. Avoidance of foods with high oxalate content is of limited value in preventing oxalate stones but is generally recommended; such foods include cabbage, rhubarb, spinach, tomatoes, celery, black tea, and cocoa. High fluid intake is required to dilute urine. An alkaline-ash diet (high in vegetable and fruit content, low in protein) is used for cystine or uric acid stones; a low-purine diet (avoidance of meat) may be helpful for patients with uric acid stones.

108. (E) Chronic urethritis is a very common problem and is often called the urethral syndrome of the female. The patient may complain of burning on urination, frequency, nocturia, and urethral discomfort and stenosis. The urine examination may show no abnormalities, although it is often caused by *Ureaplasma urealyticum* (sensitive to tetracyclines) or *Chlamydiae* (sensitive to sulfonamides or tetracyclines).

109. (D) Corneal annulus (arcus senilis) appears as an annular, hazy, gray ring about 2 mm in width in the periphery of the cornea. It is commonly seen in the elderly without any symptoms. If it is seen in the young (arcus juvenilis), it is usually associated with hypercholesterolemia (hyperlipidemia type II), and further work-ups are necessary.

110. (E) The most common cause of exophthalmos is Grave's disease (hyperthyroidism). Other causes include trauma, orbital cellulitis, cavernous sinus thrombosis, aneurysms, dermoid cysts, rhabdomyosarcoma, fibroma, paralysis of the recti muscles, macrophthalmos, lymphoma, leukemia, and high myopia.

111. (E) Necrotizing papillitis (papillary necrosis) is often due to the complications of pyelonephritis; however, it is also often associated with vesicoureteral reflux, diabetes, cirrhosis, sickle cell traits, and prolonged use of analgesics, such as aspirin or phenacetin. There may be fever, oliguria, renal tenderness, pyuria, bacteriuria, azotemia, and shock. Appropriate antibiotics may be used and underlying diseases controlled.

112. (D) Rhinitis medicamentosa is a common problem. Although nose drops may shrink the engorged nasal turbinates, compensatory relaxation will occur in the turbinate vessels. Thus, after temporary relief of the nasal obstruction by the nose drops, the nose becomes more stuffy (rebound congestion) with subsequent doses. The treatment is the discontinuation of the nose drops.

113. (D)

114. (E)

115. (C)

116. (A)

117. (B) Granuloma annulare occurs more frequently in diabetics and resembles a rheumatoid nodule. Scleroderma usually involves the face (mask-like) and hands (stiff); systemic forms involve the esophagus, kidneys, and lungs (sclerosis). Discoid lupus erythematosus is characterized by localized erythema, adherent scales, patulous follicles with follicular plugs, telangiectasia, and atrophy. Emotional stress may precipitate lichen planus, which causes pruritus with angularity of the circumscribed margin. Pemphigus may start in the mouth with blisters.

118. (C)

119. (D)

120. (B)

121. (A) Acanthosis nigricans is characterized by a gray-black, rough, or papillomatous epidermoid hypertrophy. The benign form is related to developmental and endocrine abnormalities. The malignant form is usually associated with internal malignancy, mainly adenocarcinoma of the stomach or pelvic organs. Lichen planus is a chronic inflammatory disease associated with emotional stress in adults. There are gray lines on the flat surface of each papule (Wickham's striae). The eruptions are commonly seen along a linear scratch mark (Köbner's phenomenon). Pellagra is due to niacin deficiency and low tryptophane intake. The sun-exposed areas of the body may develop erythematous vesiculation and hyper-pigmentation. Depression and psychosis may also develop. The Mongolian spot is a dusky blue pigmentation in the lumbosacral area of oriental or black infants that usually disappears during childhood.

122. **(B)**

123. **(A)**

124. **(C)** Hirradenitis suppurativa is a painful inflammatory disease of the apocrine glands in the axillas and groins, frequently caused by staphylococci. Dermatomyositis involves chiefly the striated muscle and skin. The onset is insidious, with the appearance of an unusual erythema of the eyelids and periorbital areas. Other symptoms include muscle weakness and skin change. In adult patients it is frequently associated with internal malignacy, especially bronchogenic carcinoma. Pruritus may result from inflammations (scabies), allergic reactions (contact dermatitis), sweat retention (miliaria), atopic dermatitis, metabolic abnormality (diabetes, uremia), and malignancies (Hodgkin's disease, lymphomas, and leukemias).

125. **(C)**

126. **(B)**

127. **(A)** Erythema nodosum is a deep, nodular, inflammatory reaction that appears mostly on the anterior legs and thighs. It is frequently caused by coccidioidomycosis, histoplasmosis, tuberculosis, *Streptococcus*, sarcoidois, ulcerative colitis, and reactions to drugs such as sulfonamides, salicylates, and progestogens. Stevens-Johnson's syndrome is a variation of erythema multiforme. It begins with a sudden febrile onset and involves subepidermal vesiculations which become ulcerated in the mucous membranes of the lips, buccal cavity, eyes and genitalia. Pneumonia and arthritis may also be present. Tinea versicolor is a superficial fungal infection of the skin, caused by *Malassezia furfur*. Involved areas are brown on untanned skin, pale on tanned skin.

128. **(C)**

129. **(D)**

130. **(B)**

131. **(A)** Sarcoidosis is a noncaseating granulomatous disease of unknown etiology that involves the reticuloendothelial system and can affect all organs. The Kveim test is positive in 70% of cases. Erythema nodosum, bilateral hilar lymphadenopathy, anemia, elevated serum calcium, increased gamma-globulins, and ocular involvement are usually present. Vitiligo has a strong familial tendency and is frequently associated with thyroid disease, adrenocortical insufficienty, scleroderma, alopecia areata, and pernicious anemia. The lesions are startlingly white, contain no pigment, and are frequently seen on periorbital areas, hands, axillas, perineum, and neck. Systemic lupus erythematosus is frequently precipitated by hydralazine hydrochloride (Apresoline), phenylbutazone, phenytoin (Dilantin), reserpine, trimethadione (Tridione), and mephenytoin (Mesantoin). Pemphigus is characterized by bullae; Nikolsky's signs are often positive and corticosteroids often helpful.

132. **(C)**

133. **(C)**

134. **(B)**

135. **(D)** Plane xanthomas are often associated with melanoma, leukemia, and liver disease. Xanthelasma and xanthoma tuberosum are associated with Types II and III hyperlipoproteinemia. The Type II entity is familial hypercholesterolemia, a hereditary disorder. Beta-lipoproteins are elevated, plasma triglycerides are normal, and the plasma is not milky. The Type III entity is carbohydrate-induced hyperlipoproteinemia (Types III, IV, and V), which causes elevated plasma cholesterol, triglycerides, and pre-beta-proteins. The serum is turbid and the glucose tolerance test is abnormal. Type I is essential familial hyperlipemia, which delays the clearance of chylomicrons from the serum. Xanthelasma is common. The serum is milky, plasma triglycerides are elevated, and the serum cholesterol is normal.

136. **(C)**

137. **(D)**

138. (B)

139. (A)

140. (E)

141. (F) The fundus changes typical of severe anemia (blotchy hemorrhage and "cotton wool" exudates) are not specific, seem not to occur in children, and seem to occur when the hemoglobin level falls to 50% of normal. Sickle cell retinal changes frequently occur in the peripheral temporal vessels (hemorrhages and retinal detachment). A level of hyperlipemia over 2.5% has been shown to give a pale, whitish look to the retinal vessels. Still's disease is frequently associated with uveitis, bilateral iridocyclitis, and band keratitis. Rheumatoid arthritis may associate with scleritis or even scleromalacia perforans. The spontaneous appearance of arterial pulsation on ophthalmodynamometer measurement signifies glaucoma, aortic insufficiency, aortic arch syndrome, and/or carotid stenosis.

142. (B)

143. (E)

144. (C)

145. (A)

146. (D) Congenital toxoplasmosis is characterized by chorioretinitis. *Trichinella spiralis* occasionally localizes in the extraocular muscles to produce conjunctivitis, lid edema, eosinophilia, fever, and muscle pain. Marfan's syndrome includes congenital heart disease, subluxation of the lens, high myopia, spider extremities, and increased length of the long bones. Sarcoidosis is a chronic granulomatous disease with multiple cutaneous and viscerous nodules. Thirty percent of cases are complicated by chronic bilateral arterial uveitis. Avitaminosis A frequently causes night blindness, xerophthalmia, and keratomalacia.

147. (B)

148. (C)

149. (A) Sturge-Weber's syndrome is characterized by port wine hemangioma on one side of the face following the distribution of the trigeminal nerve. Unilateral infantile glaucoma with choroid hemangioma may develop. Rosacea is associated with marginal corneal ulcers and blepharoconjunctivitis. Funduscopic changes in hypertension include vessel spasm, retinal edema, hemorrhages, cotton-wool patches, and papilledema; these are relatively reversible.

150. (C)

151. (A)

152. (B)

153. (D)

154. (E) Frequently the visual field defects are used to identify the intracranial lesions. Optic tract lesions cause incongruous (dissimilar) homonymous hemianopsia; temporal lobe lesions cause quadrantonopsias. Monocular field defects result from retinal or optic nerve lesions.

155. (B)

156. (A)

157. (D)

158. (C) Rickets and osteomalacia usually cause similar syndromes due to hypovitaminosis D, although rickets are frequently seen in children.

159. (B)

160. (A)

161. (C) Osteochondrosis involves the secondary ossification centers of virtually every bone. Like Legg-Perthes' disease (usually affecting those five to eight years of age), osteochondrosis represents disturbances in the vascular supply to the ossification centers. Osgood-Schlatter's disease is frequently seen in children 12 to 15 years of age, and x-ray shows irregular fragmentation of the tibial tuberosity.

162. (B)

163. (A)

164. **(D)**

165. **(C)** Bone spicules are perpendicular to the normal cortical surface ("sunburst" effect) in osteogenic sarcoma. Ewing's sarcoma may cause diffuse osteosclerosis of the cortex with fusiform configuration and subperiosteal lamination ("onion peel").

166. **(B)**

167. **(C)**

168. **(A)**

169. **(E)**

170. **(D)** Lateral epicondylitis (tennis elbow) is a tear in the extensor tendon, resulting in pain upon extending the wrist against resistance. The patient with frozen shoulder cannot actively abduct the arm more than 80 degrees away from the side. The thoracic outlet syndrome is caused by the compression of brachial plexus nerve roots by a cervical rib, scalenus muscle, or the clavicle, causing a burning pain radiating from the neck through the shoulder and down the arm. Patients with trigger finger (de Quervain's disease) have pain over the long abductor and short extensor tendons to the thumb around the radial styloid. The carpal tunnel syndrome is characterized by pain starting at the wrist and radiating into the fingers, innervated by median nerves. It is associated with pregnancy, gout, rheumatoid arthritis, and tenosynovitis—often associated with trauma.

171. **(B)**

172. **(A)**

173. **(C)**

174. **(D)** Polyarteritis nodosa may cause fever, weakness, anorexia, myalgia, arthralgia, hypertension, and glomerulosclerosis. Periarteritis of the gallbladder may cause cholecystitis and perforation. Wegener's granulomatosis causes nonbacterial rhinorrhea, sinusitis, otitis media, hilar enlargement, myalgias, arthralgias, purpura, and glomerulonephritis, often leading to terminal uremia. Dermatomyositis is often associated with scaling eczematoid dermatitis, bronchogenic carcinoma, and thymoma. Serum creatine phosphokinase and aldolase are elevated. Resection of the primary tumor may lead to complete disappearance of dermatomyositis. Chondrocalcinosis is associated with hyperparathyroidism, acromegaly, hemochromatosis, osteoarthritis, diabetes, and gout.

175. **(B)**

176. **(A)**

177. **(C)** Peyronie's disease is fibrosis of the covering sheaths of the corpora cavernosa, which occurs without known cause, usually in men over 45 years of age. Reiter's syndrome is characterized by conjunctivitis (or iritis), arthritis, and urethritis. The discharge is usually free of bacteria; the agent is possibly *Chlamydia*. Antiglomerular basement membrane nephritis (Goodpasture's syndrome) includes acute glomerulonephritis with pulmonary hemorrhage.

178. **(C)**

179. **(A)**

180. **(B)**

181. **(D)** Pyelonephritis is characterized by pyuria and bacteriuria; "sterile" pyuria is found in urinary tuberculosis. Acute glomerulonephritis is characterized by hematuria without casts or crystals; urinary stones also cause hematuria, but there are casts and crystals in the sediment.

182. **(C)**

183. **(B)**

184. **(D)**

185. **(A)** Parotitis is associated with mumps orchitis. Epididymitis is rare before puberty and is usually accompanied by pyuria. Torsion of the testicle causes sudden severe pain, edema, swelling, and elevation of the testicle. Pain is increased by lifting the testicle up over the symphysis; however, this maneuver usually alleviates the pain from the epididymitis.

186. (C)

187. (A)

188. (A)

189. (B) Dermatitis herpetiformis is associated with gluten-sensitive enteropathy, IgA skin deposits, HLA B8, and HLA DW3, and is dramatically responsive to sulfones (dapsone) and sulfonamides. Erythematous vesicles are often seen symmetrically in the elbows, knees, and buttocks in adults, with intense itching. Transient acantholytic dermatosis is a benign disease of discrete papulovesicles occurring in the chest, back, and thighs following sun exposure.

190. (B)

191. (D)

192. (C)

193. (A) Noise exposure includes hearing loss in the high frequency range, beginning at 1000 Hz, with a characteristic 4000 Hz notch. At 8000 Hz, the hearing loss is less. Ménière's disease causes tinnitus, whirling vertigo, and sensorineural hearing loss. Hearing loss is in the low tones, with fairly good high-tone hearing. Both Ménière's disease and noise exposure involve sensorineural loss which causes no air-bone gap. Carhart's notch is seen in the bone conduction curve (at 2000 Hz) of otosclerosis.

194. (C)

195. (C) Glaucoma is associated with diabetes mellitus, central vessel occlusion, steroid therapy (systemic and topical), Grave's disease (hyperthyroidism), and hemodialysis. Cataracts are associated with diabetes mellitus, galactosemia, Down's syndrome, myotonic dystrophy, hypophosphatemia, hypocalcemia, atopic dermatitis, gargoylism, hypothyroidism, and hypoparathyroidism. Cataracts can also be caused by the long-term use of drugs, including steroids, ethanol, phenothiazines, busulfan, and echothiophateiodide (a strong miotic used for the treatment of glaucoma).

196. (D)

197. (B) Systemic lupus erythematosus is associated with circulating DNA antibodies, which may produce occlusive vasculitis in the retina, causing "cotton wool" spots (i.e., cytoid bodies) in the eye ground. Retinal artery embolism may be caused by cholesterol, calcific, or platelet emboli due to valvular heart disease, polycythemia, sickle cell disease, or carotid artery stenosis.

198. (E)

199. (C) Sjögren's syndrome is a chronic autoimmune disease characterized by keratoconjunctivitis sicca, xerostomia, and rheumatoid arthritis. It is associated with human leukocyte antigen (HLA) DW_3 or DW_4. Ankylosing spondylitis is characterized by chronic backache in young men with x-ray findings of "bamboo spine." It is associated with rheumatoid arthritis, but the rheumatoid factor is negative. It is also associated with uveitis, psoriatic arthritis, and chronic inflammatory bowel disease.

200. (E)

201. (C)

202. (B) Subacute bacterial endocarditis may cause calcified or platelet emboli, which may generate Roth spots (retinal infarctions). Xanthopsia (yellow vision) can be caused by the use of digitalis or chlorothiazide. Gout usually results in acute uveitis. Hypervitaminosis D may cause band keratopathy due to calcium deposits in the cornea. Administration of tranquilizers may result in ocular irritation by decreasing tear production. Dilated pupils and pigmentary retinopathy may occur with the administration of phenothiazines, particularly chlorpromazine (Thorazine) and thioridazine (Mellaril).

203. (C)

204. (D)

205. (E)

206. (A)

207. (B)

Urine Sediments	
Cells	
RBC (more than 5/HPF)	Cystitis, glomeru-lonephritis, trauma, tumor
WBC (more than 5/HPF)	Infection (pyelonephritis, cystitis), tubular degeneration
Casts	
Hyaline	Fever, chronic renal disease
Granular	Renal disease
RBC	Acute glomeru-lonephritis
WBC	Chronic pyelonephritis
Bacterial	Pyelonephritis
Crystals	
Uric acid	Hyperuricemia, gout
Calcium oxalate	Urolithiasis
Cystine	Cystinuria
Bacteria	
E. coli (Gram stain)	Cystitis, pyelonephritis
M. tuberculosis (acid-fast stain)	TB
Gonococcus (intracel-lular diplococci)	Gonorrhea
Yeast	*Candida albicans*
Trichomonads	Trichomoniasis

208. (C)

209. (B)

210. (A) Normal hearing depicts the superimposed bone and air conduction curves on or within 20 db of the zero decibel line. Senile deafness (presbycusis) is a perceptive high-frequency hearing loss (4000-8000 cps). Congenital rubella syndrome and neomycin toxicity cause sensorineural hearing loss. Otosclerosis, otitis media, and the perforation of the tympanic membrane cause conductive deafness, with the sound heard better on the bone. Audiogram presentation is not characteristic for a patient with petit mal epilepsy. An EEG study usually shows three per second spikes.

211. (D)

212. (A) Hordeolum is staphylococcal infection of the lid gland. When the Meibomian gland is affected, the disease is called internal hordeolum. Sty is the external hordeolum involving Zei's or Moll's glands. Chalazion is a sterile granulomatous inflammation of unknown cause at a Meibomian gland, with no signs of acute inflammation (redness and pain). Recurrent chalazions require biopsy to rule out malignancy.

213. (B)

214. (A)

215. (C)

216. (D)

217. (E) Diabetes causes formation of new vessels on the surface of the iris (rubeosis iridis), microaneurysm, hemorrhage, and retinal detachment and cataract. Gargoylism (Hurler's syndrome) is due to accumulation of mucopolysaccharides, which results in grotesque facial appearance, mental deficiency, dwarfism, corneal opacities, deformed bone shape, and heart failure. To prevent retrolental fibroplasia, the oxygen concentration should be kept below 40%, particularly for premature babies. Myasthenia gravis is characterized by easy fatigability of striated muscles, with unilateral ptosis and diplopia. Osteogenesis imperfecta includes multiple fractures, blue sclera, and deafness.

218. (D)

219. (B)

220. (A) Senile lentigines are flat brown-to-black colored spots ("liver spots") on the dorsum of the hands, face, and neck in later age. These are benign lesions and can be treated with liquid nitrogen applications. Heat urticaria is induced by heat, exercise, or stress, with a tiny wheal on the base of a large erythema. Administration of acetylcholine will reproduce the reaction to make the diagnosis. Oncholysis is often the prominent sign of pustular psoriasis.

221. (E)

222. (C)

223. (B) Marfan's syndrome is characterized by kyphoscoliosis, excessive length of arms and legs, lens dislocation, myopia, retinal detachment, aortic regurgitation, and aortic dilatation and dissection. Marfan's syndrome is transmitted by an autosomal dominant trait; propranolol is used to reduce the risk of aortic dissection. Malignant hyperthermia is an autosomal dominant disease causing hyperthermia and muscle rigidity by administering anesthetic agents (halothane, succinylcholine, or methoxyflurane). Some patients with homocystinuria are responsive to vitamin B6 (pyridoxine-responsive homocystinuria). Gardner's syndrome includes fibromas, epidermal cysts, and increased risk of colon cancers. Colorectomy is recommended. Hemochromatosis is associated with cirrhosis, cardiomegaly, diabetes, and brownish slate-gray pigmentation. Deferoxamine, a chelating agent, is useful.

224. (D)

225. (B)

226. (A) Retinitis pigmentosa causes night blindness, gun barrel vision, and ring scotoma (loss of the peripheral visual field) and may be associated with abeta-lipoproteinemia, cataract, and glaucoma. Central scotoma may be associated with optic neuritis and macular degeneration. Optic neuritis is associated with diabetes mellitus, multiple sclerosis, pernicious anemia, methanol, tobacco, quinine, lead, and salicylate. It is characterized by loss of vision and central scotoma. Glaucoma may cause arcuate scotoma in the early stage and progress to peripheral constriction later. A left anterior temporal lobe lesion may cause right-upper quadrant hemianopsia. A left parietal lobe lesion may cause right-inferior quadrant hemianopsia.

227. (B)

228. (C)

229. (E) Synovial fluid analysis yields very useful diagnostic information and should be analyzed when there is an accessible effusion. Traumatic arthritis shows gross bloody effusion. Fat droplets represent a fracture communicating with the joint. Septic arthritis may show very low glucose content, more than 50,000 polymorphonuclear (PMN) cells, and positive Gram-stain or culture. In rheumatoid arthritis (RA), many phagocytic inclusions of PMNs (RA cells) with reduced complement level can be seen. Phagocytosis of leukocytes by macrophages is seen in Reiter's syndrome. Pseudogout presents with calcium pyrophosphate crystals, whereas gout presents with urate crystals.

230. (F)

231. (F)

232. (F)

233. (F)

234. (F)

235. (F)

236. (F)

237. (F)

238. (F)

239. (T)

240. (F)

241. (T)

242. (F)

243. (T)

244. (T)

245. (T)

246. (T)

247. (T)

Although the curbstone consultation is often unavoidable, however, you should insist that the mother brings the baby to your office to form a professional relationship and to provide needed comprehensive and continuous total health care for the entire family members. Acute otitis media is often diagnosed upon clinical findings and the selection of antibiotics is usually based upon epidemiological experiences. *Streptococcus pneumoniae* is often the most common pathogen followed by *Hemophilus influenzae*. Thus oral ampicillin 50-100 mg/kg/day in four divided doses or amoxicillin 20-40 mg/kg/day in three divided doses are usually initiated for 10 days. Nonresponsive patients may be caused by beta-lactamase producing ampicillin-resistant strains of *H. influenzae* and cefaclor (ceclor), trimethoprim-sulfamethoxazole (septra or Bactrim) can be used. Oral decongestants, antihistamines, analgesics, antipyretics are tried by some clinicians with variable results.

248. **(F)**

249. **(F)**

250. **(F)**

251. **(T)**

252. **(T)**

253. **(T)**

254. **(T)**

255. **(T)**

Although this patient is probably suffering from "honeymoon cystitis," detailed history taking and physicals are in order to differentiate with many conditions including irritation of genitalias, vaginitis (in fact this patient was also found to harbor trichomanads), cervicitis, emotional stresses, and pyronephritis. When acute cystitis is the probable cause of the presenting genitourinary symptoms, urinalysis is mandatory to identify the causal microorganisms in selecting appropriate antibiotics. *E. coli* is by far the most common pathogen and the single-dose therapy amoxicillin or trimethoprim-sulfamethoxazole (Septra DS 2 tablets) is often effective. Urine culture and antimicrobial drug sensitivity test should be ordered. If bacteriuria (10^5 or more colonies) persists in 3 to 4 days, a 10-day course of ampicillin (250 mg q.i.d.) or Sepra (1 D S tablet b.i.d.) may be continued. For those patients with pyuria and sterile culture, *Chlamydia trachomatis* is the likely pathogen and doxycyline (Vibramycin) 100 mg b.i.d. for 10 days can be prescribed. Persistent bacteriuria and recurrent UTIs require thorough work-ups to identify structural or functional abnormalities of urinary organs and to determine current pathogens (such as candidiasis or schistosomiasis) or other etiological factors (including sexual activities) for provision of continuity of care.

Chapter 6

Community Medicine

Directions: Each of the questions or incomplete statements below is followed by five suggested answers or completions. Select the BEST answer in each case.

1. The most common cause of illness-induced absenteeism in the working population is

   A. respiratory conditions
   B. injuries
   C. industrial illnesses
   D. heart conditions
   E. parasitic infestations   (41:127)

2. The lowest blood alcohol concentration which most states recognize as showing that persons are legally intoxicated is (in mg/100 ml)

   A. 600
   B. 300
   C. 150
   D. 30
   E. 5   (43:603)

3. What kind of bacteria are used as criteria to check the safety of drinking water?

   A. *Salmonella*
   B. *Shigella*
   C. cholera
   D. *E. coli*
   E. *Pseudomonas*   (41:984)

4. If a community is to double its population size in 23 years, the expected annual rate of increase is approximately

   A. 1%
   B. 3%

C. 5%
D. 10%
E. 25%   (41:760)

5. When a disease lasts two to three weeks with a fatality rate of 80%, then

   A. its incidence is higher than its prevalence
   B. its incidence is equal to its prevalence
   C. its incidence is lower than its prevalence
   D. its incidence has no relationship to its prevalence
   E. all of the above   (40:127)

6. In planning a chronic disease control program, which of the following measurements furnishes the most useful information?

   A. incidence of the disease
   B. fatality of the disease
   C. prevalence of the disease
   D. mortality of the disease
   E. life expectancy of the disease   (40:127-128)

7. Three members of a family became ill over the course of several hours. History and physical examination suggest a diagnosis of botulism. Which of the following statements reflects our epidemiological knowledge?

   A. botulism results from the ingestion of the microorganism *Clostridium botulinum*, which can be found in many meat products prior to heating
   B. *Cl. botulinum* is a normal inhabitant of the gastrointestinal tracts of animals and man

C. *Cl. botulinum* can be found in many virgin soil specimens and can be transferred from soil to certain food products

D. the aerobic requirements of *Cl. botulinum* for production of toxin are high

E. while several types of *Cl. botulinum* have been identified, the toxins elaborated are antigenically identical   (*43:478*)

8. The number of deaths that occurred in a city of 10,000 in 1985 was 98. The conventional expression of the crude death rate for this city is

A. 9.8 per 1000 population
B. 0.98%
C. 98
D. 980 per 100,000 population
E. none of the above   (*44:24*)

9. A local health department has responsibility for all of the following *except*

A. control of communicable diseases
B. supervision of the milk supply
C. inspection of meat for interstate shipment
D. supervision of swimming pools
E. enforcement of health ordinances (*43:815*)

10. When measles virus is introduced into an isolated community which has had no known cases for 50 years, which of the following might be expected?

A. sporadic cases largely limited to children
B. sporadic cases involving both children and adults
C. an epidemic largely involving children, sparing adults
D. an epidemic involving children and adults under 50 years of age
E. a completely unpredictable situation
          (*40:27*)

11. If the sensitivity of a screening test for a defined disease is 95%, then it may be expected that

A. the test will be positive in 95% of individuals with the disease
B. the test will be negative in 95% of individuals without the disease
C. of the positive individuals, 95% will have the disease
D. of the negative individuals, only 5% will have the disease
E. none of the above   (*40:245*)

12. The family physician is one who

A. serves as the physician of first contact and provides the patient a means of entry into the health care system
B. evaluates the patient's total health needs and provides medical care within the sphere of his own competency
C. assumes the responsibility of total health care of the patient and his family within the medical community
D. all of the above
E. none of the above   (*50:5*)

13. Medicaid is

A. a modern version of the Red Cross
B. an emergency medical service
C. a means test-based program
D. health insurance for the aged
E. none of the above   (*44:263-264*)

14. Medicare is

A. a modern version of the Red Cross
B. an organized home health service
C. a program to pay health care costs for a certain age group
D. a program to pay health care costs for a certain income group
E. all of the above   (*44:264-265*)

15. Health Maintenance Organizations (HMOs)

A. evolved from prepaid group practices
B. are limited to prepaid group practices
C. provide only preventive services
D. provide multiphasic screening services only
E. none of the above   (*41:1683*)

16. PSROs are a means for

A. oppressing physicians
B. reducing paperwork
C. peer review
D. outside review
E. hospital auditing   (*46:358*)

17. The effects of air pollution include

A. damage to human health
B. damage to vegetation
C. damage to property
D. annoyance to the human senses
E. all of the above   (*41:1246*)

18. The possible effects of high levels of pollution can be seen in

A. increased mortality during periods of increased pollution

B. increased hospital admissions, particularly for those with asthma, emphysema, and other lung diseases

C. increased complaints of eye and nose irritation

D. all of the above

E. none of the above   (41:1246)

19. Which method of solid waste disposal is least acceptable today?

A. landfill
B. pyrolysis
C. pulverization and compaction
D. open-dump burning
E. incineration   (41:960)

20. Causality in the etiology of disease

A. requires a specific single agent
B. can be explained as due to multiple factors
C. cannot be determined by observational studies
D. can be determined by clinical impression only
E. must be determined before the disease can be controlled   (45:419)

21. Diseases are usually developed by

A. the agent only
B. the evil spirit
C. the interaction of agent, host, and environmental factors
D. the yin-yang forces
E. random chance   (40:28)

22. The standard deviation is

A. a measure of location
B. equivalent to the range
C. a measure of normality of the data
D. a measure of the variability
E. a measure of central tendency   (47:104)

23. Suppose the hemoglobin value of a population is normally distributed; then a laboratory hemoglobin value of 15 mg/100 ml with a standard deviation of 1.5 mg/100 ml means

A. the hemoglobin value ranges from 13.5 to 16.5 mg/100 ml
B. the value reported is not significant
C. 95% accuracy within 13.5 to 16.5 mg/100 ml

D. 5% error beyond 13.5 to 16.5 mg/100 ml
E. 68% of hemoglobin values lie between 13.5 and 16.5 mg/100 ml   (47:38-39)

24. The period during pregnancy when large dosages of abdominal irradiation are most likely to cause serious abnormality in the newborn is

A. the first three months
B. months three through six
C. months six through nine
D. before conception
E. no hazardous effect during pregnancy   (48:237)

25. Ciguatera poisoning

A. is prevented by cooking the fish in a microwave oven
B. may cause the reversal of cold to hot sensation in touch and taste
C. can be treated with an antidote
D. is caused by the action of histamine
E. is caused by the toxins concentrated in the gonads (ichthyotoxic)   (107:103-105)

Directions: For each of the incomplete statements below, ONE or MORE of the numbered completions is correct. In each case select:

A. if only 1, 2, and 3 are correct
B. if only 1 and 3 are correct
C. if only 2 and 4 are correct
D. if only 4 is correct
E. if all are correct

26. The problem-oriented medical record is simply a convenient way of displaying the patient's problems. This record is implemented when

1. a defined data base is completed
2. a numbered and titled problem list is kept
3. a problem list is placed at the front of the record and regularly updated
4. progress notes are numbered and titled for each problem   (45:36, 53)

27. The advantages of the retrospective study as compared to the prospective study include

1. lower relative costs
2. relatively small sample requirements
3. ease in selection of controls

4. use in the study of rare diseases   (40:324)

28. Multiple screening programs are effective and justified when

1. the screening test is simple, specific, reasonably cheap, and sensitive
2. methods and facilities are available to confirm the diagnosis and to manage the disease
3. incidence of the disease is sufficiently high
4. the screening test uncovers an appreciable number of new cases   (49:920)

29. A new group of "physician extenders" is now being trained and formed in the United States. It includes such personnel as

1. occupational therapists
2. physical therapy assistants
3. licensed practical nurses
4. family health nurse practitioners   (49:926)

30. The responsibilities of a public health nurse include

1. coordinating community health activities
2. giving treatment in the home
3. health guidance to individuals and families
4. keeping problem-oriented records   (43:817)

31. The characteristic triangular, broad-based pattern of the population pyramid in developing countries indicates

1. high birth rate
2. high death rate
3. young median age
4. high proportion of older people
    (40:216-218)

32. The increase in the frequency of chronic diseases has principally been a result of

1. control of communicable diseases
2. a greater population of elderly persons
3. improved treatment of cardiovascular diseases
4. common occurrence of noninfectious diseases in the elderly   (41:1135)

33. The following programs are useful in reducing dental cavities

1. restriction of sweet foods
2. good mouth hygiene
3. use of fluoride solution
4. regular visits to dentists   (44:153-154)

34. Epidemiology is concerned with

1. frequency distribution
2. factors influencing observed distribution
3. causes of the disease
4. population characteristics   (42:1)

35. A patient with hypertension is at risk of developing

1. congestive heart failure
2. cerebral vascular accident
3. myocardial infarction
4. hepatic failure   (78:280-281)

36. Risk factors of atherosclerosis include

1. diabetes mellitus
2. hypertension
3. hypercholesterolemia
4. moderate alcohol intake   (73:283)

37. A positive family history is often present in the patient with

1. atherosclerosis
2. peptic ulcer
3. polycystic kidney disease
4. diabetes mellitus   (73:283, 634, 684, 1321)

38. Which of the following diseases may show family predisposition?

1. epilepsy
2. schizophrenia
3. febrile seizures
4. alcoholism   (78:1237)

39. A problem is

1. a symptom complex
2. a specific diagnosis
3. a working impression
4. an abnormal physical sign   (45:38)

Directions: Each of the questions or incomplete statements is followed by five lettered options. For each option, indicate "T" if the option is true; indicate "F" if the option is false.

40. In your practice there are 40 hypertensive patients; you found 31 of them (almost 80%) drink more than two glasses of orange juice a day. You will now:

A. conclude that hypertension is caused by orange juice consumption

B. conclude that orange juice consumption is a risk factor for hypertension
C. advise all your patients to stop drinking orange juice
D. advise only those of your hypertensive patients to stop drinking orange juice
E. none of the above

41. Which of the following are the priority areas of preventive medicine commonly practiced by family physicians?

A. provision of immunizations
B. treatments of hypertensive patients
C. performing breast plastic surgery
D. control of gonorrhea
E. all of the above   (73: 35-36)

42. Which of the following statements about midlevel primary care practitioners are correct?

A. there are more physician assistants than nurse practitioners in the United States
B. physician assistants are available only in developing countries
C. the total number of nurse practitioners are decreasing drastically in the past few years
D. all of the above
E. none of the above   (41:1732)

43. Concerning physican manpower, which of the following statements are correct?

A. the national average physician/population ratio is about 1 and 1000
B. "overabundance" of physicians has been seen in other countries
C. the number of osteopathic physicians is drastically declining in the recent years
D. 90% of physicians are engaged in primary care
E. none of the above   (41:1732)

44. The crude death rate of the conmunity A is 6.8/1000; that of the community B is 8.6/1000. The likely explanations include:

A. the death data many be more complete in the community B
B. the population of the community A may be much younger than the population of the community B
C. the population size of the community B may be smaller
D. community A enjoys a higher health status than community B

E. all of the above   (40:135)

45. Infant mortality rate is measured by:

A. the deaths of the infants under 1 month of age
B. the deaths of the infants under 6 months of age
C. the deaths of the infants under 12 months of age
D. the deaths of the infants under 18 months of age
E. none of the above   (44:24)

46. DRGS:

A. it is a retrospective payment system
B. all physicians are employed by a fixed salary under this system.
C. It stands for Diagnosis Related Groups
D. it considers only principal procecdures for its classification
E. it adopts ICD-7-CM for coding

47. Asbestosis:

A. can be prevented by cigarette smoking
B. Adriamycin is effective in 80% of the patients
C. shipyard workers may be at a higher risk
D. may cause methothelioma
E. is protective for lung cancer
          (73:2283-2284)

Directions: Each group of numbered words or phrases is followed by a list of lettered statements. MATCH the lettered statement most closely associated with the numbered word or phrase.

Questions 48 to 52

48. Used to test null hypothesis of "independence" for the two classifications of a contingency table   (47:72)
49. Hypothesis to be accepted if the null hypothesis is rejected   (47:4)
50. Three groups of patients are randomly assigned for three treatment plans   (47:198)
51. Two groups of infants are compared for the effect on weight change of two different family counseling methods   (47:155)
52. Strength of association between two variables   (42:52)

A. T-test
B. Chi-square test

C. Analysis of variance
D. Product moment correlation
E. Alternative hypothesis

Questions 53 to 55

53. Five blocks are selected randomly from 50 homogeneous blocks; 20 households are then selected randomly from each of these five blocks for household interviews to determine the health needs of the family members
54. One hundred families are drawn from the problem-oriented records of a family physician's office on the basis of a randomly selected last digit of the family number
55. One hundred households are selected from the entire 2500 households in the area on the basis of a table of random numbers
                                        (47:220-221)

A. Area-cluster sampling
B. Systematic sampling
C. Simple random sampling

Questions 56 to 59

56. Covers hospital cost
57. Covers physician services in the hospital
58. Closed physician panels
59. Group practice setting

A. Blue Cross/Blue Shield
B. Prepaid medical group
C. Both
D. Neither   *(44:254-255)*

Questions 60 to 63
The trends of death rates for females in the United States during the period 1930 to 1967 for selected cancer sites are as follows:

60. Breast cancer
61. Cervical cancer
62. Lung cancer
63. Stomach cancer   *(41:1149)*

A. Increased
B. Decreased
C. Stationary

Questions 64 to 66
64. Neonatal death rate
65. Cause-specific death rate

66. Infant mortality rate

A. Newborn deaths within one month per 1000 live births
B. Infant deaths under one year of age per 1000 live births
C. Total deaths per 1000 population
D. One year deaths with pneumonia
                                        (44:25-26)

Questions 67 to 70

67. Staphylococcus   *(44:90)*
68. Chlorine   *(41:1012)*
69. Phosphatase test   *(41:947)*
70. Aluminum sulfate   *(41:993)*

A. Milk sanitation
B. Food poisoning
C. Swimming pool sanitation
D. Public water supply

Questions 71 to 74

71. New cases
72. Recurrent cases
73. Point in time
74. Time period

A. Incidence
B. Prevalence
C. Both
D. Neither   *(40:127)*

Questions 75 to 79

75. Lung cancer
76. Skin cancer
77. Bladder cancer
78. Leukemia
79. Sinus cancer

A. Beta-naphthylamine
B. Benzene
C. Arsenic
D. Nickel
E. Fluoride   *(41:1157)*

Directions: This part of the test consists of a situation followed by a series of incomplete statements. Study the situation and select the best answer to complete each statement that follows.

Sixty people attended a picnic at which the following foods were served: fried chicken, fruit salad, rolls, butter, coffee with cream and sugar, ice cream, and custard-filled pastry. Drinking water came from a spring adjacent to a river. Between two and five hours after the meal, 45 of the people became ill with nausea, vomiting, abdominal cramps, diarrhea, or a combination of these symptoms. Stools were watery, with some containing mucus but no blood. Temperatures ranged from 37.0°C (98.6°F) to 38.0°C (100°F). Attacks lasted for 24 to 72 hours. Recovery was uneventful in all cases.

80. Which of the following was the most likely cause of the epidemic?

   A. sewage pollution of the water
   B. *Staphylococcus* enterotoxin
   C. arsenic poisoning
   D. *Salmonella*
   E. *Shigella*   (*44:90*)

81. Which of the following laboratory examinations would be most likely to determine the causative agent?

   A. chemical analysis of the food

   B. bacteriological examination of the drinking water
   C. bacteriological culture of the leftover foods
   D. stool cultures of the people who became ill
   E. stool cultures of the people who prepared the food   (*44:90*)

82. Which of the following was the most likely source of the epidemic?

   A. an intestinal carrier of a pathogenic organism
   B. contamination of the spring by sewage
   C. an insecticide
   D. an attendant's common cold
   E. a pustular lesion on the hand of the baker   (*44:90*)

83. Which of the following was most likely infected?

   A. drinking water
   B. ice cream
   C. fried chicken
   D. custard-filled pastries
   E. rolls   (*44:90*)

Answers and Explanations

1. **(A)** Ninety percent of the causes of the days of absence among the working population are due to nonoccupational illness and accidents, while 0.1% are due to industrial diseases and about 2% to occupational injuries. Approximately six work days per person per year are lost as a result of illness or injury. Respiratory ailments are by far the most common cause of sickness-absenteeism, followed by digestive disorders and other infections. Among the chronic diseases, cardiac conditions, digestive disorders, and mental and nervous conditions are among the more common causes of absenteeism from work.

2. **(C)** Approximately one-half of crashes fatal to vehicle occupants and one-fifth of crashes in which vehicle occupants were injured result at least in part from alcoholic use. The increased risk begins with blood alcohol concentrations of 30 mg/100 ml (0.03% by weight), commonly reached with one or two drinks in most individuals. All individuals are affected at or below 100 mg/100 ml. Concentrations of 100 or 150 mg/100 ml are usually regarded as evidence of alcohol influence in most states.

3. **(D)** Bacteriological techniques are available to identify the water-borne pathogens which cause typhoid, cholera, and dysentery. However, the test for the presence of a single group of organisms—the coliform group—is used almost exclusively as a bacteriological index of the degree of pollution.

4. **(B)** Neglecting migration (population growth is determined by the difference between immigration and emigration), the rate of population growth is expressed as the difference between the crude birth and death rates. A useful approximation is: years to double equals 70 divided by annual percentage increase.

5. **(A)** The prevalence (P) is related to both incidence (I) and duration (d) of disease: $P \cong I \times d$. When d is short (acute) or there is a high fatality rate, then prevalence is low as compared to incidence. In chronic diseases, the duration is long and the prevalence will be relatively large in relation to incidence. If the incidence and duration have both been stable over a long period of time and the population is also stable, then $P = I \times d$, where d is mean duration.

6. **(C)** The relative importance of certain diseases in the population is not reflected in the mortality data, and prevalence is important in determining work load, particularly in chronic diseases, in which it is a useful tool for the planning of facilities and manpower needs. Incidence is also an important measurement in planning.

7. **(C)** Most botulism outbreaks in the United States are due to toxin from Type A or B organisms and a few from Type E (smoked white fish and canned tuna). Toxin is produced in improperly processed foods, mostly

from home-canned vegetables. Pimientos, olives, and mushrooms have been prime offenders. Symptoms are acute toxic encephalitis with paralysis of ocular and pharyngeal muscles without diarrhea. Polyvalent antitoxin is used for treatment, although the fatality rate is 60%.

8. **(A)** The crude death rate is the number of deaths reported in a calendar year per 1000 population (estimated as of the middle of the year).

9. **(C)** The basic six functional areas of the local health department include: vital statistics, sanitation, communicable disease control, laboratory services, maternal and child health, and health education. Recently, evaluation, research, teaching, planning, and coordination activities, as well as provision of direct personal health service, have become important functions of the local health unit.

10. **(D)** The organism and the level of immunity of the population are crucial for the development of illness. The introduction of measles (or mumps) into a virgin population (i.e., one in which an organism has not been present for many years, if ever) will affect adults as well as children. The upper age limit is determined by the number of years since the virus last circulated in the community.

11. **(A)**

Result of screening test	Disease state	
	Disease	No disease
Positive	True positive (TP)	False positive (FP)
Negative	False negative (FN)	True negative (TN)

Sensitivity $= \dfrac{TP}{TP + FN}$ Specificity $= \dfrac{TN}{TN + FP}$

Sensitivity is the percentage of people with the disease who are detected by the test; specificity is the percentage of people without the disease who correctly labeled by the test as not diseased.

12. **(D)** In addition, the family physician is oriented to care for the whole family and the whole patient. He or she guides rehabilitation, practices preventive medicine, and is a medical advocate for his or her families. He or she assumes continuing responsibility for the health care needs of the family and provides comprehensive health care and disease management for all of the family members. Family practice is a useful way to meet community health needs.

13. **(C)** Medicaid is a grant-in-aid program in which the federal and state governments share the costs of medical care for people of all ages with low income. The state sets up a program for eligible people to receive necessary medical services. Means tests are used to determine the eligibility. However, it was estimated in 1970 that only about a third of the 30 to 40 million indigent and medically indigent who could potentially be covered were, in fact, able to receive services.

14. **(C)** In 1965, the Medicare Act provided a two-part insurance program for persons aged 65 and over covered by Social Security. This provided a basic program of hospital and related benefits to be financed through Social Security taxes. Benefits included 90 days of hospital care, 100 days of nursing home care, 100 home nursing visits, and hospital outpatient services, all subject to some deductibles and coinsurance features. Over 20,000,000 persons 65 and over were covered for hospital charges. In 1975, Medicare patients accounted for about 30–40% of all bed-days in general hospitals.

15. **(A)** HMOs carry full responsibility for health services to individuals for a fixed annual payment. The emphasis is frequently on ambulatory care (both curative and preventive) instead of hospital services to lower the cost of medical care.

16. **(C)** The Professional Standards Review Organization (PSRO) implements a peer review mechanism to control the utilization of services to assure their appropriateness in controlling program costs. In conducting its review activities, each PSRO will apply professionally developed norms of care, diagnosis, and treatment which, in turn, will be based on typical patterns of practice in its region.

17. **(E)** The effects of air pollution on health are mainly associated with irritations to the respiratory tract and eyes. Air pollution is suspected to be associated with Yokohama asthma and hay fever. The monetary loss due to air pollution has been estimated at four to eleven billion dollars per year in the United States.

18. **(D)** The three most famous and well documented episodes of acute illness and death due to general atmospheric pollution are the Mense Valley (Belgium) disaster in December 1930; the Donora (Pennsylvania) disaster in October 1948; and the London experience in December 1952.

19. **(D)** Air pollution from uncontrolled burning dumps and overloaded incinerators is common and apparent to near neighbors. The most renowned is the Kenilworth dump outside Washington, D.C. Its smoky, malodorous pall has made itself known in motion pictures and television broadcasts.

20. **(B)** The generally accepted concept of the etiology of disease is multiple causation of illness. The concept maintains that illness is the result of a basic imbalance in a person's adaptation to the multiple short- and long-term physical and emotional stresses within the environment. A more precise terminology for multiple causation might be a "chain of causation" or a "web of causation." Epidemiological studies (descriptive, analytic, and experimental) are conducted to determine the causal factors of the disease. Control of the disease is often successfully achieved long before the etiology of the disease is found. For example, although the exact cause of lung cancer is still unknown, the control of cigarette smoking will possibly lower the risk of developing lung cancer.

21. **(C)** When a factor must be present for a disease to occur, it is called the agent of that disease (e.g., influenza virus is the agent of influenza). However, an agent is considered to be a necessary but not sufficient cause of disease, because suitable conditions of the host (intrinsic factors) and environment (extrinsic factors) must also be present for disease to develop. Host factors affect susceptibility to disease, and factors in the environment influence exposure and often indirectly affect susceptibility. The interactions of these two factors determine whether or not disease develops.

22. **(D)** The standard deviation is the square root of the variance, which is the average squared deviation around the mean:

$$SD = \sqrt{\frac{\Sigma(\chi - M)^2}{N}}$$

However, the sample standard deviation is

$$S = \sqrt{\frac{\Sigma(\chi - \bar{\chi})^2}{N}}$$

The standard deviation measures the variability and dispersion, while the mean (average value) measures the central tendency. The mean is the sum of total value from all items divided by the number of items:

$$M = \frac{\Sigma X}{N}$$

23. **(E)** Assuming a normal curve, the proportion of observations that lies within one standard deviation from the mean is 68.27%; that which lies between two standard deviations from the mean is 95.45%. The percentage of hemoglobin values that are more than plus and less than minus two standard deviations from the mean is 4.55%.

24. **(A)** Irradiation before two to three weeks of gestation or after 30 weeks of gestation is not likely to produce gross abnormalities. Irradiation between four and 11 weeks of gestation would lead to severe abnormalities of many organs in most or all fetuses. Thus, during the first trimester, radiographic diagnostic procedures for pregnant women should be reserved only for cases of absolute necessity.

25. **(B)** Ciguatera poisoning is caused by the toxin derived from migratory reef fish, especially grouper, jack, snapper, and barracuda. The toxin is called ichthyosarcotoxic because it is in the body parts (musculature, viscera, skin, and mucus) of fish. Cooking cannot prevent the poisoning, and the cignatoxic fish cannot be identified by odor or color. It usually causes nausea, vomiting, diarrhea, and abdominal pain within 36 hours after

ingestion and the patient may develop numbness and tingling of the lips, hands, and feet; reversal of cold to hot sensations in touch and taste; and arthralgia and myalgia of the legs and thighs. Emesis, gastric lavage, and cathartic administration are used to remove unabsorbed toxin; atropine and intravenous fluids are administered for symptomatic relief. There are no antidotes available yet.

26. **(E)** Problem-oriented Records (POR) are very useful in record keeping for ambulatory patient care services. Thus many family practice centers are adopting POR as the record keeping system. Progress notes frequently include Subjective and Objective observations, Assessment, and Plans (SOAP). Plans should include diagnoses to be ruled out. The format of a flow sheet is frequently used for the progress notes.

27. **(B)** In a retrospective study, people diagnosed as having a disease (cases) are compared with persons who do not have the disease (controls). Relative risk is then calculated by dividing the incidence rate among the exposed (cases) by the incidence rate among the nonexposed (controls). In a prospective study, a group of people (cohort) who are free of disease are classified by exposure or lack of exposure to a factor and followed for the development of disease. In addition to relative risk, the attributable risk is also calculated by the absolute difference in incidence rates between an exposed group and a nonexposed group.

28. **(E)** Multiple screening programs are designed for the community-wide testing of individuals for several diseases at the same visit. Such programs are expensive and evaluation of the cost/benefit ratio is in order.

29. **(D)** The task of health care is broken into its component parts according to the skills needed to do each part, in order to train paramedical personnel to do jobs normally done by physicians and nurses. The most rapid increase, now and possibly in the future, is likely to occur in the relatively new groups of personnel with shorter training periods. Now in training is a new and mixed group of "physician extenders," to be called by such names as physician assistants and

nurse practitioners. Many family practice residencies have employed family health nurse practitioners and physician assistants to provide direct patient care in ambulatory family practice centers. Thus family physicians may inevitably have to spend more time on supervision.

30. **(E)** Public health nursing occupies a central role in the delivery of ambulatory and home health services. The public health nurse (PHN) is both community- and family-oriented and directs her or his attention to prevention and to the care of well families, the nonhospitalized sick, and groups of persons at special risk. PHNs will certainly play important roles in family practice residencies.

31. **(A)** The determinants of population dynamics—births, deaths, and migration—can be shown pictorially by a population pyramid which presents the population of an area or country in terms of its composition by age and sex at a point in time. The shape of the pyramid reflects the major influences on births and deaths, plus any changes due to migration, over the three to four generations preceding the date of the pyramid. The population pyramids of developing countries frequently show triangular, broad-based patterns reflecting high birth and death rates. Only a small proportion of persons have survived into the older age groups, so the median age is relatively young.

32. **(C)** The increase in the frequency of chronic diseases has principally been a result of the greater number of individuals who survive into the older age groups of the population, where the chronic noninfectious diseases are more common.

33. **(E)** The use of topical fluoride directly applied to the teeth appears to be of considerable value in reducing dental cavities. Fluoridation of public water supplies with one part per million (ppm) fluoride is effective in reducing dental cavities by as much as 60%. However, the long-term side-effects of fluoridation are not yet clear.

34. **(E)** Epidemiology is defined as the study of the distribution and determinants of disease frequency in man. However, the epidemiolog-

ical principles can be used to study the extent and the determinants of any specific characteristics in a population under investigation. The specific characteristics include diseases, injuries, or behaviors (e.g., cigarette smoking). The study population can be composed of humans, animals, or plants; it can also be a group of items of interest to the investigator.

35. **(A)** The control of hypertension decreases the risk of developing complications, including malignant hypertension, congestive heart failure, cerebral vascular accident, renal insufficiency, and myocardial infarction. All patients with diastolic blood pressure of 105 mmHg or greater should be treated with antihypertensive drugs. The patients with diastolic pressure of 90 to 104 mmHg should evaluate the risk factor to decide on the need of treatment. Those patients with a positive family history of premature coronary heart diseases or premature cardiovascular deaths and those patients with target organ involvement need to be treated.

36. **(A)** Risk factors of atherosclerosis include aging, male sex, hypertension, diabetes mellitus, obesity, hyperlipidemia, cigarette smoking, sedentary activity, type A behavior (enhanced aggressiveness, ambitiousness, competitive drive, and chronic sense of time urgency), and a positive family history. Moderate alcohol intake may reduce the risk of myocardial infarction due to a favorable HDL:LDL ratio (high-density lipoprotein: low-density lipoprotein); alcohol intake may increase the HDL level.

37. **(E)** Many illnesses and diseases are clustered in certain families—some are genetically determined through inheritance (hereditary illnesses) and some show familial aggregation without a definite inheritance pattern. In these instances, the family should be the unit of care to provide preventive and counseling services for other members of the family who are not ill (but who are at risk of developing similar diseases). A detailed family history of these diseases with familial predisposition should be recorded.

38. **(E)** Epilepsy is not a hereditary disease, but it does show familial predisposition. Schizo-

phrenia has a hereditary predisposition. Febrile seizures show a familial disposition. Alcoholism is not hereditary; however, family members of alcoholics are at increased risk of becoming alcoholics.

39. **(E)** Problems are selected and identified from the analysis of the currently available data base. Thus sometimes a general term such as "head pain" will appear on the problem list. The objective evidence obtained from subsequent studies may change the problem into a specific diagnosis, such as "conversion reaction, head pain," or the problem may remain on the problem list until resolved.

40. **A-F, B-F, C-F, D-F, E-T**
In an investigation of etiological factors in disease, it is necessary to study not only the cases of the disease, but non-ill individuals (controls) from the same environment as well. This is termed the denominator principle in epidemiology.

41. **A-T, B-T, C-T, D-F, E-F**
In 1979 Surgeon General's report urged 15 national priority areas: smoking, nutrition, physical fitness, alcohol abuse, immunization; control of hypertension, sexually transmitted diseases, toxic agents, occupational safety and infectious disease; family planning, pregnancy and infant health, dental health; and prevention of injuries caused by accidents and violence. These areas are currently practiced by most family physicians.

42. **A-F, B-F, C-F, D-F, E-T**
At present, the number of nurse practitioners is around 38,000, comparable to the total number of family physicians and is far exceeding the number of physician assistants (22,000). Midlevel practitioners are rapidly growing in the recent year in the United States.

43. **A-F, B-T, C-F, D-F, E-F**
In 1983, the physician/population ratio was 1:430, 5% of physicians are osteopathic physicians who show steady growth in number during recent years. There were 85,000 family and general practitioners representing 17% of total physician force. "Overabundance" of physicians has been seen in other countries; many physicians engage in nonmedical activities (such as taxi-drivers), and many migrate to other countries.

44. A-T, B-T, C-T, D-T, E-T
Although the crude death rate is the readily obtainable health statistics, it's not a sensitive measurement of the health status of a community due to its influence by the age composition of the population. The elderly has a relative higher risk for death and a community comprises a higher proportion of the elderly may show a higher crude death rate.

45. A-F, B-F, C-T, D-F, E-F

$$\text{Infant mortality rate} = \frac{\text{No. of deaths in first year}}{\text{Live births during same year}} \times 1000$$

46. A-F, B-F, C-T, D-F, E-F
The type of hospitalized patients (called "case mix") can be grouped into 467 categories of diagnoses or procedures (including additional 3 DRGs of ungroupable records, a total of 470 DRGs) according to principal diagnosis and procedure, secondary diagnosis and procedure, age, sex, complications and discharge status.

There are 23 major diagnostic categories in DRGs and it adopts ICD-9-CM (International Classification of Disease, 9th Revision, Clinical Modification) for its reporting upon which a predetermined (i.e. Prospective) payment schedule is reimbursed for an average length of hospital stay.

47. A-F, B-F, C-T, D-T, E-F
High risk groups for asbestos exposure include miners, shipyard workers, insulation and construction workers. The patient may develop exertional dyspnea, nonproductive cough, and pulmonary fibrosis. Treatment is symptomatic; dust control and avoidance of inhaling asbestos fibers are important preventive measures. Asbestosis is associated with methothelioma and bronchogenic cancer, particularly in smokers.

48. (B)

49. (E)

50. (C)

51. (A)

52. (D) Correlation coefficient is used for studying the degree of linear relationship between two variables. Analysis of variance is used for comparing two or more sample means. T-test is used to compare group means in two independent samples. Chi-square is used in tests of significance on qualitative data.

$$\chi^2 = \Sigma \frac{\left(\frac{\text{Observed number}}{} - \frac{\text{Expected number}}{}\right)^2}{\text{Expected number}}$$

If it is very unlikely that the observed outcome could occur if the null hypothesis (that no true difference exists) were true, then the null hypothesis is rejected and the alternative hypothesis (that a true difference exists) is accepted.

53. (A)

54. (B)

55. (C) Systematic sampling is the most frequently used sampling procedure in record analysis. If the last digit of the family number is assigned on the basis of a selective factor (e.g., income level, ethnicity, or residence), then there will be a bias. Simple random sampling usually will result in a fairly representative sample; however, the required traveling to the scattered sample households makes it expensive. The area-cluster sampling is frequently employed in the household health need survey in a large homogeneous area due to less traveling expense.

56. (C)

57. (C)

58. (B)

59. (B) Blue Cross/Blue Shield plans are nonprofit medical care prepayment insurance plans provided on an individual or on a group basis to cover hospital costs (Blue Cross) and physicians' services in hospitals (Blue Shield). They do not usually cover physicians' office services or home calls. The prepaid medical groups, such as Health Insurance Plan of Greater New York and the Kaiser Foundation Health Plan, provide their members with comprehensive coverage of health services at home, in the physician's office, and in the hospital. Usually the patients have to go to offices and hospitals which were contracted or owned by the prepaid medical groups. A few plans cover dental care as well.

60. (C)

61. (B)

62. (A)

63. (B) The mortality trend of stomach cancer has declined in both sexes, while that of lung cancer has increased. The death rate from cancer of the uterus has been steadily declining; that of breast cancer has remained stable.

64. (A)

65. (D)

66. (B) The crude death rate is the number of deaths in a calendar year per 1000 population (estimated as of the middle of the year). A cause-specific death rate is the number of deaths in a selected age group per 1000 population in that same age group.

67. (B)

68. (C)

69. (A)

70. (D) The phosphatase test is used for detecting the contamination of raw milk because 96% of the enzyme monophosphoesterase is destroyed in properly pasteurized milk. The water in public pools is chlorinated with 1.0 ppm or more of residual chlorine. The most common food poisoning is with staphylococcal organisms. Coagulation by aluminum sulfate is a common procedure in the purification of water.

71. (C)

72. (B)

73. (B)

74. (A) Incidence rate is the number of new cases divided by the population at risk during a specific period of time (i.e., the study period);

prevalence rate (point prevalence) is the number of existing cases divided by the population at risk at a point in time. The existing cases include new and chronic cases as well as recurrent cases.

75. (D)

76. (C)

77. (A)

78. (B)

79. (D) Several occupations have been found to be associated with an increased risk of lung cancer: uranium mining, nickel refining, chromate manufacturing, asbestos manufacturing, and gas and tar work. Inhalation of asbestos is also associated with mesothelioma of the pleura and peritoneum. Chronic exposure to nickel carbonyl has been shown to produce bronchogenic, nasal, and sinus carcinomas in industrial workers. It is believed that arsenic compounds can produce skin cancer. Exposure to high concentrations of benzene has been reported to produce leukemia in men. Ionizing radiation has also been found to be associated with leukemia.

80. (B)

81. (C)

82. (E)

83. (D) The most common food poisoning in the United States is by enterotoxin of the staphylococcus organism. This disease is characterized by acute nausea, vomiting, and diarrhea which occur two to four hours after ingestion of contaminated food. The patient usually recovers after 24 hours. It is usually due to contamination of food from infections existing on the body of the food handler, typically boils on the hands or other body surfaces. The food implicated includes milk, milk products, and custard- or cream-filled pastries.

Chapter 7

Medicine

Directions: Each of the questions or incomplete statements below is followed by five suggested answers or completions. Select the BEST answer in each case.

1. The major difficulty in limiting the use of influenza virus vaccine has been the

   A. inability to purify vaccine
   B. inability to grow virus to high titer
   C. inability of patients to make high titers of antibody
   D. inability to obtain enough of the appropriate virus to make effective vaccine
   E. severe side-effects of vaccine   (85:300-301)

2. A patient with chronic otitis media and mastoiditis develops meningitis caused by *Bacteroides fragilis*. The antimicrobial agent of choice in the treatment of this patient is

   A. penicillin G
   B. ampicillin
   C. chloramphenicol
   D. clindamycin
   E. tetracycline   (73:1583)

3. Which of the following patients are *not* recommended for influenza immunizations?

   A. pregnant patients with heart diseases
   B. patients with cystic fibrosis
   C. patients with Guillain-Barre's syndrome
   D. elderly patients with chronic obstructive pulmonary diseases
   E. cancer patients receiving cytotoxic chemotherapy   (73:1704)

4. A 24-year-old has had four recurrences of pyelonephritis in the past two years. She now develops pyuria, fever to 101°F, and *E. coli* greater than 10^5 in her urine. She is treated with ampicillin 500 mg PO four times a day and her symptoms improve after two weeks. To prevent recurrences, you would treat her with

   A. ampicillin 250 mg PO four times a day for two more weeks
   B. cranberry juice, one juice glass twice a day for one year
   C. Pyridium (phenazopyridine) twice a day for three months
   D. Mandelamine (methenamine mandelate) chronically for one year
   E. sulfamethoxazole and trimethoprim one tablet PO every day for one year   (73:622)

5. Rifampin, a semisynthetic antibiotic which acts through the inhibition of RNA synthesis, has been found clinically effective in the treatment of

   A. nasopharyngeal carriers of *Neisseria meningitidis*
   B. *Mycobacterium tuberculosis*
   C. *Mycobacterium kansasii* (Group I atypical mycobacteria)
   D. trachoma
   E. all of the above   (73:597)

6. A nurse develops a large boil on her right thigh which is fluctuant and red. She has a temperature of 101°F. After incision and drainage, which of the following would *not* be appropriate therapy?

A. oral phenoxymethyl penicillin
B. oral cephalexin in adequate doses
C. oral dicloxacillin
D. oral oxacillin
E. oral erythromycin   (73:1550)

7. Which is *not* an example of antibiotic synergy?

A. sulfamethoxazole and trimethoprim
B. penicillin and aminoglycoside against enterococci
C. penicillin and tetracycline against streptococci
D. INH and ethambutol against tuberculosis
E. pyrimethamine and sulfur against *Pneumocystis* spp.   (73:1527)

8. A 17-year-old high school student notes the onset of severe sore throat, malaise, and fever of 102°F of one day's duration. On physical examination, he has bilateral enlarged tonsils with several white plaques and diffuse erythema. There are several 1 cm submandibular nodes and postcervical nodes. As a child, he developed wheezing and urticaria following penicillin therapy. When you see him, you do a throat culture and decide he looks sick enough to begin antibiotics. You would treat him with

A. clindamycin 300 mg PO four times per day for 10 days
B. tetracycline 250 mg PO four times per day for 10 days
C. tetracycline 500 mg PO four times per day for 10 days
D. erythromycin 500 mg PO four times per day for 10 days
E. oral cephalexin 500 mg PO four times per day for 10 days   (73:1527)

9. A 50-year-old nurse with chronic bronchitis develops influenza and then develops an acute patchy bronchopneumonia. Gram stain of the sputum grows Gram-positive cocci in clusters. Antibiotic therapy should be

A. oral phenoxymethyl penicillin
B. aqueous penicillin, 2,000,000 units every six hours
C. benzathine penicillin G, IM 2,400,000 units
D. oxacillin, 2 g IV every six hours
E. chloramphenicol, 0.5 g IV every six hours   (73:1701)

10. During "flu" season, a 25-year-old pregnant woman develops fever and sore throat and then suddenly develops acute dyspnea and nonproductive cough. She is found to be extremely hypoxic. She most likely has

A. pneumococcal pneumonia
B. staphylococcal pneumonia
C. influenza viral pneumonia
D. *Pseudomonas* pneumonia
E. streptococcal pharyngitis   (73:1702)

11. Examples of drug incompatibilities involving antimicrobial agents and other drugs, conditions, or antibiotics, include all of the following *except*

A. penicillin G and food
B. streptomycin and tetracycline
C. tetracyclines and milk
D. combined intravenous gentamicin and carbenicillin
E. oral tetracyclines and ferrous sulfate   (39:953)

12. The most common reason for antibiotic failure is

A. gross overuse for viral or nonbacterial illnesses
B. inappropriate route of administration
C. prolonged time intervals between administered doses
D. inadequate dosage
E. patient noncompliance   (39:952)

13. For which one of the following surgical procedures is the use of prophylactic antibiotics indicated (normal heart)?

A. insertion of indwelling catheters
B. cesarean section
C. cystoscopy
D. vascular surgery involving grafts
E. all of the above   (39:976-977)

14. An antibiotic that achieves high concentration in the nonobstructed gallbladder and has been used with some success in the treatment of chronic carriers of *Salmonella typhosa* is

A. cephalexin
B. carbenicillin
C. chloramphenicol
D. ampicillin
E. minocycline   (73:1589)

15. A patient who is being treated with tetracycline for beta-hemolytic streptococcal tonsillitis develops coincidental oral thrush. One should then

A. continue tetracycline and add nystatin rinses
B. discontinue tetracycline, start penicillin, and add nystatin rinses
C. discontinue tetracycline
D. continue tetracycline and add amphotericin B irrigation 50 µg/ml
E. discontinue tetracycline and start Mysteclin-F (tetracycline plus amphotericin B)   (39:960)

16. Failure to treat peritonitis for anaerobic infection leads to a higher risk of

A. endotoxemia
B. bacteremia
C. ileus
D. abdominal abscess
E. mesenteric phlebitis   (39:966)

17. A 25-year-old man develops onset of fever and hacking cough of five days' duration. His cough comes in uncontrolled paroxysms. He has a fever of 101°F. Chest examination reveals minimal scattered rales at the left-lower lung. Chest x-ray shows bilateral alveolar and interstitial infiltrates in the left-lower end and right-middle lung fields. After culturing his sputum, you would

A. treat him with 1,200,000 units per day of aqueous or procaine penicillin in appropriate divided doses for 10 days
B. administer erythromycin, 500 mg four times per day for one week
C. administer clindamycin, 300 mg PO four times per day if he was penicillin allergic
D. administer erythromycin, 500 mg four times per day for three weeks
E. none of the above   (73:1506)

18. Which antibiotic does not readily cross the inflamed brain barrier?

A. chloramphenicol
B. sulfur compounds
C. penicillin
D. INH
E. cephalothin   (54:46)

19. The *least* likely skeletal radiological change in hemophilia and other related disease is

A. hemarthrosis
B. epiphyseal overgrowth
C. pseudotumor formation
D. premature fusion of growth plates
E. thickening and sclerosis of the cortices of the vertebral end plates   (70:1387)

20. Which of the following concerning Burkitt's lymphoma is *least* likely?

A. it frequently starts in the mandibular region
B. long bones may be affected with an appearance resembling round cell tumor involvement
C. a facial mass is usually the presenting finding
D. retroperitoneal involvement is common
E. it may be of spirochetal origin, perhaps related to yaws   (73:1000)

21. Multiple myeloma *least* likely presents

A. in patients between 45 and 70 years
B. with small osteolytic lesions with sharp, punched-out margins
C. sclerosis of bone
D. as a development of plasma cell myeloma (plasmocytoma)
E. as an associated secondary finding of osteoporosis, soft tissue mass, and spinal cord compression; amyloidosis is often seen   (73:1016)

22. The most common cause of anemia in the adult is

A. poor diet or reducing diet
B. inflammatory disease
C. pernicious anemia
D. blood loss
E. renal failure   (73:872)

23. An 18-year-old girl acutely ill with fever, headache, joint pain, and widespread purpura is found to be bleeding profusely from venipuncture sites. Gram-negative cocci are observed on a smear of cerebrospinal fluid. The most likely cause of the hemostatic failure is

A. thrombocytopenia
B. disseminated intravascular coagulation (DIC)
C. hepatic failure
D. primary fibrinolysis
E. circulating anticoagulant   (83:1215)

24. An elevated titer of carcinoembryonic antigen (CEA) is detected in your adult patient
whose symptoms are nonspecific. Which
statement is most accurate?

A. the patient probably has carcinoma of the
colon with metastases to the liver
B. CEA is not specific for colon cancer but
indicates the presence of some type of
malignancy
C. CEA is not specific for malignancy
D. CEA has no association with cancer in
adults, but only with "embryonic" tumors
in young children
E. none is accurate   (55:998)

25. Which of the following is *not* thought to be a
predisposing lesion, greatly increasing the
risk of developing colon carcinoma?

A. hereditary familial polyposis
B. villous adenoma of the colon
C. ulcerative colitis
D. adenomatous polyp
E. none has any relation to colon carcinoma
                                  (55:994-995)

26. Which is correct with respect to diverticular
disease of the colon?

A. the initiating or primary factor appears to
be increased muscular tone and colonic
muscular hypertrophy
B. congenital weakness in colonic musculature is primary
C. fecal impaction is the underlying etiological cause
D. predisposes to development of villous
adenoma
E. none is correct   (58)

27. Ulcerative colitis and so-called Crohn's disease of the colon differ clinically and morphologically in several respects. Which is a
morphological feature distinguishing them
on biopsy or at resection?

A. full-thickness involvement of the colon
wall
B. presence of granulomas
C. extent of fibrosis (marked)
D. association with fistulas
E. all of the above   (59)

28. With respect to the liver biopsy morphology
in hepatitis, which is correct?

A. HAA-positive and HAA-negative hepatitis
are readily distinguished by their microscopic characteristics
B. "councilman bodies" represent the etiological viral particles
C. polymorphonuclear leukocytes are the
prominent cell type in acute viral hepatitis
D. lymphocytes are the predominant inflammatory cell infiltrating the damaged liver
E. more than one of the above   (55:1039-1044)

29. The liver changes associated with alcohol
abuse may include which of the following?

A. fatty change
B. alcoholic hyalin
C. fine, delicate, fibrous connective tissue
strands separating uniform-sized, small
nodules of hepatocytes
D. variation in size of nodules, with some
broad bands of fibrous tissue
E. all are associated   (55:1051-1054)

30. Spastic bowel may lead to

A. cancer
B. ulcerative colitis
C. lactose intolerance
D. diverticulosis
E. intestinal obstruction   (64)

31. Lactose deficiency has been observed in

A. Eskimos
B. Japanese
C. African blacks
D. Swedes
E. all of the above   (65)

32. Lactose intolerance may be due to

A. peptic ulcer
B. milk-protein allergy
C. hypermotility
D. regional enteritis
E. acute appendicitis   (65)

33. Dissolution of gallstones may be caused by

A. cholesterol
B. lithogenic agents
C. cholic acid
D. chenodeoxycholic acid
E. vitamin E   (68)

34. Diverticuli are most frequently located in
the

A. cecum
B. ascending colon
C. transverse colon
D. sigmoid
E. descending colon   (86:1747)

35. Which of the following roentgenographic signs most likely suggests a malignant ulcer?

A. greater curvature location
B. antral location
C. Carman's sign
D. Hampton's sign
E. smooth mound of tissue around the ulcer
                                       (94:359)

36. Nonembolic cerebral infarction may be seen

A. in atherosclerotic occlusion of the internal carotid artery
B. following trauma to the carotid artery
C. in patients with Fallot's tetralogy
D. all of the above
E. none of the above   (73:779)

37. Transient ischemic attacks most often

A. are microembolic
B. are small clots blocking carotids
C. are related to blood pressure fluctuations
D. occur with syncope
E. are due to occlusion of the intracranial arteries
                                       (73:2097)

38. The most common site of occlusion of blood vessels to the head is

A. carotid
B. middle cerebral artery
C. anterior cerebral
D. anterior choroidal
E. postcerebral   (73:2097)

39. A finding useful in differentiating partial (focal) seizures with secondary generalization from grand mal seizures is

A. urinary incontinence
B. postictal confusion
C. a positive response to treatment with phenytoin
D. postictal hemiparesis
E. loss of consciousness   (73:2151-2153)

40. A 55-year-old man has been admitted for an acute myocardial infarction with uneventful recovery. The morning of contemplated discharge from the hospital, he complains of precordial pain as well as pain over the left anterior part of his chest, aggravated by breathing. He is mildly febrile and has a pericardial friction rub. The most likely diagnosis is

A. the postmyocardial infarction syndrome
B. pulmonary infarction
C. congestive heart failure
D. recurrent myocardial infarction
E. shoulder-hand syndrome   (76:1442)

41. A 52-year-old man is admitted to the hospital with an acute myocardial infarction of the anterior wall. On the third hospital day he suddenly experiences severe dyspnea, diaphoresis, and hypotension. A new systolic murmur is heard at the left sternal border and a thrill is palpated in the same region. A roentgenogram of the chest discloses pulmonary edema. The most likely cause of these findings is

A. rupture of a papillary muscle
B. acute aortic dissection
C. rupture of the ventricular septum
D. rupture of a mitral chordae tendineae
E. pulmonary embolism   (67:1209)

42. When an acyanotic middle-aged adult has roentgenographic evidence of enlarged pulmonary arteries and increased lung markings, the most likely diagnosis is

A. ventricular septal defect
B. coarctation of the aorta
C. pulmonary valvular stenosis
D. an atrial septal defect (ASD)
E. truncus arteriosus   (76:1079)

43. A 20-year-old white male medical student has been seized with severe chest pain, radiating down the back, tearing in nature. On examination he is found to have a diastolic murmur at the base and a BP of 200/90 mmHg; pulses are felt in both arms. He is admitted to the emergency room of your community hospital. The electrocardiograph showed nonspecific S-T segment changes. Which one of the following is your conclusion?

A. The patient has a dissecting aneurysm and should immediately be started on hypertensive therapy.
B. The patient should be admitted to a CCU and monitored carefully.

C. The patient should be given nitroglycerine as a therapeutic trial.

D. Because pulses are present, it is unlikely that the patient has dissecting aneurysm.

E. This is a case of rheumatic mitral stenosis, and digitalis is indicated.   (76:1180)

44. Angina pectoris can occur in the presence of normal coronary arteries. Which of the following statements in respect to the condition is *not* true?

A. it is more common in females
B. it can occur with aortic valve disease
C. it commonly leads to a myocardial infarction
D. it can occur with hypertrophic subaortic stenosis
E. treatment is similar to that with patients having coronary artery disease
(73:284-288)

45. Major renal vein thrombosis is *least* likely to occur in

A. dehydration in infancy
B. carcinoma of the kidney
C. renal trauma
D. amyloidosis
E. chronic pyelonephritis   (38:352)

46. A patient comes into the hospital and states that he has had severe, crushing mid-chest pain present for 30 minutes, unrelieved by nitroglycerine. He has a previous history of angina. His pulse is 110, his blood pressure is 110/70 mmHg, and he appears quite anxious. His electrocardiogram shows regular sinus rhythm. The first drug to administer is

A. propranolol, 1 mg IV push
B. morphine sulfate, 2-20 mg IV titrated to relieve pain
C. atropine
D. morphine sulfate, 15 mg IM
E. anticoagulants   (73:294)

47. Which of the following terms most precisely identifies the commonly encountered alteration of the aorta in advancing age?

A. Mönckeberg's medial calcific sclerosis
B. arteriolosclerosis
C. arteriosclerosis
D. atherosclerosis
E. calcification   (55:598)

48. "Onionskin-like" thickening of an arteriole, in which concentric, laminated thickening of the vessel wall occurs, accompanied by luminal narrowing is characteristic of

A. arteriosclerosis in normotensive individuals
B. mild hypertension
C. severe hypertension
D. atherosclerosis
E. syphilitic involvement of vessels   (55:612)

49. In acute myocardial infarction, rupture of the myocardium is most likely to occur during the first seven days after the onset of infarction. The morphological substrate which leads to this propensity is best characterized as

A. hemorrhage into the pericardial sac
B. replacement of myocardial cells by fibroblasts
C. dissolution of myocardial fibers with presence of lipid-rich cell debris and macrophages
D. exudate composed solely of polymorphonuclear leukocytes
E. none of the above is appropriate
(55:655-659)

50. In rheumatic heart disease, the microscopic lesion considered pathognomonic for the disease is the Aschoff's body. Which element is *not* an expected component of the Aschoff's body?

A. polymorphonuclear leukocytes
B. Anitschkow myocytes
C. multinucleate giant cells
D. fibrinoid
E. none of the above is correct   (55:668)

51. Which is *not* a generally expected late consequence of multiple episodes of acute rheumatic endocarditis and valvulitis and their healing process?

A. valvular stenosis
B. valvular insufficiency
C. fused chordae tendinae
D. ruptured chordae tendinae
E. shortened chordae tendinae   (55:668-671)

52. A patient with a known diagnosis of infective (bacterial) endocarditis develops hematuria. One possible cause would be renal

infarction due to dislodgment of fragments of vegetation. Another possibility is "focal glomerulitis" or "glomerulonephritis." This is thought to be due to

A. small emboli derived from the vegetation lodging in kidney
B. septic infarcts extending to involve glomeruli
C. viable streptococci lodging in the glomerular tufts
D. an immunological reaction
E. none of the above   (55:681-683)

53. A 46-year-old woman complains of pain in her left leg of two days' duration. There is no peripheral edema. Examination shows redness, increased warmth, and tenderness which is confined to a narrow area (3-5 cm in width) on the medial side of the leg from the ankle almost to the knee. Pressure on the posterior aspect of the calf and dorsiflexion of the foot produce no pain. A blood count shows a slight increase in the number of leukocytes. The most likely diagnosis is

A. deep venous thrombophlebitis
B. phlegmasia cerulea dolens
C. lymphangitis
D. superficial venous thrombophlebitis
E. acute obstruction of the superficial femoral artery   (73:363)

54. Propranolol may be of use in the following conditions:

A. control of blood pressure
B. aortic dissection
C. management of angina pectoris
D. supraventricular arrhythmias
E. all of the above   (73:93)

55. A 65-year-old man has angina pectoris for six weeks. The electrocardiogram reveals a left anterior hemiblock. This patient most likely has

A. triple-vessel disease
B. disease of the right coronary artery and circumflex artery
C. single-vessel disease of the left anterior descending artery
D. disease of the left coronary artery
E. none of these   (62)

56. A 40-year-old man enters the hospital with congestive heart failure. The history reveals atypical chest pain. The electrocardiogram reveals left bundle branch block. Fluoroscopy reveals an enlarged heart and coronary artery calcification. The diagnosis is

A. cardiomyopathy
B. arteriosclerotic heart disease
C. a selective coronary angiogram is necessary for diagnosis
D. valvular heart disease
E. SBE   (63)

57. Where on the adult chest would you place the heel of your hand in order to perform chest compression?

A. two or three fingers above the lower end of the sternum
B. on the upper third of the sternum
C. where the sternum and collarbone meet
D. on the middle of the sternum
E. on the xiphoid process   (53:845)

58. What too frequently happens to an unconscious person when he is lying on his back with a pillow under his head?

A. he aspirates vomitus into his airway
B. his tongue falls back in his throat and blocks his airway
C. it is the position easiest to start effective mouth-to-mouth breathing
D. he clears his airway better
E. his whole body is easily exposed for close observation   (53:841)

59. A 26-year-old nurse who previously had a negative PPD (intermediate strength) skin test is found to have a positive PPD skin test three months after inhospital exposure to a patient with active tuberculosis. The nurse is asymptomatic and a roentgenogram of the chest discloses no abnormalities. Sputum concentrates for *Mycobacterium tuberculosis* are negative. The most appropriate management would consist of

A. repeat roentgenograms of the chest at annual intervals
B. administration of isoniazid for 12 months
C. administration of rifampin for three months
D. administration of isoniazid and ethambutol for 12 months
E. repeating roentgenograms of the chest

every three months and institution of treatment if roentgenographic evidence of tuberculosis appears   *(76:1028)*

60. A 32-year-old pregnant woman is admitted to the hospital because of severe dyspnea and cyanosis. The patient has had a skin rash for the past five days. Her two children had a febrile exanthem for 14 days and nine days, respectively, prior to the patient's illness. Which of the following is the most likely diagnosis?

    A. lupus erythematosus
    B. varicella pneumonia
    C. amniotic fluid emboli
    D. staphylococcal pneumonia
    E. mycoplasmal pneumonia   *(75:287)*

61. A patient is suspected of having allergic alveolitis secondary to inhalation of thermophilic *Actinomyces* (farmer's lung). Useful diagnostic findings would include

    A. demonstration of serum-precipitating antibody to an extract of *Blastomyces*
    B. a specific histological reaction evident on a biopsy of the lung
    C. production of dyspnea, fever, and pulmonary infiltrates five to six hours after an inhalation challenge with thermophilic *Actinomyces*
    D. reduction in diffusing capacity with a normal vital capacity
    E. an increase in diffusing capacity with a normal vital capacity   *(75:401)*

62. The arterial blood CO_2 tension can be expected to be elevated in all of the following conditions *except*

    A. scleroderma of the lung
    B. radiation fibrosis
    C. asthma
    D. pulmonary emphysema
    E. obesity   *(75:405)*

63. The following conditions are commonly seen in psychological hyperventilation:

    A. a low blood arterial P_{CO_2} and normal blood P_{O_2}
    B. both low arterial CO_2 and P_{O_2}
    C. high arterial CO_2 and low arterial P_{O_2}
    D. high arterial CO_2 and P_{O_2}
    E. low arterial CO_2 and high arterial P_{O_2}
    (71:67)

64. A half hour after insertion of an intravenous feeding catheter into the right subclavian vein, the patient complains of dyspnea and tightness in the chest. The most likely cause is

    A. pulmonary embolus
    B. acute coronary occlusion
    C. pneumothorax
    D. anxiety
    E. pneumonia   *(71:983)*

65. Lung abscess is usually caused by

    A. *Mycobacterium* tuberculosis
    B. *Fusobacterium nucleatum,* anaerobic streptococci, and *Bacteroides fragilis*
    C. *Bacteroides melaninogenicum* and actinomycosis
    D. *Peptococcus*
    E. *E. coli*   *(73:420)*

66. Hereditary deficiency of alpha-antitrypsin is

    A. the cause of most cases of panlobular emphysema
    B. the cause of only a small portion of cases of emphysema, most often of centrilobular (centriacinar) pattern
    C. associated with emphysema in animal experimental models, but not seen in man
    D. the cause of chronic bronchitis in some individuals, but not related to emphysema
    E. none of the above   *(57)*

67. Twenty-four hours after admission, intubation, and the institution of mechanical ventilation in a man of 70 with COPD, hypotension occurs, "coffee-ground" material comes from the nasogastric tube, and his HCT falls to 28%. The most likely cause is

    A. cirrhosis of the liver
    B. chronic peptic ulcer
    C. stress ulcer
    D. pulmonary tuberculosis
    E. peptic esophagitis   *(51:1547)*

68. Twelve days after the successful treatment of an episode of acute respiratory failure in a 60-year-old man with COPD, he begins to cough up a purulent sputum, he develops a temperature of 104°F, and chest x-ray reveals an area of consolidation in the right–lower lobe. The most likely complication encountered at present is

    A. pulmonary infarction

B. congestive heart failure
C. staphylococcal empyema
D. *Pseudomonas* pneumonia
E. *E. coli* septicemia   *(51:1547)*

69. Although many laboratory studies may be suggestive of pulmonary embolism, with or without infarction, the most helpful diagnostic finding is

A. an arterial Po_2 lower than normal
B. abnormalities on a perfusion lung scan
C. a serum glutamic oxaloacetic transaminase (SGOT) concentration higher than normal
D. abnormalities on a pulmonary arteriogram
E. a serum lactic dehydrogenase (LDH) concentration higher than normal
          (76:1564)

70. Which of the following clinical features is *least* likely to occur in classical Cushing's syndrome?

A. purple striae
B. hypotension
C. diabetic glucose tolerance curve
D. osteoporosis
E. menstrual disturbances   *(74:1230)*

71. A 45-year-old male complains of back pain. The serum calcium is found to be 15 mg/100 ml, serum phosphorus 1.3 mg/100 ml, and alkaline phosphatase 14 Bodansky units. X-ray of the spine shows demineralization. The most likely diagnosis is

A. osteitis deformans
B. osteoporosis
C. hyperparathyroidism
D. hyperthyroidism
E. hypothyroidism   *(74:962-980)*

72. The impairment of pancreatic function in thyrotoxicosis is evidenced by

A. calcification in the pancreas seen on abdominal x-ray
B. an increase of serum amylase
C. hypoglycemic episodes of weakness
D. a decrease in glucose tolerance
E. an increase of free fat in the stool
          (74:176-208)

73. A 65-year-old executive with a history of duodenal ulcer has had epigastric pain and frequent vomiting for five days. On the day he visits the emergency room, he has weakness, thirst, and drowsiness. Physical examination reveals: blood pressure 100/70, pulse 112, decrease of skin turgor, epigastric tenderness, no edema. Lab values are as follows: HCT 50; BUN 48; Na^+ 115; K^+ 2.1; Cl^- 70; HCO_3^- 32. His acid-base status is best described as

A. metabolic acidosis
B. normal
C. metabolic alkalosis
D. respiratory alkalosis
E. respiratory acidosis   *(72:386-390)*

74. A patient presents with lethargy. His serum chemistries reveal Na^+ 150; Cl^- 100; K^+ 3.0; CO_2 40; albumin 3.5 g/100 ml; pH 7.55. He displays 3$^+$ pitting edema of the extremities. This situation is caused by

A. secondary aldosteronism due to diuretics
B. vomiting
C. primary aldosteronism
D. ingestion of alkali
E. licorice ingestion   *(73:542)*

75. A 60-year-old man presents with weakness of several days' duration. Serum chemistries reveal Na^+ 135; K^+ 2.5; Cl^- 115; CO_2 10; pH 7.30. The first step in correction of the electrolytes in this patient is administration of

A. $NaHCO_3$
B. NaCl
C. KCl
D. sodium lactate
E. D5W   *(39:35)*

76. An 18-year-old girl has developed nausea, vomiting followed by cramping abdominal pain, floating, and diarrhea with mucus and blood in the stool. She has also experienced fever. There is no evidence of dehydration; however, the stool culture has identified *Salmonella enteritidis*. The choice of drug is

A. chloramphenicol
B. ampicillin
C. sulfamethoxazole and trimethoprim (Septra or Bactrim)
D. all of the above
E. none of the above   *(106:112-117)*

77. A patient is suspected of having Rocky Mountain spotted fever. You would now

A. perform a blood culture
B. order a Weil-Felix test
C. perform bone marrow aspirations
D. order a CT scan of the skull
E. order an HLA test   (76:1067)

78. A 22-year-old college girl developed tingling and burning in the back of the neck radiating to the upper back, arms, and front of the chest 20 minutes after eating at a Chinese restaurant. She also complains of throbbing pain in the temples and infraorbital region. The most likely cause of her symptoms is

A. monosodium glutamate
B. monosodium urate
C. monosodium pyrophosphate
D. monosodium oxalate
E. monosodium citrate   (73:782)

79. Influenza epidemics and pandemics occur again and again because the virus

A. changes its cell size
B. maintains its antigenicity with no change
C. can shift the antigens on its surface
D. can attack different host cells
E. none of the above   (73:1700)

80. A 40-year-old man, diabetic since age 25, has previously been stable on insulin. His blood chemistries have been normal. Six days before admission, he developed fever and nausea with continuous vomiting. Three days before admission, he stopped taking insulin. He continued to urinate six to eight times a day. On the day of admission, he became lethargic. Physical examination reveals: blood pressure 95/70, pulse 115, respiration 28, mental dullness, and decreased skin turgor. Lab values are as follows: HCT 52, BUN 60, blood sugar 560, Na^+ 152, K^+ 5.2, Cl^- 108, HCO_3^- 16. Urine studies revealed: 50 ml/hour, specific gravity 1.020, glucose 4+, ketones 2+, protein 2+. His acid-base status is best described as

A. metabolic acidosis
B. normal
C. metabolic alkalosis
D. respiratory alkalosis
E. respiratory acidosis   (78:74)

81. Cirrhosis of the liver is a recognized complication of each of the following diseases except

A. hemochromatosis

B. Wilson's disease
C. hypertension
D. alpha-antitrypsin deficiency
E. syphilis   (73:835)

82. A hypertensive patient on hydrochlorothiazide (Hydrodiuril) for three years is found to have a serum calcium level of 12.6 mg%. The patient has no complaints and the physical examination is within normal limits. Now you would

A. order IVP
B. change hydrochlorothiazide (Hydrodiuril) to chlorothiazide (Diuril)
C. start mitomycin therapy
D. order a further work-up for hyperparathyroidism
E. reassure the patient of the laboratory error   (73:210)

83. Spirometric tests provide useful quantitative information in

A. obstructive airway disease
B. sleep apnea
C. pneumonia
D. alveolar-capillary diffusion blocks
E. lung cancer   (104:994-997)

84. An elderly patient on thiazide therapy for hypertension was found to have a low serum sodium level of 120 mEq/liter. The preferred treatment is

A. potassium-restriction diet
B. high-purine diet
C. zinc-restriction diet
D. fluid-restriction diet
E. high-carbohydrate diet   (78:794-796)

85. All of the following statements concerning bronchopulmonary aspergillosis are true except

A. significant eosinophilia is usually present
B. serum precipitins are frequently found against *Aspergillus fumigatus*
C. patchy infiltrates may be seen on the chest x-ray
D. patients often expectorate small brown plugs in the sputum
E. *Aspergillus fumigatus* is always isolated from sputum   (78:397)

86. A 30-year-old female complains of a sore throat lasting two days. Physical examina-

tions reveal an infected pharynx without any other findings. You would now

A. prescribe oral penicillins
B. order SMA-14
C. order a chest x-ray
D. give a penicillin shot
E. none of the above   (73:1696)

87. Legionnaire's disease is caused by:

A. a Gram-negative bacterium
B. sexual activities of Legionnaires
C. chronic noise exposure
D. *Chlamydia psittaci*
E. *Aspergillus funigatus*   (78:1035)

88. Recurrent genital herpes may be treated with:

A. bretylium
B. acyclovir
C. propanolol
D. metronidazole
E. erythromycin   (73:1090)

89. Diagnosis of herpes simplex can be done by:

A. dexamethasone test
B. tensilon test
C. Tzanck test
D. Weil-Fleix test
E. CT scan of the pelvic region   (73:1090)

90. Which of the following is the angiotensin converting enzyme inhibitors:

A. clonidine
B. prazosin
C. minoxidil
D. captopril
E. lopressor   (73:293-294)

91. A 24-year-old female received a normal pre-employment physical, however, the screening laboratory test revealed a total serum bilirubin level of 1.7 mg/dl with an indirect level of 1.0 mg/dl. You ordered liver enzymes (GOT, GPT) and serum alkaline phosphatase, all of them were within normal limits. HBs Ag was also negative. The most likely condition is:

A. liver cirrhosis
B. acute cholecystitis
C. hepatocellular adenoma
D. Gilbert's syndrome
E. cytomegalovirus disease   (78:804-805)

Directions: For each of the incomplete statements or questions below, ONE or MORE of the numbered answers is correct. In each case select:
A. *if only 1, 2, and 3 are correct*
B. *if only 1 and 3 are correct*
C. *if only 2 and 4 are correct*
D. *if only 4 is correct*
E. *if all are correct*

92. Which of the following is true about isoniazid?

1. it produces hepatitis, especially in people with underlying liver disease
2. it produces a rheumatoid arthritis-like syndrome
3. it is safe to use during pregnancy
4. it produces a psychosis in the elderly   (73:1203)

93. Which of the following statements is true?

1. clindamycin can cause serious life-threatening diarrhea
2. minocycline can cause dizziness and unsteady gait
3. methicillin in high doses causes interstitial nephritis
4. tetracycline can cause acute yellow atrophy of the infant's liver when given during pregnancy   (54:97-127)

94. At initial presentation, nonspecific complaints of weakness, fever, skin and gum bleeding, and pallor are common in acute nonlymphatic leukemia; for the diagnosis, which of the following must also be found?

1. splenomegaly and abnormal white cells in the peripheral blood
2. hepatosplenomegaly and skin lesions
3. peripheral leukocytosis and normal bone marrow
4. blast cells in the peripheral blood and an increase in blast cells in bone marrow   (73:989)

95. Thrombocytosis is commonly detected in patients with which of the following?

1. malignancy
2. chronic infection
3. inflammation
4. myeloproliferative disorders   (83:1129)

96. Thrombocytopenia may be caused by which of the following?

1. folic acid deficiency

2. excessive alcohol ingestion
3. administration of quinidine
4. administration of aspirin   *(83:1111)*

97. The sickle cell trait may cause which of the following?

   1. hematuria
   2. pulmonary infarction
   3. hyposthenuria
   4. abundant sickle cells in the blood
                                    (83:855-856)

98. The following features are frequently associated with Hodgkin's disease:

   1. lymph node biopsy usually shows characteristic Reed-Sternberg giant cells
   2. herpes zoster
   3. pruritus
   4. pain in the region of enlarged lymph nodes after drinking alcohol   *(73:1060)*

99. Cerebral hemorrhage is often seen in patients with which of the following conditions?

   1. hypertension
   2. childhood leukemia
   3. arteriovenous malformations
   4. obesity   *(73:271)*

100. In patients with amyotrophic lateral sclerosis, which of the following commonly occur?

   1. atrophy and fasciculations in the upper extremities
   2. spastic weakness of the legs
   3. involvement of the facial and oropharyngeal muscles
   4. involvement of the extraocular muscles
                                    (84:557)

101. The subclavian steal syndrome is characterized by which of the following features?

   1. vertigo and diplopia caused by arm exercise
   2. difference of blood pressure
   3. stenosis or occlusion of innominate artery
   4. strong radial pulse   *(39:280)*

102. Berry aneurysms are frequently associated with which of the following features?

   1. congenital defects in the media of cerebral vessels

2. most commonly seen in the junction of the posterior communicating artery and internal carotid
3. commonly occur in hypertensive patients
4. familial clustering   *(73:2103)*

103. Which of the following isolated valvular lesions in adults is almost always caused by rheumatic fever?

   1. aortic valvular stenosis
   2. mitral regurgitation
   3. aortic regurgitation
   4. mitral stenosis   *(76:1403)*

104. The etiology of aortic regurgitation includes which of the following?

   1. hypertension
   2. Marfan's syndrome
   3. rheumatoid spondylitis
   4. blunt trauma to the chest   *(76:1414)*

105. Which of the following statements concerning oral contraceptives is correct?

   1. administration of combinations of estrogen and progesterone may cause an increase in blood pressure
   2. the blood pressure may return to normal after discontinuing administration of estrogen-progesterone combinations
   3. the administration of estrogen-progesterone combinations may worsen pre-existing hypertension
   4. the progesterone component is responsible for the elevation of blood pressure
                                    (76:1478)

106. Idiopathic hypertrophic subaortic stenosis often includes the following clinical features:

   1. an increase in the intensity of the murmur while standing
   2. deep Q-waves in Leads II, III, and aVF
   3. postexertional syncope
   4. propranolol is useful in therapy   *(76:1304)*

107. Chronic constrictive pericarditis may be caused by which of the following?

   1. Coxsackie B viral infections
   2. mediastinal irradiation
   3. pneumococcal infections
   4. uremia   *(73:334)*

108. Prinzmetal angina pectoris is a variant form of angina pectoris. Which of the following statements is true about Prinzmetal angina pectoris?

1. associated with an increase CPK and SGOT serum enzyme
2. risk of myocardial infarction is reduced
3. hypertension is usually present in the majority of patients
4. associated with S-T elevation on the EKG
   (73:285)

109. Which of the following statements concerning patients with moderate hypertension (diastolic pressures between 95 and 120 mmHg) is correct?

1. reduction of blood pressure in patients with persistent moderate hypertension reduces the mortality from congestive heart failure
2. the incidence of cerebrovascular accidents is increased
3. the incidence of myocardial infarction and ruptured aortic aneurysm is increased
4. morbidity from drug therapy is too great to justify treatment
   (76:1475)

110. Severe dyspnea due to a decrease in the compliance of the lung occurs in which of the following?

1. the shock lung syndrome
2. radiation fibrosis
3. scleroderma
4. pulmonary emphysema
   (71:630)

111. Isoproterenol could be expected to be of value in

1. asthma
2. scleroderma
3. chronic bronchitis
4. kyphoscoliosis
   (71:158, 431)

112. The use of intubation and mechanical ventilation can be expected to decrease the arterial P_{CO_2} in the following entities:

1. pulmonary emphysema
2. chronic bronchitis
3. kyphoscoliosis
4. asthma
   (75:384)

113. A 40-year-old patient is admitted in status asthmaticus. A routine arterial blood gas (ABG) reveals a P_{O_2} of 65 mmHg and a P_{CO_2}

of 48 mmHg. Which of the following statements is true?

1. most patients in status asthmaticus have a low P_{O_2} and a low P_{CO_2}
2. vigorous and repeated nasotracheal suctioning is necessary to prevent acute worsening of the blood gas abnormalities
3. syndrome of acute diffuse bronchial mucous occlusion is a complication of status asthmaticus
4. conventional therapy of bronchodilators and steroids alone is adequate for patient management   *(51:1545-1546)*

114. A 70-year-old male with moderately severe COPD had a cholecystectomy for cholelithiasis yesterday. Today he is somewhat dyspneic and coughing up yellow sputum. His x-ray shows no pneumonia, and his ABG reveals a P_{O_2} of 50 mmHg and a P_{CO_2} of 65 mmHg, with a pH of 7.33. Which of the following statements is correct?

1. this degree of hypercapnea is not important in a man with COPD and is probably the same as his preoperative value
2. when hypoxemia is severe enough, it may produce metabolic acidosis due to cellular hypoxia, anaerobic state, and lactic acid production
3. he is in acute respiratory failure and the first step should be intubation and mechanical ventilation
4. he should be vigorously suctioned, bedside fiberoptic bronchoscopy should be used if necessary, and low-flow oxygen should be administered with serial ABG measurements in an attempt to make intubation and mechanical ventilation unnecessary
   (51:1542)

115. Three days after a severe automobile accident in which both femurs were fractured, a 20-year-old male begins to complain of dyspnea. Soft alveolar shadows are seen in both lung fields. The following statements are true:

1. a P_{O_2} of 45 mm Hg on room air and a P_{CO_2} of 38 mm Hg would not be unexpected
2. administration of 100% oxygen by face mask might raise the P_{O_2} to only 50 mmHg
3. an increase in free fatty acids in the blood would not be surprising

4. if the patient were intubated, the lungs would be found to be stiff—i.e., to have a low compliance—and a pressure-limited ventilation would be adequate to assure greatly improved oxygenation

(51:1544-1545)

116. A 40-year-old male with diffuse influenzal pneumonia and adult respiratory distress, or stiff lung syndrome, has been intubated and mechanical ventilation has been started. The following statements are true:

1. if 100% oxygen and minute ventilation using IPPB doesn't raise the P_{O_2} to over 40 mmHg, PEEP should be used
2. when the patient improves so that the vital capacity is 10 cc/kg and his negative effort is 30 cm of H_2O, he is ready for weaning
3. palpation of subcutaneous emphysema in the suprasternal notch in this patient suggests the need for a chest tube on the right side
4. four hours of increasing dyspnea and hypoxemia and right chest pain while on PEEP probably mean a nosocomial infection and pleurisy

(51:1545-1547)

117. The therapy for shock lung syndrome includes which of the following?

1. high doses of corticosteroids
2. maintenance of oxygenation by inspired oxygen mixtures
3. assisted ventilation
4. positive end-expiratory pressure (PEEP)

(51:1542-1543)

118. The habitual intravenous self-administration of narcotics produces which of the following?

1. foreign-body embolism
2. interstitial granulomas in the lung
3. decreased pulmonary diffusing capacity
4. obstructive pulmonary disease   (71:867)

119. Five days ago, a 60-year-old man underwent surgical removal and drainage of empyema of the gallbladder. You are asked to recommend therapy for a serum sodium of 115 mEq/liter. His BUN is 40 and Una 15 mEq/liter. Physical exam reveals: BP 110/60, pulse 100, anasarca, no visible neck veins, and no S3 gallop. You would conclude that

1. the patient is dehydrated
2. the patient has intravascular volume depletion
3. the patient has renal disease
4. the serum albumin is less than 2.0 mg/100 ml   (72:91)

120. A 60-year-old man presents with weakness of several days' duration. Serum chemistries reveal Na^+ 135, K^+ 5.4, Cl^- 115, CO_2 10, pH 7.30. Points in the history that would be of importance to the cause of acidosis would include

1. ingestion of chloride salts
2. diarrhea
3. nocturia and polyuria
4. ingestion of phenformin   (72:229)

121. A 60-year-old man presents with shortness of breath, 3+ edema, neck vein distention and an S3 gallop. Serum sodium is 115 mEq/liter; Una is 20 mEq/liter. You would

1. administer 0.9% saline
2. restrict NaCl and H_2O
3. order a high water intake
4. give furosemide (Lasix)   (73:525)

122. A 50-year-old woman presents with severe muscle weakness. She has been taking chlorothiazide. Serum chemistries reveal Na^+ 132, K^+ 1.8, CO_2 38, Cl^- 80, BUN 42, pH 7.55. You would

1. give KCl
2. correct alkalosis slowly, since serum K^+ may fall rapidly
3. volume-expand the patient with NaCl solutions
4. administer NH_4Cl (73:543)

123. Which of the following statements is true concerning immunoglobulins?

1. IgG comprises approximately 80% of normal serum gamma-globulin; this group includes most of the acquired antibodies
2. IgA makes up approximately 15%, exhibited with a variety of antimicrobial activities, and is the principal type of antibody present in external secretions
3. IgM, comprising perhaps 5%, includes such antibodies as heterophil
4. IgE antibodies appear responsible for immediate hypersensitivity reactions such as atopic dermatitis and allergic asthma

(73:1848)

124. The following clinical features are characteristic of craniopharyngioma:

1. bitemporal hemianopsia
2. growth retardation
3. diabetes insipidus
4. normal skull x-ray   (88:105-106)

125. Chronic alcoholism may produce which of the following clinical features?

1. megaloblastic anemia
2. Wernicke's encephalopathy
3. Mallory-Weiss' syndrome
4. increased productivity   (76:1288)

126. Lactic acidosis is often caused by

1. DBI (phenformin)
2. endotoxic shock
3. isoniazid
4. leukemia   (73:540)

127. A 25-year-old female has complained of palpitation and headache. Her T4 was found to be high. You would now

1. order T3 resin uptake
2. order radioiodine uptake
3. order TSH
4. take a contraceptive history   (73:1283)

128. Adriamycin may cause

1. congestive heart failure
2. myelosuppression
3. stomatitis
4. hematuria   (78:633)

129. Vincristine may cause

1. foot drop
2. alopecia
3. inappropriate antidiuretic hormone syndrome
4. severe bone marrow depression   (78:632)

130. Vitamin D deficiency may be associated with

1. biliary cirrhosis
2. postgastrectomy status
3. short bowel syndrome
4. small bowel resection   (12:229)

131. Tetany may be caused by

1. alcoholism
2. hyperventilation syndrome
3. acute pancreatitis
4. hyperparathyroidism   (39:673)

132. Diazoxide may cause

1. tachycardia
2. hypertension
3. hyperuricemia
4. hypoglycemia   (78:294)

133. Antiplatelet agents include

1. aspirin
2. sulfinpyrazone (Anturane)
3. dipyridamole (Persantine)
4. ergonovine (Ergotrate)   (78:521)

134. Cis-platinum has been associated with

1. nephrotoxicity
2. severe nausea and vomiting
3. hearing loss
4. severe hematologic suppression   (78:636)

135. Hypophosphatemia is commonly associated with

1. insulin treatment in diabetic ketoacidosis
2. alcoholism
3. respiratory alkalosis
4. hypoparathyroidism   (73:913)

136. A 55-year-old housewife complains of a lump in the right side of her neck which, on physical examination, turns out to be a slightly enlarged thyroid with prominence of the right lobe. No nodes or tenderness are present. Now you would

1. order T4
2. order TSH
3. order a thyroid scan
4. order antithyroid antibody titers   (76:633)

137. Crohn's disease is associated with

1. pyoderma gangrenosum
2. renal calculi
3. colon cancer
4. vitamin B2 deficiency   (73:741)

138. Ulcerative colitis is frequently associated with

1. toxic megacolon
2. sclerosing cholangitis
3. hemolytic anemia
4. lung cancer   (73:2263)

139. Chronic pancreatitis is frequently associated with

1. diabetes mellitus

2. peptic ulcer
3. pseudocyst
4. hypoparathyroidism   (73:775)

140. Acromegaly is characterized by

1. cardiomegaly
2. extreme body height
3. excessive perspiration
4. clubbing of fingers   (87:67)

141. Alcoholics are at higher risk of developing

1. riboflavin deficiency
2. folic acid deficiency
3. pyridoxine deficiency
4. niacin deficiency   (78:1485)

142. Coccidioidomycosis

1. is associated with erythema nodosum
2. may produce arthralgia
3. may show a coin lesion on the chest x-ray
4. may cause cough, chest pain, and fever
                                         (73:1762)

143. Complications of prosthetic heart valves include

1. infection
2. hemolytic anemia
3. thromboembolism
4. heart failure   (78:220)

144. Protamine

1. is an anticoagulant
2. is strongly acidic
3. is an antidote to heparin
4. is an enzyme   (78:517-518)

145. Bronchogenic carcinoma may be associated with

1. erythema multiforme
2. inappropriate antidiuretic syndrome
3. clubbing of digits
4. myasthenic syndrome   (78:374)

146. Peptic ulcer may be associated with

1. stress
2. cigarette smoking
3. aspirin ingestion
4. hot spices   (73:684-685)

147. A middle-aged housewife with recurrent abdominal pains was found to have acute inter-

mittent porphyria. Now you would inform the patient that the following drugs may precipitate subsequent abdominal pains:

1. griseofulvin
2. steroids
3. estrogen
4. hematin   (73:1156)

148. Galactorrhea can be caused by the ingestion of

1. alpha-methyldopa
2. phenothiazines
3. reserpine
4. progesterone   (73:198-1399)

149. Polycythemia may be associated with

1. hypernephroma
2. hepatoma
3. uterine myoma
4. pheochromocytoma   (78:560)

150. Asthma may be induced by

1. ibuprofen
2. toluene-di-isocyanate (TDI)
3. exercise
4. epinephrine   (78:392-397)

151. Pancreatitis is associated with the use of

1. estrogen
2. furosemide
3. thiazide
4. ethanol   (76:1837)

Directions: Each of the questions or incomplete statements below is followed by five lettered options. For each option, indicate "T" if it is correct; indicate "F" if it is incorrect.

152. Cardiac myxomas:

A. may lead to embolism
B. may present with syncope
C. is the metastatic tumor of the breast
D. marked decrease of gamma globulin level is pathognomic
E. 95% arise from right ventricle
                                         (78:356-357)

153. Following agents may cause QT widening in EKG:

A. quinidine

B. procainamide
C. tocainide
D. disopyramide
E. calcium   (73:322-324)

154. Side effects of neuroleptics include:

A. akathisia
B. tardive dyskinesia
C. hypoprolactinemia
D. increase of libido
E. orthostatic hypotension   (78:1378)

155. In a patient with subarachnoid hemorrhage and no primary cardiac disease, which of the following electrocardiographic changes may occur?

A. elevated S-T segments
B. a prolonged Q-T interval
C. marked right axis deviation
D. inverted T waves
E. large, wide Q waves   (78:1290)

156. The managament of patients with *Campylobacter fetus* gastroenteritis includes:

A. symptomatic treatment
B. replacement of water loss
C. correction of any electrolyte imbalance
D. administration of nitrofurantoin
E. administration of vancomycin   (78:10607)

157. Hypokalemia may be caused by:

A. HCTZ
B. spirolactone
C. furosemide (Lasix)
D. metoprolol (Lopressor)
E. carbenicillin (Geocillin)   (73:532)

158. NSAIDS:

A. enhance prostaglandin synthesis
B. may cause upper GI bleeding
C. may be useful in the treatment of osteoarthritis
D. may cause headache
E. they are muscle relaxants   (78:1163)

159. Traveller's diarrhea:

A. is caused by high zinc content of the water
B. is caused by the enterotoxin producing *E. coli*
C. is treated by amphoterecin B
D. is treated by penicillin K

E. is prevented by immunizations prior to travel   (73:716-717)

160. Reflux esophagitis:

A. may cause substernal pain
B. symptoms usually relieved by recumbency
C. consumption of alcohol improves the symptoms
D. weight gain improves symptoms
E. metoclopramide (Reglan) inhibits gastro-esophageal motility   (39:362-363)

161. Influenza:

A. may cause pneumonia
B. often present with fever (102°F and 103°F) and chills
C. amantadine (Symmetrel) can be used for chemoprophylaxis
D. amantadine (Symmetrel) can shorten the symptoms
E. can be prevented by vaccines
                                  (73:1703-1704)

162. Management of peptic ulcer:

A. proximal gastric vagotomy is tha management of choice for all patients
B. subtotal gastrectomy is the current standard management procedure for all patients
C. bland diet is the first line therapy
D. milk may strongly stimulate acid secretion
E. smoking definitely promotes ulcer healing
                                  (73:688-693)

163. Following medications are commonly used for patients with peptic ulcer:

A. sucralfate (Carafate)
B. cimetidine (Tagemet)
C. diphenhydramine (Benadryl)
D. ranitidine (Zantac)
E. sodium bicarbonate   (73:688-689)

164. Following statements concerning the use of drugs in the elderly are true:

A. the dosage of tetracyclines should be increased 1.5 times of the usual dose
B. diazepam may prolong the elimination half-life in the elderly
C. increased digoxin dosage may take 2 weeks to show the effect
D. the lidocaine dosage needs to increase

two-fold because of the increase in liver clearance

E. the sensitivity to CNS depressants is increased   *(73:78)*

165. Following side-reactions are commonly seen in the lipid-lowering drugs:

A. clofibrate (Atromid-S) may cause flu-like syndrome
B. gemfibrozil (Lopid) may cause anemia
C. nicotinic acid (Nicolar) results in hypertension
D. resins (Colestid) may cause bleeding
E. probucol (Lorelco) may prolong QT interval in the EKG   *(78:924-925)*

166. Calcium channel blockers:

A. are "fast channel blockers"
B. are effective antidotes in hypercalcemic crisis
C. may result in hypotension
D. may worsen congestive heart failure
E. are used to treat patients with sick sinus syndrome   *(78:325-326)*

Directions: Each group of numbered words or phrases is followed by a list of lettered statements. MATCH the lettered statement most closely associated with the numbered word or phrase.

Questions 167 to 169
167. *Pseudomonas* pneumonia   *(73:1510)*
168. *Bacteroides* pneumonia   *(73:1583)*
169. *Klebsiella* (Friedlander's) pneumonia
                                      (73:1569)

A. Lobar pneumonia
B. Massive foul-smelling empyema often present
C. Arteritis frequently seen histologically
D. Urinary tract often the source
E. Erythromycin therapy effective

Questions 170 to 173
170. Iron deficiency
171. Azotemia
172. Malabsorption syndrome
173. Multiple myeloma

A. Normocytic normochromic anemia

B. Hypochromic microcytic anemia
C. Hyperchromic macrocytic anemia
                                      (73:870-876)

Questions 174 to 176
174. Vascular headache
175. Unilateral headache very common
176. Without prodromes

A. Classic migraine
B. Common migraine
C. Both
D. Neither   *(50:1161)*

Questions 177 to 180
177. Anterior infarct
178. Posterior infarct
179. LVH
180. RBBB

A. S-T elevation and Q in V_1 and V_2
B. S-T depression and large R in V_1 and V_2
C. S in V_1 and R in V_5
D. RR' in V_1 or V_2
E. notched P   *(92:245-249)*

Questions 181 to 184

	pH	PCO_2	HCO_3^-
181.	7.10	80	24
182.	7.70	40	48
183.	7.10	40	12
184.	7.70	20	24

A. Metabolic acidosis
B. Normal status
C. Respiratory alkalosis
D. Respiratory acidosis
E. Metabolic alkalosis   *(72:167-170)*

Questions 185 to 187
185. Riedel's thyroiditis
186. Hashimoto's thyroiditis
187. DeQuervain's thyroiditis

A. High titers of thyroid autoantibody
B. Very low ^{131}I uptake; high ESR
C. Low titer of thyroid autoantibody; normal ^{131}I uptake   *(74:239-243)*

Questions 188 to 190
188. Hypothyroidism

189. Grave's disease
190. Thyroid cancer

    A. Cold nodule
    B. Generalized decrease in radioactivity
    C. Enlarged homogeneous radioactivity
                           (90:140)

Questions 191 to 194
The numbered responses are observed during carotid sinus massage. Match the response with the most likely lettered arrhythmia.
191. Rate gradually falls from 130 to 112
192. Abrupt change in rate from 160 to 75
193. Drop in rate from 150 to 75 with rapid return to a rate of 130
194. No perceptible change in apical rate

    A. Atrial fibrillation
    B. Sinus tachycardia
    C. Atrial tachycardia
    D. Atrial flutter   (73:300-329)

Questions 195 to 198
Match the numbered atrial rate with the most likely lettered arrhythmia.
195. 45
196. 140
197. 180
198. 280

    A. Paroxysmal atrial tachycardia
    B. Sinus bradycardia
    C. Sinus tachycardia
    D. Atrial flutter   (73:300-329)

Questions 199 to 204
Match the numbered EKG change with the lettered drug or electrolyte abnormality inducing it.
199. U-waves
200. S-T depression
201. Tall peaked T-waves
202. Widened QRS complex
203. Shortened Q-T interval
204. Prolonged Q-T interval

    A. Hyperkalemia
    B. Hypocalcemia
    C. Hypokalemia
    D. Hypercalcemia
    E. Pronestyl (procainamide) and quinidine
    F. Digitalis   (92:230-239)

Questions 205 to 209
Match the lettered pulmonary opportunistic infections with the appropriate numbered characteristic roentgen pattern.
205. Ill-defined nodular infiltrates   (71:197)
206. Shaggy nodule appearance   (71:245)
207. Diffuse alveolar appearance   (71:210)
208. Fistulae tracheobronchial invasion   (71:249)
209. Infiltrative or nodular lesion with cavitation
                         (71:242)

    A. *Pneumocystis carinii* pneumonia
    B. Nocardiosis
    C. *Phycomycetes* pneumonitis
    D. Cytomegalovirus pneumonia
    E. Aspergillosis

Questions 210 to 213
210. Capable of reducing gastric acid throughout the nights
211. In the fasting state, this produces acid reduction of less than one hour duration
212. Leads to increased healing rate of duodenal ulcer
213. Leads to acid reflux from the stomach into the esophagus

    A. Cimetidine (Tagamet)
    B. Antacids
    C. Both
    D. Neither   (73:683)

Questions 214 to 216
214. Erythropoietin
215. Hypoglycemia
216. ACTH

    A. Neoplasm of the liver
    B. Retroperitoneal fibrosarcoma
    C. Both
    D. Neither   (103:407-408)

Questions 217 to 219
217. Postprandial pain, worse on lying down
218. Heartburn, improved by standing upright
219. Epigastric hunger pain relieved by food, unchanged by motion

    A. Hiatal hernia
    B. Peptic ulcer
    C. Both
    D. Neither   (73:687-688)

Questions 220 to 222
220. Tyramine-restricted diet
221. Alcohols
222. Low-sodium diet

A. Phenylketonuria
B. Monoamine oxidase inhibitors
C. Gout
D. Hypertension
E. Celiac disease   *(73:37, 689)*

Questions 223 to 225
223. Ventricular fibrillation
224. Digitalis tachyarrhythmias
225. Atrial tachycardia

A. Phenytoin (Dilantin)
B. Lidocaine (Xylocaine)
C. Bretylium (Bretylol)
D. Procainamide (Pronestyl)
E. Quinine (Quinamm)   *(78:322)*

Questions 226 to 230
226. XY
227. XX
228. XO
229. XXY
230. XXX

A. 0 Barr body
B. 1 Barr body
C. 2 Barr bodies
D. 3 Barr bodies
E. 4 Barr bodies   *(39:1033)*

Questions 231 to 235
231. Decreased CSF glucose
232. Increased CSF protein
233. First zone colloidal gold curve in CSF
234. Elevated CSF gamma-globulin
235. Mononuclear cells in CSF

A. Paretic neurosyphilis
B. Crypotococcal meningitis
C. Both
D. Neither   *(78:1337)*

Questions 236 to 237
236. Primary recognition of antigen
237. Production of immunoglobulin

A. Monocytes
B. Histiocytes
C. Lymphocytes

D. Plasma cells
E. Erythrocytes   *(91:11-16)*

Questions 238 to 239
238. Hypernatremia
239. Transient vertigo

A. Carbenicillin
B. Gentamicin
C. Minocycline
D. Erythromycin estolate (Ilosone)
E. Trimethoprim-sulfamethoxazole (Septra)
          (39:962-965)

Questions 240 to 241
240. Potassium iodide
241. Triple sulfonamides

A. Nocardiosis
B. Blastomycosis
C. Cutaneous sporotrichosis
D. Tubercle bacilli
E. Venereal warts   *(85:393, 422, 727)*

Questions 242 to 243
242. Plasma ACTH decreased
243. Plasma aldosterone decreased

A. Primary (hypoadrenal) adrenocortical insufficiency
B. Secondary (pituitary) adrenocortical insufficiency
C. Both
D. Neither   *(87:213-215)*

Questions 244 to 245
244. Segmental involvement with normal skip areas in x-rays
245. Continuous serration and pseudopolyposis in x-rays

A. Ulcerative colitis
B. Granulomatous colitis
C. Both
D. Neither   *(73:2263)*

Questions 246 to 247
246. Postural hypotension
247. Hemolytic anemia

A. Methyldopa (Aldomet)
B. Prazosin (Minipress)
C. Both
D. Neither   *(73:276-280)*

Questions 248 to 251
248. Hypertrichosis
249. Adynamic ileus
250. Hyperkalemia
251. Rebound hypertension

    A. Clonidine
    B. Spironolactone
    C. Chlorothiazide
    D. Minoxidil
    E. Trimethaphan   *(78:293-295)*

Questions 252 to 254
252. CPK of 600
253. BUN/creatinine ratio of 17
254. Positive EB virus antibodies

    A. Hashimoto's thyroiditis
    B. Infectious mononucleosis
    C. Dehydration
    D. Acute hepatitis
    E. Duchenne's (pseudohypertrophic) muscular
       dystrophy   *(39:848, 1091)*

Questions 255 to 257
255. Elevated LDH
256. Elevated LDH_1/LDH_2 ratio
257. Elevated CPK MB

    A. Acute myocardial infarction
    B. Rheumatoid arthritis
    C. Hepatic congestion
    D. Acute appendicitis
    E. Gouty arthritis   *(78:261)*

Questions 258 to 260
258. Aspiration pneumonitis
259. Tendinous xanthomas
260. Creamy plasma

    A. Familial hypercholesterolemia
    B. Familial fibrocystic dysplasia
    C. Familial polyposis coli
    D. Familial hyperchylomicronemia
    E. Familial dysautonomia   *(78:917-918)*

Questions 261 to 263
261. Holosystolic murmur heard best at the apex
    with radiation to the left axilla
262. Crescendo-decrescendo systolic murmur
    heard at right second interspace, transmitted
    to the neck and apex
263. Middiastolic rumbling at the apex

    A. Mitral stenosis
    B. Mitral regurgitation
    C. Innocent murmur
    D. Aortic stenosis
    E. Aortic regurgitation   *(78:212)*

Questions 264 to 266
264. Midsystolic click
265. Opening snap
266. S4 gallop

    A. Mitral stenosis
    B. Pericarditis
    C. Mitral valve prolapse
    D. Atrial septal defect
    E. Acute myocardial infarction   *(78:212)*

Questions 267 to 269
267. Auer rod
268. Atypical lymphocyte
269. Hypersegmented neutrophils

    A. Infectious mononucleosis
    B. Pernicious anemia
    C. Acute myeloblastic leukemia
    D. Lupus erythematosus
    E. Hodgkin's disease   *(73:940-960)*

Questions 270 to 272
270. Increased megakaryocytes
271. Increased immature plasmacytes
272. A great increase of immature leukocytes

    A. Aplastic anemia
    B. Spherocytosis
    C. Idiopathic thrombocytopenic purpura (ITP)
    D. Acute leukemia
    E. Multiple myeloma   *(73:940-960)*

Questions 273 to 275
273. ST elevation
274. Notched P
275. Right axis deviation

    A. Mitral stenosis
    B. Pericarditis
    C. Wenckebach's phenomenon
    D. Wolff-Parkinson-White's syndrome
    E. Cor pulmonale   *(73:170-175)*

Questions 276 and 277
276. Stimulate beta-1-adrenergic receptor
277. Vasodilator

A. Propranolol
B. Dobutamine
C. Atropine
D. Hydralazine
E. Disopyramide (Norpace)   (76:412)

Questions 278 and 279
278. Myasthenia gravis
279. Multiple sclerosis

A. B27
B. B8
C. B18
D. B12
E. BW17   (91:138)

Directions: Each of the questions or incomplete statements below is followed by four or five suggested lettered options. For each of these lettered options, indicate "T" if the option is true, indicate "F" if the option is false.

A 27-year-old male complained of sore throat, nonproductive cough, nausea, anorexia, occasional epigastric discomfort and general malaise for a week. He worked as an engineer in a government agency for 2 years; 3 months ago a new adminstrator arrived with multiple new directives which gave him a lot of stress. He has been married for a year and his wife was in the second trimester of pregnancy. Physical examinations were unremarkable and he was supported with compassion and encouragement. One week later, the patient returned with dark urine and yellow skin. Liver was enlarged and tender, GOT and CPT were in the range of 1000 I.U with positive HBs Ag.

The appropriate treatments include:

280. administration of corticosteroids
281. megadose acetaminophen
282. metrotrexate 15 mg IM b.i.d. for 10 days
283. high-protein high-fat low carbohydrate diet during acute phase

The patient's colleagues at work:

284. are at higher risk to develop hepatitis D
285. all need to receive HBIG
286. all need to receive hepatitis B vaccine

The patient's wife was found to be HBs Ag positive and HBe negative. You should recommend:

287. the wife to receive 3 doses of hepatitis B vaccine 40 mg
288. the newborn baby to receive HBIG and hepatitis B vaccine   (78:816-817)

Answers and Explanations

1. **(D)** The influenza virus vaccine is prepared in eggs that have been rendered noninfective by formaline or ultraviolet. A broad spectrum of protective immunity to influenza can be engendered by the proper administration of polyvalent (A₁, A₂, B) vaccine. The duration of protective immunity is about three to six months. In the U.S., the vaccinations should be completed before November.

2. **(C)** *B. fragilis* is sensitive to clindamycin, metronidazole, and chloramphenicol; chloramphenicol is sensitive to all anaerobes, with only rare strains resistant, and is very effective clinically. It penetrates the central nervous system wall.

3. **(C)** Influenza immunizations are recommended for the elderly over age 65, for patients with heart diseases, chronic bronchopulmonary diseases, renal diseases, diabetes mellitus, chronic liver diseases, Addison's diseases, sickle cell anemia, chronic anemias, and neoplastic diseases. Pregnancy is not an absolute contraindication against the influenza immunization because pregnant women are at higher risk to develop influenza pneumonias. Pregnant women with above-mentioned conditions may need influenza immunizations. Influenza immunizations may increase the risk of developing the Guillain-Barre's syndrome.

4. **(E)** Recent studies show this to be a very effective agent in preventing recurrent pyelonephritis. Megaloblastic anemia may develop while on trimethoprim therapy.

5. **(E)** Rifampin may cause jaundice by interfering with hepatic uptake of bilirubin. It may produce light-chain proteinuria and leukopenia.

6. **(D)** Since the patient is a nurse, the most likely offending organism would be a penicillin-resistant *Staphylococcus aureus*. The treatment of choice is oxacillin. Cephalexin is also used for staphylococcal infections. Other hospital-acquired infections are frequently caused by *Candida, Pseudomonas,* and *Serratia* spp.

7. **(C)** Penicillin and tetracycline in combination give an example of antagonism.

8. **(D)** Erythromycin is the drug of choice in penicillin-allergic patients with probable streptococcal sore throat. Oral clindamycin, though effective, has a serious side-effect of pseudomembranous enterocolitis. Tetracycline-resistant strains of streptococci are now being reported. Oral cephalexin offers an expensive way of treating strep throat.

9. **(D)** Bacterial pneumonia complicating influenza most often occurs on day five; early treatment of influenza with antibiotics usually does not prevent bacterial pneumonia. Pneumonia is commonly due to bacterial infection with pneumococci or staphylococci. As a nurse, the patient most likely has a penicillin-resistant *S. aureus* pneumonia.

10. **(C)** The incubation period is from 24 to 72 hours, and 1% of patients with influenza will

develop pneumonia. Bacterial pneumonia is frequently a complication for pregnant patients. However, the definite diagnosis of influenza viral pneumonia is frequently made by serial determination of complement-fixing and hemagglutination-inhibiting antibody titers.

11. **(B)** Oral absorption of tetracyclines is impaired when taken with milk products or drugs containing calcium, magnesium, aluminum, and iron. Carbenicillin will inactivate the effect of gentamicin.

12. **(A)** The first step in utilizing antibiotics is to determine whether the patient has a microbial infection that can be influenced by antimicrobial drugs.

13. **(D)** Recommendations on the use of prophylactic antibiotics in surgery include use when heavy contamination is very likely, when prolonged surgery is anticipated, and when the patient's resistance to injection may be severely compromised. The shorter the duration of use, the better.

14. **(D)** Chloramphenicol is more effective than ampicillin in the treatment of acute typhoid fever, but the incidence of relapses and post-treatment carriers is greater. Ampicillin, not chloramphenicol, is usually used against the chronic carrier state.

15. **(B)** The treatment of choice for streptococcal tonsillitis is penicillin. Thrush of the mouth is due to outgrowth of *Candida albicans,* usually caused when the balance of the oral flora is disturbed by antiinfective therapy, particularly tetracyclines. Specific therapy consists of nystatin mouth rinses, 500,000 units three times daily (100,000 units/ml in a flavored vehicle).

16. **(D)** The most frequent sequel of peritonitis is abscess formation in the pelvis, in the subphrenic space, between the leaves of the mesentery, or elsewhere in the abdomen. Antibiotic therapy may mask or delay the appearance of localizing signs of abscess. When fever, leukocytosis, toxemia, or ileus fails to respond to the general measures for peritonitis, a collection of pus should be suspected. This usually requires surgical drainage.

17. **(D)** This man most likely has mycoplasmal pneumonia. Erythromycin is now considered the drug of choice in this infection and is best used for three weeks. Tetracycline is also effective. *Mycoplasma pneumoniae* infection is often associated with bullous myringitis.

18. **(E)** Cephalothin is not effective in meningitis; in fact, several examples have been reported of meningitis occurring while on this drug.

19. **(E)** Osteoporosis is common and may cause complete loss of articular surfaces and flattening of bone ends. Hemarthrosis causes soft-tissue swelling, irregularities of the joint surface, and cystic areas in the bones. Hemophilic cysts (pseudotumors) are a rare but dangerous complication. Extensive destruction of the bones is associated with the large soft-tissue mass.

20. **(E)** An arthropod vector is suggested by its geographical and anatomical distribution. It seems to be caused by EB (herpes-like) virus, also the agent of infectious mononucleosis. Tumors are peculiarly multiple and bilateral and develop very rapidly.

21. **(C)** X-rays of bones in patients with multiple myeloma show rounded, punched-out, or mottled lesions. New bone formation is lacking. Sometimes there is diffuse osteoporosis, which frequently leads to pathological fractures.

22. **(D)** The most common cause for anemia in the adult is blood loss by menstruation; the next most common is gastrointestinal bleeding. The resulting anemia is usually of the iron-deficiency type.

23. **(B)** Acute DIC manifests itself with bleeding. Generalized ecchymoses, petechiae, and bleeding from previously intact venipuncture sites or around indwelling intravenous needles or catheters are present in many patients. In patients with meningococcemia (such as this patient), cutaneous hemorrhage may be striking. It is also the pathophysiological process of pseudomembranous enterocolitis, postoperative enterocolitis, and necrotizing enterocolitis.

24. **(C)** A variety of nonneoplastic processes are associated with the abnormal presence of CEA in adults. Though it was originally thought rather specific for colon carcinoma, irrespective of liver metastases, other neoplasms are now recognized to also result in its elevation. "Embryonic" refers to the normal presence of this antigen in the fetus, not to the morphology of the tumor.

25. **(D)** The pedunculated adenomatous polyp frequently occurs in the adult population with a different distribution in the large bowel than is favored by carcinoma. This is one of several lines of evidence suggesting that this common lesion does not particularly predispose the patient to colon carcinoma.

26. **(A)** The underlying process is no longer thought to be defects in the colonic wall through which mucosal outpouching occurs. Fecal impaction in the sometimes narrow-necked diverticulum prompts inflammatory response and subsequent peridiverticular fibrosis, but is not felt to be primary. Villous adenoma is not related to this disease process.

27. **(E)** All the features listed are those of Crohn's disease of the colon (or regional ileocolitis) and serve to separate it morphologically from idiopathic ulcerative colitis.

28. **(D)** Lymphocytes, not polys, are the characteristic cell involved in many types of viral (or probably viral) infections, including hepatitis. The liver appearance in HAA-positive and HAA-negative hepatitis is indistinguishable under the microscope. Though "viral particles" have reportedly been observed in livers in hepatitis (by electron microscopy), the councilman body is much larger, being visible with the light microscope. It is thought to represent residue of damaged cellular organelles.

29. **(E)** A, B, and C, are characteristic, but D may also occur in late stages. End-stage cirrhotic livers, damaged by excessive alcohol intake, may gradually, with evolution of the scarring and regeneration, lose their distinctive morphological features and assume a less characteristic pattern with large and small nodules and broad as well as fine bands of collagen.

30. **(D)** It is now believed that prolonged spasm of the empty bowel, as may be seen in the spastic bowel syndrome, can cause diverticulosis due to the high intracolonic pressures present.

31. **(E)** Lactose deficiency occurs in about 10% of Anglo-Saxons.

32. **(D)** Inflammatory disease of the small bowel may cause lactose deficiency by destruction of the cells lining the jejunum.

33. **(D)** Medical therapy for gallstones has been devised using daily oral doses of chenodeoxycholic acid, one of the bile acids, to increase the ratio of bile acid to cholesterol in bile. Clinical studies have proved that this does occur and that bile which previously has been supersaturated with cholesterol can be made undersaturated. When this happens, cholesterol crystals go back into solution and gallstones decrease in size. In patients treated this way, approximately 50% of cholesterol stones have decreased 50% in size within one year and many stones have disappeared completely.

34. **(D)** Ninety-five percent of patients· with colonic diverticula have involvement of at least the sigmoid colon; the prevalence of diverticula in the more proximal colon is progressively less but increases with the duration of the disease.

35. **(C)** The most important single sign of malignant ulceration is the presence of a mass. Occasionally, during stomach examination with special compression techniques, barium cannot be displaced from an ulcer crater and the niche maintains a lens-like configuration. This trapping of barium by a cuff of tumor is known as the Carman-Kirklin meniscus complex (Carman's sign) and is a sign of malignant ulceration within a mass.

36. **(D)** Nonembolic cerebral infarction is usually caused by atherosclerosis, dissecting aneurysm, arteritis, neck injury, tumor, inflammatory lymphadenopathy, polycythemia, sickle cells, thrombocytopenia and disseminated intravascular coagulation.

37. **(A)** Neurological symptoms without infarction, often manifested as transient ischemic attacks, most often arise from embolization

of small fragments from areas of proximal arterial disease (microemboli) to the cerebral cortex. Momentary weakness or numbness of the contralateral arm or leg and temporary partial or complete loss of vision of the ipsilateral eye or both eyes (amaurosis fugax) are common manifestations.

38. **(A)** The lesion is often located in the extracranial arteries in segmental distribution. The areas most often involved are the common carotid bifurcation, the origin of the verterbral artery, and the intrathoracic segments of the aortic arch branches.

39. **(D)** Focal seizures are usually developed by adult patients. The initial discharge comes from a focal unilateral area of the brain with pathology of trauma, tumor, vascular infarct, or congenital hippocampal sclerosis. Jacksonian motor seizure begins as a repetitive movement of a distal portion of an extremity and then spreads by a march of the clonic contractions up the extremities toward the trunk. Focal sensory seizure is the marching of abnormal sensations such as numbness and tingling spreading up an extremity. Grand mal seizures are the true epileptic seizures which are characterized by postictal state.

40. **(A)** Shoulder-hand syndrome is the pain and stiffness of the left arm and shoulder following MI. Early ambulation is indicated. The postmyocardial infarction syndrome is possibly due to an antoimmune pericarditis, pleuritis, and pneumonitis, which respond well to steroid.

41. **(C)** The clinical presentation is CHF with pansystolic murmur of ventricular septal defect. The signs of CHF in acute MI include S3 gallop, rales, congestion by chest x-ray, peripheral edema, and neck vein distention.

42. **(D)** Patients with ASD are usually asymptomatic until the fourth decade. The symptoms developed include pulmonary hypertension, atrial arrhythmias, bidirectional and then right-to-left shunting of blood, and cardiac failure.

43. **(A)** Medical therapy with hypotensive agents may halt the progress of dissection. Drugs that decrease the cardiac contractile

force, such as propranolol (Inderal), are useful. The drug of choice is trimethaphan. Progressive aortic regurgitation may require surgical treatment.

44. **(C)** The condition occurs predominantly in young women, who amount to 5-10% of patients referred for angiography. Angina can be a complication of hypertrophic subaortic stenosis. It is possible that some patients may not have angina of cardiac origin. Many patients are heavy smokers and the angina may be caused by spasm of the patent coronary artery.

45. **(E)** Renal vein thrombosis is rare in adults. In infants, it is frequently due to a complication of ileocolitis. Renal venography will reveal the thrombus.

46. **(B)** Sedation must be adequate to relieve pain. Morphine is the drug of choice (good sedation in addition to good analgesia). The IV route is preferred over the IM route, since the absorption is erratic and may cause false elevation in serum enzymes. Anticoagulants are used for the prevention of phlebitis and mural thrombosis. Atropine is used for bradycardia or complete heart block. Propranolol is used for continuing angina in the immediate postinfarct period that is unresponsive to analgesics and sedation.

47. **(D)** While arteriosclerosis is also correct, it is a more general term and properly includes both A and B as well as D. Calcification is a common complication, but is not the fundamental process.

48. **(C)** Mild hypertension produces hyaline thickening, with dense pink material deposited in the vessel wall. The basic lesion of atherosclerosis is the fibrous fatty subintimal plaque, not concentric layering. Syphilis produces an endarteritis, which may affect the vasa vasora of the aorta and be responsible for aortic damage, but concentric layering is not a feature.

49. **(C)** Dissolution of necrotic myocardial fibers, with influx of macrophages and the presence of lipid-rich debris, are prominent during the second portion of the first week of postinfarction. The infarct is weakest during this period. Earlier, when the exudation of polys is

at its peak, dissolution of fibers is not yet prominent. Fibroblast ingrowth begins to again restore some of the lost tensile strength, though the infarcted zone remains akinetic and may even suffer aneurysmal dilatation. Hemopericardium is, of course, the consequence of, not the substrate for, rupture.

50. **(A)** Polymorphonuclear leukocytes are not a component of this essentially mononuclear (including giant-cell) response which surrounds a focus of fibrinoid necrosis, typically in a perivascular location in the myocardium.

51. **(D)** Rupture of chordae tendinae is not expected in rheumatic heart disease, which tends to render chordae shortened, fused, and thickened. These scarred chordae are not prone to rupture. Of course, valvular insufficiency is in part the result of the altered chordae not permitting the leaflets to close. Stenosis results from the fusion of valve commissures as well as fibrous thickening (scarring) and calcification of the leaflet. Conditions where rupture of chordae occur include infective endocarditis and alterations of connective tissue, as in patients with ballooning valve leaflets. Myocardial infarction may be responsible for rupture of a papillary muscle, but not usually of the chordae themselves.

52. **(D)** An immunological mechanism is implicated. This serves to explain the observed occurrence of "focal glomerulitis" (previously misnamed "focal embolic glomerulonephritis") with right-sided endocarditis.

53. **(D)** The features of superficial thrombophlebitis include: mass or cord purpura, rubor, edema, dolor, history of trauma, and pre-existing varicose veins. The treatment consists of application of an elastic bandage or stocking from the toes to the knee and continued ambulatory activity.

54. **(E)** In addition, propranolol may be of use in idiopathic hypertrophic subaortic stenosis, hypertrophic obstructive cardiomyopathy, and asymmetrical septal hypertrophy. The main use of propranolol is for the therapy of angina pectoris by the mechanism of decreased contractility and decreases in heart rate. Major complications of propranolol therapy include fatigue, A-V block, and bronchospasm; it should be used with caution in patients with CHF and cardioversion.

55. **(C)** Isolated left anterior hemiblock, in the absence of a prior myocardial infarction and with angina for less than one year, strongly suggests single-vessel disease of the left anterior descending artery.

56. **(B)** Congestive heart failure and/or cardiomegaly with LBBB indicates double- or triple-vessel disease and always indicates significant disease of the left anterior descending artery. In the absence of coronary disease, coronary artery calcification is uncommon under the age of 55.

57. **(A)** The rescuer feels the tip of the xiphoid and places the heel of his hand on the lower half of the sternum about 1-1½ inches away from the tip of the xiphoid and toward the victim's head for chest compression. The depth should be 1½-2 inches and the ratio to be used for adult CPR is 15 compressions with two ventilations. The contraindication of CPR is if the patient has numerous rib fractures and a "flail" chest. To start cardiac compression, the patient should be put on a firm surface, such as a floor.

58. **(B)** The most common cause of airway obstruction is from the tongue. Thus tilting the head back to hyperextend the patient's head adequately is important in order to lift the tongue away from the back of the throat.

59. **(B)** Chemotherapy with isoniazid for a year has been shown to reduce the risk of the development of dormant infection into active tuberculosis by 75%. Close contacts of an infectious tuberculous patient and persons whose tuberculin conversion has occurred within the previous year or two should be put on chemoprophylaxis.

60. **(B)** Varicella pneumonia may cause hemoptysis. Extensive bilateral nodular opacities of the lung are usually seen on chest x-rays of severely ill patients. Respiratory failure should be avoided, for the mortality is 10-25% if untreated.

61. **(C)** There is a fall in lung compliance, vital capacity, and P_{O_2}.

62. **(A)** Scleroderma, like all diffuse fibroses, is characterized either by a normal or low P_{CO_2}; the latter is partly caused by hyperventilation.

63. **(A)** Psychogenic hyperventilation is frequently seen in patients with acute anxiety or neurocirculatory asthenia.

64. **(C)** Frequent iatrogenic causes of pneumothorax include subclavian puncture, thoracentesis, pleural biopsy, tracheostomy, and artificial ventilation.

65. **(B)** The treatment of choice is penicillin, combined with aminoglycosides. Postural drainage is also an important modality of treatment. Pneumonia caused by *S. aureus* or *Klebsiella* spp. may also be complicated by abscess formation.

66. **(E)** The genetically determined homozygous recessive, severe deficiency of serum alpha-antitrypsin occurs relatively rarely, in less than 0.1% of the general population. It accounts for only a very small proportion of clinically encountered cases of pulmonary emphysema. The heterozygous intermediate deficiency is not rare, occurring in 6-14% of the general population, but its association with increased incidence of emphysema is less clear. The anatomical pattern of emphysema associated with severe deficiency has usually been panlobular rather than centrilobular and tends to be severest in the lower lobes. It occurs at an earlier age (symptomatic onset may occur in the thirties), with equal sex incidence and independent of smoking history or of chronic bronchitis; in fact, these features distinguish patients with this particular, unusual process from the ordinary emphysema victim.

67. **(C)** Stress ulcers of the stomach and duodenum, with hemorrhage, develop frequently in patients with severe acute respiratory failure. Bleeding may be massive, frequently leading to shock that is difficult to overcome even with large volumes of infused blood. If in the first 12 to 16 hours after the onset of bleeding, the patient has several episodes of shock or remains in shock in spite of blood replacement, celiac axis angiography should be performed to find the bleeding site. This should probably be followed by surgery consisting of subtotal gastrectomy, bilateral vagotomy, and, if one large bleeding area is present, ligation of its blood supply. Unfortunately, the period of protracted hypotension sometimes causes acute renal failure, which, when severe, requires peritoneal dialysis or hemodialysis. Mortality is unfortunately quite high in patients with these multiple complications.

68. **(D)** Hospital-acquired pulmonary infections caused by Gram-negative organisms (especially *Pseudomonas*) are very common and probably result in part from contaminated respiratory therapy equipment. The danger of Gram-negative *Pseudomonas* pneumonia stems from the frequent complication of septicemia, with endotoxin shock, disseminated intravascular coagulation, and, later, renal failure. Since hospital-acquired Gram-negative infections are major complications of treatment for acute respiratory failure, and since Gram-negative septicemia has a 50% mortality, it is essential that everything possible be done to prevent these infections.

69. **(D)** Pulmonary angiography is the only means for providing anatomical information about the pulmonary vasculature. Electrocardiogram may also show no change, right axis deviation, nonspecific T-wave change, right bundle branch block, or Q-waves in Lead III. Arterial P_{O_2} is frequently in the vicinity of 50 mmHg. Pulmonary edema may occur in the following situations: on exposure to high altitude, in the presence of a traumatic hypothalamic lesion, with heroin overdosage, and with pulmonary embolism.

70. **(B)** Due to hypercortisolism or excessive secretion of associated steroids, the majority of patients with Cushing's syndrome have high blood pressure.

71. **(C)** Hyperparathyroidism is usually associated with back pain, renal stone, hypercalcemia, hypophosphatemia, and hypercalcuria.

72. **(D)** The oral glucose tolerance curve is often abnormal in patients with thyrotoxicosis and varies from one in which the peak glycemia is increased and somewhat delayed to one that is frankly diabetic in form. Plasma insulin concentration is increased, suggesting insulin antagonism.

73. **(C)** His arterial pH is close to 7.48 and the serum osmolarity is low. He apparently has lost H^+, K^+, and Cl^- ions during the course of the episode. The intravenous replacement therapy includes KCl, 5% dextrose, and isotonic saline solution.

74. **(D)** This is a condition of metabolic alkalosis. Diuretics should be used with water replacements of urine losses (D5W).

75. **(C)** Serum K^+ is elevated by acidosis and depressed by alkalosis due to anion shift. Thus a pH of 7.30 with K^+ of 2.5 means the patient's K^+ is depleted. Serum K^+ should be replaced while correcting acidosis to prevent its sudden fall.

76. **(E)** *Salmonella* gastroenteritis is commonly caused by eating uncooked food (such as homemade ice cream made of eggs or meats) contaminated with *Salmonella*. The symptom usually develops in 8 to 48 hours. The treatment is symptomatic. Antidiarrheal agents (paregoric or Lomotil) are used only for severe cases to relieve diarrhea and abdominal pain. Intravenous fluid replacement is indicated when dehydration is significant (10% of body loss in children). Antibiotics are not indicated because they do not shorten the course of illness and they may actually prolong the bacterial colonization; they are reserved only for bacteremia (chloramphenicol or ampicillin). Chloramphenicol is the drug of choice for typhoid fever (caused by *Salmonella typhi*); ampicillin and Bactrim are alternative drugs. Ampicillin is also used to eradicate the carrier state of typhoid fever.

77. **(B)**

Disease	Pathogen	Vector	Positive Weil-Felix test
Rocky Mountain spotted fever	*R. rickettsii*	Ticks	OX19, OX2
Epidemic typhus	*R. prowazekii*	Body lice	OX19
Scrub typhus	*R. tsutsugamushi*	Mites	OXK
Endemic typhus	*R. mooseri*	Fleas	OX19

78. **(A)** Chinese restaurant syndrome is probably caused by monosodium glutamate used as seasoning in Chinese food. The symptoms are usually self-limited and last for 45 minutes to two hours. Reassurance can be provided for the patient.

79. **(E)** One of the possible major sources of viral recombination occurs in animals. The major antigenic change in the virus usually makes previously acquired immunity ineffective against the new virus. However, the exact mechanism is still unknown.

80. **(A)** His arterial pH is close to 7.30, with high serum osmolarity. During the period of acute illness he has sustained losses of Na^+, K^+, and HCO_5^-. Hypopotassemia is common.

81. **(C)** In addition, cirrhosis may be caused by chronic ulcerative colitis, acute viral hepatitis, alcoholism, schistosomiasis, chronic congestive heart failure, polycystic diseases, and biliary cirrhosis.

82. **(D)** Thiazide diuretics cause transient hypercalcemia during the first few weeks of therapy in 5% of patients. Hypercalcemia with prolonged use of thiazide usually persists even when the drug is stopped. Even though the patient is asymptomatic, further evaluation may disclose the existence of primary hyperparathyroidism.

83. **(A)** Spirometry is useful in differentiating obstructive airway diseases (asthma, emphysema) from restrictive lung disease (silicosis, pulmonary fibrosis), as shown below.

Spirometric measurement	Restrictive lung diseases	Obstructive airway diseases
FVC (observed/predicted)	Reduced	
FEV_1 (observed/predicted)	Reduced	
FEF_1 25-75% (observed/predicted)		Reduced
FEV_1/FVC ratio		Reduced

84. **(D)** Syndrome of inappropriate secretion of antidiuretic hormone (SIADH) is a real pos-

sibility; work-ups include urine osmolarity, sodium excretion, and serum osmolarity. SIADH is characterized by hyponatremia with hypoosmolarity of the serum, high urine osmolarity, and high urine sodium content. SIADH is associated with oat cell lung carcinoma, gastrointestinal cancers, pancreatic carcinoma, thymoma, lymphoma, head injury, tuberculosis, pneumonia, meningitis, subarachnoid hemorrhage, psychosis, myxedema, Addison's disease, hypopituitarism, acute intermittent porphyria, vasopressin, oxytocin, vincristine, chlorpropamide (Diabinese), clofibrate, cyclophosphamide (Cytoxan), carbamazepine, and thiazide. Treatments include fluid restriction, management of the underlying causes, and administration of demeclocycline (Declomycin).

85. **(E)** Allergic bronchopulmonary aspergillosis may develop in patients with a history of asthma. It is characterized by a cough that is often productive of brownish, rubbery sputum, fever, wheezing, pulmonary infiltrates, elevation of serum IgE levels, serum precipitins against *Aspergillus fumigatus,* and occasionally, but not always, *Aspergillus fumigatus* in the sputum. Positive wheal and erythema skin test results with late reactions at six to eight hours are found. Response to corticosteroid therapy is usually excellent.

86. **(E)** Simple pharyngitis is an extremely common complaint in family practice. The cause is usually viral in origin and the treatment is symptomatic: rest, warm gargles, and adequate fluid intake. Analgesics are used when indicated. Antibiotics are prescribed when there is evidence of bacterial infections, which can be confirmed by throat culture.

87. **(A)** Legionnaire's disease is a disease caused by *Legionella pneumonia*. It is characterized by interstitial pneumonia with spread, patchy alveolar consolidation. The patients are usually middle-aged or elderly males who smoke and drink heavily. Extrapulmonary manifestations are common and include diarrhea, abdominal pain, delirium, stupor, jaundice, renal failure, and shock. Epidemics may arise from cooling towers, air conditioners, or shower heads. It is responsive to erythromycin.

88. **(B)** Acyclovir (Zovirax) is useful in genital herpes. Five percent ointment can be applied to decrease viral shedding and pruritus. Recurrent infections can be treated by 200 mg oral acyclovir capsules five times a day. Side reactions include headache, nausea, vomiting, vertigo, arthralgia, and inguinal adenopathy.

89. **(C)** Herpes simplex can be diagnosed by tissue culture, complement fixation tests and Papanicolaou smear. However, the scrapings of the ulcer base stained with methylene blue may show multinucleated giant cells which are also diagnostic. The test is called Tzanck test.

90. **(D)** Captopril (Capoten) is effective in mild to moderate essential hypertension and renovascular hypertension. Side reactions include proteinuria, agranulocytosis, impaired taste, eruptions, and reflex tachycardia.

91. **(D)** Gilbert syndrome is a benign syndrome caused by hereditary glucuronyl transferase deficiency. The patient may show slight scleral icterus but is usually asymptomatic with mild, persistent unconjugated hyperbilirubinemia. The syndrome is present in 7% of the population and is relatively common in family practice.

92. **(E)** The hyperreflexia, convulsions, and psychosis are probably related to a relative pyridoxine deficiency. Isoniazid can also reduce the metabolism of phenytoin, increasing its blood level and toxicity.

93. **(E)** Tetracyclines given during pregnancy usually cause renal tubular damage, discoloration and fluorescence of teeth in newborns, and super infection with *C. albicans, S. aureus,* and *Proteus*. Clindamycin often causes nausea and skin rashes. There are reported fatal cases of diarrhea due to clindamycin (pseudomembranous enterocolitis).

94. **(D)** Acute nonlymphatic leukemia is essentially granulocytic, monocytic, erythroid, and megakaryocytic leukemia. With combination chemotherapy, adjuvant immunotherapy with heterologous cells, BCG or MER-25 (ethamoxytriphenol), and supportive measures, complete remissions can be obtained in almost 70% of patients.

95. **(E)** Malignancies which cause thrombocytosis include Hodgkin's disease, lymphoreticular disorders, and various carcinomas. Other causes include osteoporosis, nephrotic syndrome, renal cysts, and Cushing's syndrome.

96. **(E)** Before diagnosing idiopathic thrombocytopenic purpura, secondary thrombocytopenia should be ruled out. Folic acid or vitamin B12 deficiency causes disorders of the hematopoietic system. Ethanol selectively suppresses the megakaryocyte. Quinidine provokes thrombocytopenia by an unknown mechanism.

97. **(A)** The erythrocytes of patients with sickle cell trait contain more HbA than HbS. Sickled cells are rarely found in the blood of a person with the sickle cell trait. Hyposthenuria, spontaneous hematuria, splenic infarction, renal papillary necrosis, central retinal artery occlusion, asymptomatic bacteriuria, thrombophlebitis, pulmonary disease, and diabetic vascular disease are more common in patients with sickle cell traits. However, the overall mortality is not increased.

98. **(E)** The complications of Hodgkin's disease include hemolytic anemia, intractable itching, superior vena cava obstruction, and pleural effusion.

99. **(A)** The most common causes of cerebral hemorrhage include: aneurysms, arteriovenous malformations, hypertension, coagulation defects, and idiopathic causes.

100. **(A)** The muscles of the lower half of the face in patients with amyotrophic lateral sclerosis are weak, giving an expressionless facies, but the muscles of the upper half are spared. The extraocular muscles are rarely, if ever, affected. The cause is unknown; the pathology is the degeneration of motor cells in the spinal cord and medulla oblongata, which results in atrophy and fibrillation of the somatic musculature.

101. **(A)** In this syndrome, radial pulse is absent. There is very tight stenosis or occlusion of the proximal subclavian artery. The affected upper extremity "steals" its blood supply from the carotid and other vertebral arteries, the blood flowing from the base of the

brain to the extremity via the vertebral artery of the affected side. The flow in this vertebral artery is reversed. It enters the subclavian artery distal to the point of obstruction.

102. **(A)** Berry aneurysms are rarely seen in infants and are not familial.

103. **(D)** Rarely, mitral stenosis is congenital in origin, most commonly involving the so-called parachute mitral valve. Electrocardiograph shows enlarged left atrium with notched P (P mitrale) in limb leads and diphasic P in V_1.

104. **(E)** Aortic regurgitation is most commonly of rheumatic origin. Less commonly, bacterial endocarditis may result in aortic regurgitation.

105. **(A)** The estrogen component may be responsible for secondary hypertension by stimulating hepatic synthesis of the renin substrate, angiotensinogen, which increases angiotensin and aldosterone.

106. **(E)** Idiopathic hypertrophic subaortic stenosis may be associated with Wolff-Parkinson-White's syndrome and mitral regurgitation. Prophylactic antibiotic therapy during dental extraction is indicated.

107. **(E)** Coxsackie B viral infections of the heart may cause chest pain and fever. Myocarditis is fairly common in patients who develop pericarditis. Cardiac tamponade is an uncommon complication. Pleurodynia is characteristic. Classic cases are usually due to tuberculosis. Rheumatoid arthritis often is associated with chronic constrictive pericarditis.

108. **(D)** The prognosis in variant angina is less favorable. A high incidence of myocardial infarction and sudden death has been reported.

109. **(A)** Evidence continues to mount in support of the effectiveness of antihypertensive drug therapy in improving prognosis. In a prospective study conducted by the Veterans Administration Cooperative Study Group on antihypertensive agents, the benefit of the therapy is clear-cut after five years. The

complications of hypertension include CHF, acute MI, angina pectoris, stroke, and renal failure.

110. **(A)** Emphysema is characterized by attenuation and loss of pulmonary septal tissue, which causes the loss of elastic recoil with increase in pulmonary compliance and reduction of diffusing capacity. Pulmonary fibrosis results in a reduction of diffusing capacity associated with an increased stiffness of the lung and decreased lung compliance.

111. **(B)** Isoproterenol is a beta-2-bronchodilator and is only effective for bronchial obstructions occurring in asthma and chronic bronchitis.

112. **(A)** Asthma often does not respond very well. The reason significant clinical improvement sometimes does not occur for asthma is the peripheral airway occlusion due to plugs of viscid mucus. Bronchial lavage and hydration may be helpful.

113. **(A)** Syndrome of acute diffuse bronchial mucous occlusion is the complication of status asthmaticus responsible for the 3-5% of patients who die following hospitalization for acute asthma. In most patients with status asthmaticus, increasing dyspnea is due to increasing bronchospasm alone. In a minority, however, there is obstruction of the bronchi and bronchioles with thick, tenacious mucus. Fortunately for the diagnosis of this syndrome, those patients with organic obstruction of the bronchial tree have a physiological correlate of this abnormality in a rising PCO_2. Since most patients in status asthmaticus have a low to normal PCO_2, the presence of this syndrome is suggested when the PCO_2 is 47 mmHg or above. Unless patients with organic bronchial obstruction complicating acute asthma are treated vigorously with more than conventional therapy, they may progress to severe acute respiratory failure with acute respiratory acidosis, become comatose, undergo cardiac arrest, and die.

The proper management of the hypercapnic asthmatic with this syndrome must include intrabronchial therapy as well as conventional treatments such as hydration, humidification, steroids, and bronchodila-

tors. Nasotracheal suctioning should be employed every 15 minutes; if the PCO_2 has not decreased toward normal—or has continued to rise—the patient should then have bronchoscopy and lavage under general anesthesia, or intubation and the use of a respiratory support system. Properly treated, patients with this syndrome usually have a normal PCO_2, in 12 to 24 hours.

114. **(C)** Following surgery in the upper abdomen, acute respiratory failure often develops, and is one of the major causes of postoperative morbidity and mortality. The respiratory center is frequently depressed for several hours postoperatively owing to the premedications and anesthesia. The muscular component of the neuromuscular connections may be abnormal for some time after surgery if succinylcholine was used in combination with the anesthesia. After high abdominal surgery, the pressure dressings and binders, coupled with diaphragmatic inflammation, greatly limit chest cage motion. Secretions become inspissated because of the low humidity of the anesthetic gases, leading frequently to airway obstruction. Finally, alveoli often collapse because production of surfactant is impaired by various anesthetic agents. Severe hypoxemia may result in lactacidemic metabolic acidosis.

115. **(A)** Pressure-limited machines are only satisfactory for normal or mildly diseased lungs without stiffening. Stiffened lungs require a volume-limited instrument. Fat embolism, a well defined sequela of extensive trauma, particularly fracture of the femurs, is characterized biochemically by the mobilization of various lipids into the circulation. One of the lipid components, the free fatty acids, exert a destructive effect on capillaries in the brain, skin, and lungs. In the lung, multiple areas of interalveolar hemorrhage develop, leading to decreased ventilation in areas still perfused and therefore hypoxemia.

116. **(A)** Positive end-expiratory pressure (PEEP) is a great therapeutic advance for patients with intractable hypoxemia, usually as a part of a "stiff-lung" syndrome. Gradual "weaning" from a respirator may begin when the vital capacity, measured at the bedside

using a special spirometer, is 10 cc/kg or greater. Atelectasis, owing to an endotracheal tube slipping into the right-lower lobe bronchus, pneumonia, and especially tension disorders, including pneumomediastinum and pneumothorax, are all occasional complications of the management of acute respiratory failure and indicate the importance of daily chest x-rays in all such cases. In fact, any unexplained worsening of the arterial blood gas measurements or any new symptoms developing in these patients should alert the physician to obtain a new chest x-ray immediately. The adequacy of ventilation should also be checked with an arterial blood gas measurement at least every four hours in the acutely ill patient. Leaks in the tubing component of the support system, obstruction in the endotracheal tube, secretions accumulating throughout the bronchial tree, and inadequate inspiratory pressure settings may all lead to decreased alveolar ventilation and increasing P_{CO_2} during treatment.

117. **(E)** Shock lung is seen in nonthoracic trauma and following hemorrhagic and endotoxin shock. The initial pathological lesion is interstitial edema with some capillary thrombosis; later the intactness of the alveolar capillary membrane is disrupted, with red blood cells and plasma pouring into the alveoli in many areas. As in fat embolism, the ventilation-perfusion relationship is disturbed and hypoxemia results.

118. **(A)** Heroin addicts may develop embolic pneumonia, lung abscess, and pulmonary fibrosis secondary to foreign body granulomas. The granuloma may be due to cotton particles or may be the talc granuloma seen in addicts who inject blue velvet (paregoric and PBZ [tripelenamine]). More dramatic is the acute pulmonary edema that rarely occurs after heroin injection. The pathogenesis is unknown.

119. **(C)** The loss of sodium is frequently seen in biliary lavage. Therapy for this patient includes volume replacement with colloids and slow diuresis.

120. **(A)** High serum chloride indicates metabolic acidosis due to HCO_3^- loss from diarrhea or renal tubular acidosis. Ingestion of acid chloride salts will also produce this. The first step in correcting the electrolyte imbalance is the administration of sodium bicarbonate. Hyperchloremic acidosis is due to administration of ammonium chloride (or other chloride salts), administration of carbonic anhydrase inhibitor, dilution acidosis, diarrhea or draining GI fistulas, proximal or distal renal tubular acidosis, and ureteroenterostomy.

121. **(C)** Hyponatremia is due to dilution of electrolyte by water retention. Total body sodium is usually elevated or normal; thus sodium should not be administered. Water intake should be restricted and furosemide administered to produce diuresis.

122. **(B)** This is a case of metabolic alkalosis. Volume contraction produced by diuretics is corrected by NaCl administration. Use of acid salts such as NH_4Cl is rarely necessary. Muscle weakness is due to a low serum K^+.

123. **(E)** Immunoglobulins are gamma-globulins synthesized by different classes of plasma cells. They are classified into four groups: IgG, IgA, IgM, and IgE.

124. **(A)** Approximately three-fourths of children with craniopharyngiomas show diffuse flecks of calcification in the sella or suprasellar region in plain radiograms of the skull. Increased intracranial pressure may also be seen as suture spread or demineralization of the vault or clinoid processes.

125. **(A)** Chronic alcoholism may produce megaloblastic anemia due to folic acid deficiency, ringer sideroblastic defect of bone marrow with increased serum iron concentration due to interference with pyridoxine metabolism, and Wernicke's encephalopathy due to thiamine deficiency. The incidence of peptic ulcer is exceptionally high in the alcoholic population. A less frequent but serious cause of hematemesis is the so-called Mallory-Weiss' syndrome, which is characterized by lacerations of the gastric mucosa occurring at or just below the gastroesophageal junction.

126. **(E)** Accumulation of lactic acid is a relatively common cause of metabolic acidosis. Lactic acidosis is frequently encountered in patients with circulatory failure caused by dehydration, hemorrhage, or endotoxic or cardiogenic shock. Hypoxemia shifts the aerobic metabolism of the tissue to anaerobic glycolysis, which produces lactic acid. Spontaneous lactic acidosis is usually associated with diabetes, hepatic failure, SBE, and leukemia. The cause is unknown. Phenformin therapy and accidental ingestion of 15-20 g of isoniazid may also cause lactic acidosis. Plasma expanders and sodium bicarbonate are used for treatment.

127. **(D)** T4 is elevated in hyperthyroidism, the use of birth control pills, and pregnancy. To differentiate these conditions, T3 resin uptake should be ordered. In hyperthyroidism, T4 and T3 resin uptake are both elevated; in hypothyroidism, T4 and T3 resin uptake are both depressed; in estrogen effect (pregnancy or the use of oral contraceptives), T4 is elevated and T3 resin uptake is depressed. However, a detailed history on contraceptive use and menstrual history should be obtained first to rule out the use of oral contraceptives and pregnancy. Even if T3 resin uptake is low, if there is no estrogen effect, radioiodine uptake should be ordered to search for existing hyperthyroidism. TSH is not useful in the diagnosis of hyperthyroidism but is useful for the diagnosis of hypothyroidism (high TSH indicates primary hypothyroidism; low TSH indicates secondary hypothyroidism).

128. **(A)** Doxorubicin (Adriamycin) is an antitumor antibiotic used for the treatment of Hodgkin's disease, breast cancer, and acute lymphocytic and myelocytic leukemia. It intercalates in the minor groove of helical DNA and interferes with transcription. It also inhibits DNA synthesis in high concentration. It may cause myelosuppression, nausea and vomiting, alopecia, stomatitis, hyperpigmentation in blacks, and cardiotoxicity. Cardiotoxicity is potentiated by cyclophosphamide (Cytoxan) and mediastinal radiotherapy. PVCs, ST and T changes, arrythmia, subendocardial fibrosis, and congestive heart failure may develop. The drug can turn the urine briefly red and the patient might mistakenly believe that he has developed hematuria.

129. **(A)** Vincristine (Oncovin) is derived from vinca alkaloids to use in the treatment of acute lymphocytic leukemia, non-Hodgkin's lymphoma, Hodgkin's disease, Wilms' tumor, neuroblastoma, breast tumor, and sarcoma. It rarely causes severe bone marrow depression, but it may cause severe bone marrow depression, but it may cause alopecia, abducens nerve palsy, inappropriate antidiuretic hormone syndrome (hyponatremia and high urinary sodium concentration), severe peripheral neuropathy (wrist drop, foot drop, parasthesia of fingers and toes, muscle weakness, and loss of deep tendon reflexes), and adynamic ileus. Vincristine interacts with microtubular proteins to cause mitotic inhibition through metaphase arrest.

130. **(E)** Vitamin D deficiency causes rickets. Children with malabsorption syndromes, pancreatitis, cystic fibrosis, hepatic diseases, kidney diseases, and corticosteroid administration are at higher risk of developing vitamin D deficiency. Black children and children who are rarely exposed to ultraviolet irradiation are also at high risk of developing vitamin D deficiency.

131. **(A)** Tetany results from decreased ionized calcium levels due to lowered total calcium or increased binding of calcium to albumin with alkalosis. Mild tetany with paresthesias and muscle cramps can result from hyperventilation due to anxiety (respiratory alkalosis). Leg cramps during pregnancy, neonatal tetany (maternal hypoparathyroidism), and acute pancreatitis may be present. Primary hyperaldosteronism may cause tetany, hypertension, hypokalemia, and polyuria. Magnesium depletion may cause decreased parathyroid hormone (PTH) secretion or diminished bone responsiveness to PTH, secondarily producing sympromatic hypocalcemia. This syndrome is most commonly associated with alcoholism or chronic intestinal malabsorption.

132. **(B)** Diazoxide (Hyperstat) is an antihypertensive drug which rapidly lowers the blood pressure level and is used for hypertensive encephalopathy, malignant hypertension, and preeclampsia-eclampsia. Side-reactions include hypotension, tachycardia, water and sodium retention, hyperglycemia, and hyperuricemia. Hypoglycemia caused by functioning islet cell tumor can be treated with diazoxide.

133. **(A)** Antiplatelet agents are used for the pro- phylactic treatment of thrombotic disease. Aspirin is used for prophylaxis against tran- sient cerebral ischemia (150-325 mg/day). In- dividuals at high risk for atherosclerotic cardiovascular disease can be given prophy- lactic low-dose aspirin (less than 325 mg/ day). Sulfinpyrazone may be useful in reducing thrombotic occlusions in arterio- venous communications. Warfarin (an anti- coagulant) combined with dipyridamole is useful in patients with prosthetic heart valves. Ergonovine promotes uterine con- traction to prevent postpartum hemorrhage.

134. **(A)** Cis-platinum is a soluble platinum com- pound used for testicular tumor (often in combination with bleomycin), ovarian can- cers, and melanoma. It causes little hemato- logic suppression, however, it results in severe nausea and vomiting, hearing loss and tinnitus, nephrotoxicity, and peripheral neuropathy. Its action is caused by its inter- calation with helical DNA.

135. **(A)** Hypoparathyroidism (with low calcium) often results in hyperphosphatemia; hyper- parathyroidism and hyperthyroidism cause hypophosphatemia. Reversible muscle weak- ness and paralysis as well as dysfunction of the central and peripheral nervous system, including seizures and coma, have been de- scribed with phosphates below 1.0 mg%. Re- versible congestive heart failure has been reported as well. Hypophosphatemia implies either total body depletion or intracellular shift of inorganic phosphate and occurs inde- pendently of the changes in serum calcium.

136. **(B)** Hashimoto's thyroiditis is an autoim- mune disease which is characterized by hy- pothyroidism (low T4, low T3 resin uptake), patchy scan, and high antithyroid antibody titers. Levothyroxine is often effective in causing regression of the goiter. In patients suspected of having Hashimoto's thyroiditis, T4 and T3 resin uptake tests and a thyroid scan should be ordered first to rule out a possible cold nodule (which may be carci- noma). If patchy scan is found, TSH and an- tithyroid antibody titer should be ordered.

137. **(A)** Crohn's disease is frequently associated with ankylosing spondilitis and its associ- ated HLA antigen B27. It is often associated with arthritis, iritis, enterovesical fistulas, pyoderma gangrenosum, pericholangitis, cir- rhosis, nephrolithiasis, hydronephrosis, and renal amyloidosis. The incidence of colonic and rectal cancer is increased. The involve- ment of the ileum results in failure of ileal absorption of the intrinsic factor—vitamin B12 complex and vitamin B12 deficiency may result. There is no strong association with vitamin B2 deficiency.

138. **(A)** Ulcerative colitis is associated with an- kylosing spondylitis, which is associated with HLA antigen B27. Obsessive-com- pulsive immaturity with parental depen- dency may be seen in the patient. It is often associated with arthritis, erythema nodo- sum, uveitis, hemorrhoids, sclerosing cholan- gitis, iliofemoral venous thrombosis, Coombs- positive hemolytic anemia, and impaired growth and sexual development in children. The patient with ulcerative colitis is at higher risk of developing colonic cancer—2 percent at 10 years and 10 percent at 20 years. Ulcerative colitis *per se* is not directly associated with lung cancer.

139. **(A)** Chronic pancreatitis is often associated with chronic alcoholism, narcotic addiction, diabetes mellitus, peptic ulcer, pseudocyst, pancreatic abscess, pancreatic insufficiency (steatorrhea), malnutrition, cholestatic liver disease, cholelithiasis, hyperlipidemia, and hyperparathyroidism. The association of chronic pancreatitis and pancreatic carci- noma is not clear; however, pancreatitis is often found surrounding a small carcinoma.

140. **(B)** Acromegaly causes excessive growth of bone and soft tissue, which may result in "spade hand" rather than clubbing of fin- gers. Acromegaly occurs after long bone epiphyseal closure, and height will not be increased. Cardiomegaly, hypertension, and heart disease are often associated with acro- megaly. Hepatosplenomegaly may also be noted. Hyperprolactinemia, glucose intoler- ance, degenerative joint disease, headache, and cerebrovascular disease may develop.

141. **(E)** The poor nutrition of alcoholics often results in vitamin deficiences. Niacin defi- ciency (pellagra) may cause diarrhea, der- matitis, and dementia; riboflavin (B2) deficiency may cause dermatitis, cheilosis,

and stomatitis; pyridoxine (B6) deficiency may cause sideroblastic anemia; folic acid deficiency may cause macrocytic anemia; and vitamin C deficiency (scurvy) may cause perifollicular hemorrhages and gingival hemorrhages. However, the most common vitamin deficiency of alcoholics is thiamine (B1) deficiency, which may result in Wernicke's encephalopathy (nystagmus, diplopia, abducens palsy) and beriberi (circulatory collapse, high-output heart failure).

142. **(E)** In a suspected patient, positive sputum examination with KOH and culture, a positive coccidioidin skin test result, and a rising complement fixation titer of 1:16 are helpful in establishing diagnosis. Amphoterecin B is effective.

143. **(E)** Patients with prosthetic heart valves are at high risk of developing infective endocarditis, and prophylactic antibiotics should be instituted during dental or minor surgical procedures. Homograft and heterograft valves have lowered the incidence of thromboembolism. Paravalvular leak may occur and regurgitation murmur may develop. Heart failure, syncope, angina, and embolization may occur in prosthesis malfunction. Chronic hemolysis may cause hemolytic anemia with iron deficiency.

144. **(B)** Protamine is a simple protein containing arginine and is strongly basic. Although it has an anticoagulant effect, it forms a stable salt with heparin (which is strongly acidic), and both drugs lose anticoagulant activity. It is used only via the intravenous route. It may cause a sudden fall in blood pressure, bradycardia, dyspnea, transitory flushing, and a feeling of warmth.

145. **(E)** Bronchogenic carcinoma may cause numerous clinical syndromes, including Horner's syndrome, recurrent laryngeal nerve palsy, erythema multiforme, dermatomyositis, hypercalcemia, hyperadrenocorticism, carcinoid syndrome, inappropriate antidiuretic hormone secretion (hyponatremia with urinary hypertonicity), gynecomastia, pulmonary hypertrophic osteoarthropathy, clubbing of digits, peripheral neuropathy, and myasthenic syndrome.

146. **(A)** Diet is not considered to be a causal factor in peptic ulcer, and the patient will be benefited by a well balanced diet. Peptic ulcer is associated with the group O blood type, social events which cause psychic conflicts, stresses (Curling's ulcer, Cushing's ulcer, brain injury, sepsis, burns, surgery, shock), hyperparathyroidism, chronic bronchitis, emphysema, liver cirrhosis, pancreatic cancer, alcoholism, salicylates (aspirin), indomethacin, phenylbutazone, steroids, and ibuprofen (Motrin).

147. **(A)** Drugs, steroids, starvation, and infection may convert the latent disease to a manifest disease and should be avoided. Drugs include sulfonamides, griseofulvin, and barbiturates. The short-acting barbiturate (thiopental) is the most notorious one. In the acute attack, hematin is used; a high dosage of propranolol may also be useful.

148. **(A)** Galactorrhea is caused by ingestion of birth control pills (rich in estrogen), tranquilizers, antidepressants, amphetamines, antihypertensives, and gonadotropins. Excessive estrogen (oral contraceptives with a high dosage of estrogen) may cause galactorrhea, whereas progesterone may have a restraining effect. Galactorrhea is seen in pituitary microadenoma, in which prolactin is secreted.

149. **(E)** Secondary polycythemia can be caused by congenital cardiovascular diseases, pulmonary arteriovenous fistulas, high altitude residence, Pickwickian syndrome (obesity, hypoventilation), erythropoietin-producing malignancies (ovarian carinoma, CNS malignancies, hypernephroma), renal cysts, adrenal hypercorticism, virilizing tumors, and the use of androgens, sulfonamides, nitrites, and alcohols.

150. **(A)** Asthma is a reversible obstructive airway disease due to hyperirritability of the airways caused by a variety of substances, including acetylcholine, methacholine, histamine (these substances are used in bronchial challenge tests to reproduce asthmatic symptoms in questionable cases), prostaglandin $F_2 \alpha$ bradykinin (a slow-reacting substance of anaphylaxis), and respiratory irritants. In exercise-induced asthma, strenuous exercise may precipitate asthmatic attack. This may be associated with inhalation of dry and cold air. Occupational exposure to TDI and other chemicals can produce asthmatic syndromes

in some workers. Aspirin-induced asthma is often associated with nasal polyps and hyperplastic sinusitis and may be produced by aspirin, phenylbutazone, aminopyrine, indomethacin, and ibuprofen.

151. (E) The pathogenesis of pancreatitis is still unknown. However, it is associated with hyperlipoproteinemia (types I and V), pancreatic carcinoma, duodenal ulcer, hypercalcemia, gallstones, hyperparathyroidism, abdominal surgery, abdominal trauma, Group B *Coxsackie virus* infection, mumps infection, pregnancy, alcoholism, and the administration of drugs, including corticosteroids, estrogens, furosemide, thiazide, azathioprine, and acetaminophen.

152. A-T, B-T, C-F, D-F
Cardiac tumors are mostly metastatic tumors from melanoma, leukemia, and lymphomas without significant problems. Primary tumors include myxomas, rhabdomyomas, fibromas and methotheliomas. Myxomas may cause cachexia, fever, syncope, dyspnea, arrhythmia and Raynaud's disease. The third heart sound varies in time after the second heart sound, and can be diagnosed by EKGs, chest x-rays, and echocardiograms. Ninety-five percent arise from atria with 75% from left atrium. It elevates ESR and serum gamma-globulins.

153. A-T, B-T, C-F, D-T, E-F
Quinidine, procainamide, and disopyramide are used for auricular flutter/fibrillation and ventricular arrhythmia. Quinidine may cause cinchonism, hemolytic anemia, hepatitis and thrombocytopenia. Procainamide (Pronestyl) may cause lupus syndrome and granulocytopenia; disopyramide (Norpace) may cause anticholinergic symptoms (urinary retention, dry mouth). Tocainide is used for ventricular arrhythmia; it may cause Q-T shortening in EKG, tremor, insomnia, and hallucination. Hypocalcemia may prolong Q-T interval and hypercalcemia may shorten Q-T interval in EKG.

154. A-T, B-T, C-F, D-F, E-T
Common side-effects of most neuroleptics include pseudoparkinsonism, gynecomastia-galactorrhea, dry mouth, blurred vision and impotence. Orthostatic hypotension is an important side-reaction for the elderly because of an increased risk of accidental falls. Thioridazine (Mellarill) may cause retinal degeneration, chlorpromazine (Thorazine) may cause cholestatic jaundice and photosensitivity

dermatitis. The patients with the neuroleptic malignant syndrome present with fever, striking rigidity, and confusion; these patients can be treated with dantrolene (Dantrium).

155. A-T, B-T, C-F, D-T, E-F
Intrarachnoid hemorrhage is frequently caused by ruptured congenital aneurysms located at the bifurcation of the arteries forming the circle of Willis. It often presents with a sudden onset of headaches during strenuous physical activity, altered consciousness, nuchal rigidity, bloody CSF and the presence of subarachnoid blood in the basal cisterns by the cranial computerized axial tomography. Electrocardiographic abnormalities may simulate myocardial ischemia on the precordial leads.

156. A-T, B-T, C-T, D-F, E-F
Campylobacter enteritis is usually self-limited and is treated symptomatically. In rare case correction of water and salt depletion is needed. In protracted or severe illness, a seven day course of erythromycin (50 mg/kg-1 day in four divided doses) can be administered.

157. A-T, B-F, C-T, D-F, E-T
Hypokalemia can also be caused by administration of gentamicin, amphotericin B, vitamin B12 therapy, chronic laxative ingestion and steroid administration.

158. A-F, B-T, C-T, D-T
Nonsteroidal anti-inflammatory drugs (NSAIDS) are prostaglandin antagonists to synthetase. They may cause gastric irritation, acute gastritis, peptic ulcer and upper gastrointestinal bleeding. Headache, tinnitus, and dizziness may occur also. NSAIDS are used in patients with rheumatoid arthritis, osteoarthritis, bursitis and tendinitis. Selected patients with gout or ankylosing spondylitis may also be responsive to NSAIDS.

159. A-F, B-T, C-F, D-F, E-F
Traveller's diarrhea is commonly caused by enterotoxigenic *Escherichia coli*. Other pathogens include *Shigella, Salmonella*, and *Giardia lamblia*. The illness is usually self-limited and the treatment is symptomatic. Ingestion of bismuth subsalicylate (Pepto-Bismol) 60 ml q.i.d. may reduce the incidence of the illness. Trimethoprim-sulmethoxazole (septra) may be used for chemoprophylaxis in selected cases.

160. A-T, B-F, C-F, D-F, E-F
Reflux esophagitis is characterized by heart

burns, substernal pain, and nocturnal regurgitation. Symptoms are often improved by upright position, aggravated by recumbency, alcohol consumption and cigarette smoking. Weight reduction, use of antacids, administration of H_2 blockers (such as cimetidine) or metoclopramide (Reglan) may be beneficial. Metoclopramide is a gastrointestinal stimulant which increases gastroesophageal motility.

161.   A-T, B-T, C-T, D-T, E-T
Influenza syndrome is characterized by sore throat, fever, chills, prostration, nonproductive or productive cough, headache, photophobia, myalgia (back and legs) and chest discomfort. Pneumonia, Reye's syndrome, myositis, myoglobinuria, myocarditis, pericarditis, and transverse myelitis may develop. Amantadine is administered until symptoms disappear. Flu vaccines are recommended for the elderly and for those in chronic cardiopulmonary diseases. Amantadine chemoprophylaxis may start in conjunction with vaccine administration.

162.   A-F, B-F, C-F, D-T, E-F
The standard management approach for patient with peptic ulcer is medical therapy. Subtotal gastrectomy is reserved for patients with malignant ulcers. Proximal gastric vagotomy enjoys lower operative mortality and complications (dumping, diarrhea and weight loss) but the recurrent rate is high. No specific diet is of proven benefit for ulcer healing. Patients should eat a balanced diet and avoid foods which may cause them discomfort. Milk is a strong acid stimulant and smokers may delay ulcer healing. Alcohol may damage gastric mucosa thus it should be consumed in moderation.

163.   A-T, B-T, C-F, D-T, E-F
Peptic ulcer is treated by antacids (either magnesium or aluminum hydroxide and H_2 receptor antagonists (cimetidine and ranitidine). Sucralfate may enhance mucosal defense and may also be used for therapy. Sodium bicarbonate is not commonly used because of its short duration of action and its propensity to produce sodium retention and alkalosis. Diphenhydramine is a H_1 receptor antagonist and is not used specifically for peptic ulcer diseases.

164.   A-F, B-T, C-T, D-F, E-T
In the elderly, due to decreased muscle mass a normal serum creatinine level does not guarantee that the drug clearance is normal, it usually is reduced. Thus the dosage of tetracyclines, sulfonamide and cephalosporins should be reduced accordingly. The liver clearance is decreased in the elderly and the dosage of lidocaine needs to be reduced.

165.   A-T, B-T, C-F, D-T, E-T
All lipid-lowering drugs cause GI symptoms (abdominal pain, diarrhea, flatulence, nausea and vomiting). However, resins may also cause severe constipation requiring stool softener. Clofibrate and gemfibrozil may also be associated with cardiac arrhythmias. Nicotinic acid may cause hypotension and may activate peptic ulcer diseases.

166.   A-F, B-F, C-T, D-T, E-F
Calcium channel blockers are "slow channel blockers" which selectively inhibit the transmembrane influx of extracellular calcium irons into cardiac muscle and smooth muscle without changing serum calcium concentration. They are not used for treating hypercalcemia; they are used for treating vasospastic (Prinzmetal's) angina. Calcium channel blockers may also be of value to patients with unstable angina and stable exertional angina. They may cause hypotension, worsen congestive heart failure, bradycardia and conduction blocks; thus should be avoided in patient with sick sinus syndrome. Commonly used calcium channel blockers include verapamil (Calan, Isoptin), nifedipine (Procardia), and diltiazem (Cardizem).

167.   (C)

168.   (B)

169.   (A) *Klebsiella* pneumonia is lobar pneumonia with nonputrid, homogeneous, rusty, thick sputum. *Pseudomonas* pneumonia often occurs during hospitalization, usually in patients receiving inhalational therapy. *Bacteroides* pneumonia is often caused by dental or periodontal drainage, aspiration, or pulmonary necrosis and has an indolent course. Foul-smelling sputum or pus may be found in lung abscess and necrotizing pneumonia associated with empyema. It often involves dependent pulmonary segments.

170.   (B)

171.   (A)

172.   (C)

173.   (A) Normocytic normochromic anemia is commonly associated with acute blood loss, menstruation, aplastic anemia, multiple myeloma, azotemia, and hypothyroidism. Hypochromic microcytic anemia is frequently caused by iron deficiency or a defect in iron utilization. Hyperchromic macrocytic anemia is frequently seen in pernicious anemia, liver disease, and malabsorption syndrome (sprue-like).

174. (C)

175. (A)

176. (B) Classic migraine headaches are periodic, throbbing, severe, frequently unilateral, and often over the eye with photophobia. They usually start in teenage girls, decrease during the thirties and forties, and are exacerbated around menopause. There is very frequently a family history of headache or of motion sickness as a child. Common migraine is less often unilateral.

177. (A)

178. (B)

179. (C)

180. (D) Acute posterior infarction is characterized by a large R and S-T segment depression in Leads V_1, V_2, and/or V_3. Q and S-T segment elevation in Leads V_1 and V_2, V_3, or V_4 are seen in anterior infarction. Inferior infarction is designated by Q in Leads II, III, and aVF. Lateral infarction is shown by Q in Leads I and aVL. In bundle branch block, QRS is three small square or more wide. In RBBB, there are RR' in Lead V_1 or V_2 and wide S in Leads V_5 to V_6. In LBBB, there are RR' in Leads V_5 or V_6 and wide S in Leads V_1 to V_2.

181. (D)

182. (E)

183. (A)

184. (C)

	pH	PCO_2	HCO_3^-
Normal	7.4	40	24
Respiratory acidosis	Decreased	Increased	—
Respiratory alkalosis	Increased	Decreased	—
Metabolic acidosis	Decreased	—	Decreased
Metabolic alkalosis	Increased	—	Increased

185. (C)

186. (A)

187. (B) Hashimoto's thyroiditis is familial and is commonly seen in middle-aged myxedematous women with a large symmetrical goiter that feels rubbery. Riedel's thyroiditis is a very rare disease occurring in a middle-aged woman with a moderately enlarged asymmetrical thyroid which is stone-hard. There is no enlargement of regional lymph nodes. Subacute thyroiditis (deQuervain's thyroiditis) is characterized by sudden painful thyroid which is firm, tender, and nodular with reddened, warm overlying skin. The pain is referred to the ear and jaw.

188. (B)

189. (C)

190. (A) Focal defects of thyroid scans are often caused by adenomas, cysts, neoplasms, or hemorrhage. "Hot" nodules (areas of increased radioactivity) are almost never malignant. Fifteen percent of "cold" areas (focal decreased radioactivity) are reported to be malignant.

191. (B)

192. (C)

193. (D)

194. (A) Carotid sinus massage causes sudden slowing or standstill in atrial flutter, with rapid return to the original rate on release of pressure. The ventricular rate is usually one-half of the atrial rate (2:1 block), or 150 beats/minute. In atrial fibrillation, carotid sinus massage has no effect or causes only slight slowing. Carotid sinus massage has no effect on atrial tachycardia or promptly abolishes the attack. Carotid sinus massage gradually slows sinus tachycardia.

195. (B)

196. (C)

197. (A)

198. (D) The atrial rate in sinus tachycardia is 100-160 beats/minute; in sinus bradycardia, slower than 60 beats/minute; in paroxysmal atrial tachycardia, 170-220 beats/minute. Atrial flutter (250-350 beats/minute) is best treated by DC cardioversion when no CHF is present.

199. (C)

200. (F)

201. (A)

202. (E)

203. (D)

204. (B) Hypokalemia causes sagging S-T, T depression and U elevation. Hyperkalemia causes tall, tent-shaped T-waves; wide flat P-waves; and wide QRS complex. With hypercalcemia, the Q-T interval shortens, but with hypocalcemia, the Q-T interval becomes prolonged. Digitalis causes gradual downward sloping of the S-T segment. Excess digitalis causes A-V block; digitalis toxicity may cause bigeminy, PVCs, and ventricular tachycardia. Quinidine causes notching of a wide P-wave and widening of the QRS complex. There is often an S-T depression, prolonged Q-T interval, and U-waves.

205. (D)

206. (E)

207. (A)

208. (C)

209. (B) Pneumocystosis causes diffuse mixed alveolar and interstitial pneumonitis. Radiological appearance of the lung lesion is variable in nocardiosis, but typically there are one or more areas of dense pneumonia; lesions tend to cavitate and empyema is common. Aspergillosis in lungs is termed aspergilloma, which causes a shaggy nodular appearance in chest x-ray. *Phycomycetes* (mucormycosis) may cause pulmonary infarction, cavitation, and pleural effusion.

210. (A)

211. (B)

212. (C)

213. (D) Cimetidine is a histamine H_2 receptor antagonist which inhibits gastric acid secretion. Cimetidine hastens healing of duodenal ulcer and is probably beneficial for the healing of gastric ulcer. It is effective in Zollinger-Ellison's syndrome. However, when the drug is stopped, many patients may experience recurrences. Side-reactions include gynecomastia, galactorrhea, and leukopenia. Antacids promote healing of duodenal ulcer. When they are administered one hour after meals, they prevent postprandial acid rise; however, large dosages are often required.

214. (A)

215. (C)

216. (D) When a patient presents with signs of excessive polypeptide hormone, a neoplasm must be considered in the differential diagnosis, because, if such a possibility is overlooked, a nonoffending endocrine organ may be incorrectly removed and a neoplasm may thus be left untreated. Deterioration of such a patient with signs of excessive polypeptide hormone production may be due to a treatable ectopic hormone syndrome. ACTH is often produced by oat cell carcinoma of the lung, which also causes renin production. The ectopic ACTH syndrome often results in hypokalemia and, less frequently, hyperpigmentation.

217. (A)

218. (A)

219. (B) Hiatal hernia (peptic esophagitis) is often asymptomatic. Pain and heartburn are often dull, postprandial, retrosternal, worse on lying down, and improved by sitting and standing. Pain may radiate down the inner

aspect of the arms, simulating angina pectoris. Peptic ulcer is characterized by epigastric distress one hour after meals or nocturnal pain, both of which are relieved by food, antacids, or vomiting.

220. (B)

221. (C)

222. (D) Phenylketonuria causes hyperphenylalanemia, which results in seizure and mental retardation. Affected newborns identified by screening tests should be on a phenylalanine-restricted diet. A low-purine diet may not be very helpful in preventing gout; however, alcohols are to be avoided for preventing acute attacks. Monoamine oxidase inhibitors (Parnate) are second-line medications for depression. Ingestion of tyramine-rich foods (beer, wine, cheeses, chicken livers, pickled herring, chocolate) may precipitate hypertensive crises and shoud be avoided. With the administration of chlorothiazide, a rigid low sodium diet (350 mg or less per day) is not necessary; 2g sodium per day is allowed. A gluten-free diet is useful for gluten-sensitive enteropathy in celiac disease.

223. (C)

224. (A)

225. (D) Bretylium is used for ventricular fibrillation or ventricular tachycardia. It may cause hypotension, nausea and vomiting, and tachycardia. Phenytoin is used for symptoms of digitalis toxicity, such as PVCs and bigeminy. It may cause ataxia, macrocytic anemia, nystagmus, hepatitis, and gingival hyperplasia. Procainamide is used for atrial tachycardia, atrial flutter, atrial fibrillation, and accelerated A-V conduction syndromes (WPW). It may cause Lupus-like syndrome. Quinine is used for leg cramps.

226. (A)

227. (B)

228. (A)

229. (B)

230. (C) The Barr body is a rounded chromatin mass located near or at the inner surface of the nuclear membrane. The number of the chromatin bodies in a cell is one less than the number of X chromosomes in that cell.

Sex chromosome	Number of X	Barr bodies (X-1)
XY (normal male)	1	0
XX (normal female)	2	1
XO (Turner's syndrome)	1	0
XXY (Kleinefelter's syndrome)	2	1
XXX (Triple X)	3	2

231. (B)

232. (C)

233. (A)

234. (A)

235. (B) Paretic neurosyphilis is the tertiary syphilis characterized by insidious onset of personality changes, irritability, insomnia, and decreased intellectual capabilities. Progressive dementia with periodic euphoria, tremor of the hands and tongue, and hyperactive reflexes develops. Cryptococcal meningitis is frequently associated with stupor, seizures, immunosuppressive therapy, and Hodgkin's lymphoma. Amphoterecin B is used.

236. (C)

237. (D) The lymphocyte is responsible for the primary recognition of antigen and is an immunologically specific effector cell. It produces antibody-like immunoglobulin molecules that remain fixed to the lymphocyte and serve as receptor sites for reaction with antigen. The production of immunoglobulins (antibody) for secretion is the primary function of the plasma cell. The Golgi apparatus of the plasma cell may play an active role in the secretion of immunoglobulins. Blood macrophages (monocytes) migrate into tissue, where they become tissue macrophages (histiocytes).

238. (A)

239. (C) Trimethoprim-sulfamethoxazole is used for chronic urinary tract infection (chemoprophylaxis) and *Pneumocystis carinii* infection and may cause anemia with reticulocytosis, particularly in patients with glucose-6-phosphate dehydrogenase deficiency. Erythromycin is used for *Mycoplasma* pneumonia and Legionnaire's disease and may cause jaundice or hepatitis. Minocycline is used for patients with meningococcal carriers (chemoprophylaxis) and may cause transient vertigo or ataxia. Gentamicin is used for sepsis from *Proteus, Pseudomonas,* and *Enterobacter* and may cause permanent vestibular damage and nystagmus. Carbenicillin is used for bacteremia from *Staphylococcus, Klebsiella,* or other Gram-negative organisms and may cause hypernatremia and hypersensitivity.

240. (C)

241. (A) Cycloserine is also effective for nocardiosis. Amphotericin B is effective for histoplasmosis and blastomycosis. 2-Hydroxystilbamidine, soramycetin, and hamycin are also useful for the treatment of blastomycosis. In severe cases of sporotrichosis, potassium iodide may be helpful. Presence of tubercle bacilli is usually treated with isoniazid. Venereal warts are often treated with podophyllin applications.

242. (B)

243. (A)

Plasma level	Adrenocortical hypofunction	
	Primary	Secondary
ACTH	Increased	Decreased
Aldosterone	Decreased	Normal

In primary adrenocortical insufficiency, ACTH is increased due to loss of cortisol feedback and the aldosterone level is decreased due to the impairment of all secretory zones of the adrenal. In secondary adrenocortical hypofunction, ACTH secretory capacity is lost due to pituitary impairment and aldosterone secretion is normal due to its independence of pituitary function.

244. (B)

245. (A) Ulcerative colitis and granulomatous colitis are difficult to separate. However, in ulcerative colitis, toxicity (toxic megacolon) is more common, and in Crohn's disease, perirectal fistulas and perforation are more common. Aphthous stomatitis is associated with Crohn's disease. In sigmoidoscopy, ulcerative colitis shows diffuse, friable superficial ulceration and Crohn's disease shows more discrete lesions. Ulcerative colitis may be cured by surgery, but recurrences are common in Crohn's disease. Ulcerative colitis carries a higher risk than Crohn's disease of development of colonic cancer; Crohn's disease is also associated with a small increase in the incidence of small bowel carcinoma.

246. (C)

247. (A) Methyldopa and Prazosin are both used as antihypertensives, with comparable potency. Both may cause headache and postural hypotension. Methyldopa may also cause impotence, hepatitis, and Coombs-positive hemolytic anemia.

248. (D)

249. (E)

250. (B)

251. (A) Clonidine (Catapres) may cause sedation, dry mouth, and dizziness. Severe postural hypotension with syncope may occur in the first week of treatment. Abrupt cessation of the drug may result in rebound hypertension. Spironolactone spares potassium and should not be used in renal impairment. Chlorothiazide may cause hypokalemia. Minoxidil (Loniten) may cause weight gain, edema, tachycardia, and hypertrichosis. Trimethaphan is used for dissecting aneurysm. It may cause mydriasis, urinary retention, anorexia, nausea, vomiting, and adynamic ileus.

252. (E)

253. (C)

254. (B) In infectious mononucleosis, the mononucleosis spot test is positive (more specific than the heterophil test) and the antibody of the Epstein-Barr (the causative organism) is present. Dehydration (prerenal azotemia) may cause the BUN/creatinine ratio to be greater than 15 (10 is normal). CPK is greatly elevated in myopathies.

255. (C)

256. (A)

257. (A) In both hepatic damage (acute hepatitis or hepatic congestion) and acute myocardial infarction, the LDH level is elevated. However, in hepatitis and hepatic congestion (right ventricular failure), LDH_2 (the slow-moving fraction of LDH) rather than LDH_1 is elevated. In acute myocardial infarction, both LDH_1 and LDH_2 are elevated, with LDH_1 (the electrophoretically rapid-moving isoenzyme of LDH) rises higher than those of LDH_2 ("flipped" LDH). CPK can be elevated in intramuscular injections, hypothyroidism, acute alcoholism, cerebrovascular diseases, and myopathies. However, acute myocardial infarction causes CPK MB isoenzyme to rise.

258. (E)

259. (A)

260. (D) In family practice, the family is the unit of care and screening services are offered to identify familial disease entities to provide unaffected members with needed preventive care. Familial dysautonomia is characterized by autonomic nervous system dysfunction and aspiration pneumonitis. Familial fibrocystic dysplasia is characterized by early clubbing of fingers and multiple lung cysts. Familial hypercholesterolemia is characterized by hypercholesterolemia, hypertriglyceredemia, elevated low-density lipoprotein levels, and tendinous or tuberous xanthomas with a very high risk of coronary heart disease. Patients with familial polyposis coli are at higher risk of developing colonic cancer, and periodic examinations are required; often prophylactic colectomies are performed for these patients. Familial hyperchylomicronemia is a rare disease associated with recurrent pancreatitis, eruptive xanthomas, and hepatosplenomegaly. The patients with hyperchylomicronemia are sensitive to dietary fat because of the deficient lipoprotein lipase activity.

261. (B)

262. (D)

263. (A)

Condition	Murmurs
Innocent murmur	Systolic murmur variable with respiration at the left second interspace
Aortic stenosis	Crescendo-decrescendo systolic murmur at the right second interspace transmitted to the neck and apex
Aortic regurgitation	Decrescendo diastolic murmur at the right second interspace
Mitral stenosis	Middiastolic rumbling at the apex
Mitral regurgitation	Holosystolic murmur at the apex radiated to the left axilla

264. (C)

265. (A)

266. (E) Mitral stenosis causes increased intensity of the first heart sound, opening snap and middiastolic rumbling and presystolic murmurs. Pericarditis is characteristic of friction rub. Mitral valve prolapse causes mid-to-late systolic murmur preceded by midsystolic clicks. Atrial septal defect causes wide, fixed splitting second sounds and middiastolic rumbling at the left-lower sternal border. In acute myocardial infarction, S3 and/or S4 may be present. However, gallop rhythm may be produced by anemia, pregnancy, hyperthyroidism, Paget's disease, and beriberi.

267. (C)

268. (A)

269. (B) Infectious mononucleosis shows atypical lymphocytes (round and oval nucleus with blue cytoplasm which contains many vacuoles). Pernicious anemia (vitamin B12 deficiency) shows macrocytosis, hyperchromia, and hypersegmented neutrophils. Auer rods (red rods in the granulocytes) are seen in acute leukemia. Lupus erythematosus is characteristic for LE cells (phagocytosis of another PMN's nucleus by a PMN). Sternberg-Reed cells (large multinucleoli cells) are seen in Hodgkin's disease.

270. **(C)**

271. **(E)**

272. **(D)** In aplastic anemia, bone marrow shows pancytopenia and a fatty appearance. In acute leukemia, marrow is packed with immature leukocytes even when leukopenia exists. In multiple myeloma, immature, atypical plasma cells are seen in the marrow. In ITP, marrow megakaryocytes are increased in number but are not surrounded by platelets; these abnormal megakaryocytes contain scant cytoplasms, vacuoles, and single nuclei. In spherocytosis, erythroid hyperplasia is present in bone marrow.

273. **(B)**

274. **(A)**

275. **(E)** In pericarditis, S-T elevation in all leads preserves normal upward concavity; in acute myocardial infarction, S-T elevation is concave downward or depressed. P-mitrale (mitral stenosis) is notched P, representing left atrial enlargement; P-pulmonale (cor pulmonale) shows peaked P, right axis deviation, and deep S in V_6. In Wenckebach's phenomenon, the P-R interval is progressively prolonged until P is completely dropped. In WPW syndrome, a delta wave is present and P-R is shortened.

276. **(B)**

277. **(D)** In congestive heart failure due to open heart surgery, myocardial infarction with pulmonary edema or acute heart failure without severe hypotension dobutamine (Dobutrex) may be used to increase myocardial contractility. It may precipitate tachyarrhythmia and hypertension. Hydralazine is useful in reducing afterload by arterial vasodilatation. It is used for the treatment of hy-

pertension and pulmonary edema precipitated by myocardial infarction. Hydralazine may combine with dobutamine for acute failure, but it can also be used for chronic failure.

278. **(B)**

279. **(C)** HLA B27 is associated with ankylosing spondylilitis, Reiter's disease, acute anterior uveitis, juvenile rheumatoid arthritis, psoriatic arthritis, and *Yersinia* arthritis. HLA B8 is associated with gluten-sensitive enteropathy, myasthenia gravis, dermatitis herpetiformis, and chronic active hepatitis. Multiple sclerosis is associated with HLA A3, B7, and B18; and psoriasis vulgaris is associated with HLA B12 and BW17.

280. **(F)**

281. **(F)**

282. **(F)**

283. **(F)**

284. **(F)**

285. **(F)**

286. **(F)**

287. **(F)**

288. **(T)**

The treatment of acute hepatitis B is symptomatic and the use of corticosteroids is unnecessary. Acetaminophen and methotrexate may damage liver cells and should be avoided. Diet is not critical for recovery, although low-fat and high-carbodydrate regimen is often adopted. HBV is a DNA virus (Dane particle) but delta-virus is a RNA virus sharing HBs Ag outer coat. Unless the patient's colleagues maintain a close contact (such as sexual or blood contact) with the patient they are not at an higher risk to contact either hepatitis B or D. However, if there is sufficient interest among employees an institution-wide screening for HBV can be instituted. Those individuals who are HBs AG(−) and HBs Ag(−) (preferably also HBc Ag and HBe Ag negatives) may receive hepatitis B vaccine (Heptavax B).

Hepatitis B vaccine is not contraindicated during pregnancy, however, the pregnant wife has had a positive HBs Ag and hepatitis B vaccine is not indicated. The newborn baby needs HBIG and hepatitis B vaccine to reduce vertical transmission. A patient with positive HBs Ag is at a higher risk to develop chronic acute hepatitis, liver cirrhosis, and hepatoma, thus a continuity of care is needed.

Chapter 8

Pediatrics

Directions: Each of the questions or incomplete statements below is followed by five suggested answers or completions. Select the BEST answer in each case.

1. A newborn infant is found to have had no bowel movement for its first 36 hours and is vomiting green material. The x-ray shows a bubble-like appearance in the intestinal loops. The most likely diagnosis is

   A. cystic fibrosis of the pancreas
   B. Hirschsprung's disease
   C. pyloric stenosis
   D. intussusception
   E. none of the above   *(11:285)*

2. Two hours after birth, a four pound boy developed dyspnea and cyanosis. X-ray reveals a reticulogranular appearance in the lungs. The most likely diagnosis is

   A. hyaline membrane disease
   B. asthma
   C. croup
   D. pneumonia
   E. pneumothorax   *(12:324-325)*

3. A staph epidemic occurs in the newborn nursery. Management consists of all of the following *except*

   A. admit all new babies to newly established nurseries staffed by separate uninfected personnel
   B. admit new infants to regular nurseries only after all others are discharged
   C. hexochlorophene bath for new admissions

   D. a septic technique to handle the baby admitted
   E. kanamycin prophylaxis for infants
                                    (12:410)

4. All of the following are true of Niemann-Pick's disease *except*

   A. hepatosplenomegaly
   B. severe psychomotor retardation
   C. early death
   D. accumulation of ganglioside
   E. seizures   *(12:482-483)*

5. The only child of unaffected parents has a cleft lip and palate with no other indication of abnormality. The chance that a second child will have a cleft lip and palate is approximately

   A. 1 in 1000, the same as for the general population
   B. 1 in 20
   C. 1 in 10
   D. 1 in 2
   E. unknown   *(12:882)*

6. A young woman, the sister of one of your patients who has classic hemophilia, is considering marriage. Her boyfriend has been proved to have a deficiency of erythrocyte glucose-6-phosphate dehydrogenase (G6PD). If the young woman is not a carrier of G6PD deficiency, which of the following statements about their potential offspring is correct, if she decides to marry him?

A. every daughter will be a carrier for hemophilia and G6PD deficiency
B. every son will have G6PD deficiency
C. some daughters and some sons will have G6PD deficiency
D. none of the sons will have both hemophilia and G6PD deficiency
E. none of the above are correct   (12:1244)

7. Hand-Schuller-Christian's disease is characterized by all of the following *except*

A. diabetes mellitus
B. exophthalmos
C. diabetes insipidus
D. skull defects
E. maculopapular skin rash   (11:424)

8. Evaporated milk: 6 oz
    Boiled water: 14 oz
    Carbohydrate: 3/4 oz
    The caloric content per fluid ounce of the formula shown above is approximately

A. 4
B. 8
C. 10
D. 16
E. 25   (11:31)

10. In a two-year-old child with irritability, painful extremities, pallor, coarse hair, and x-rays revealing periosteal elevation, the most likely diagnosis is

A. vitamin A deficiency
B. hypervitaminosis D
C. hypervitaminosis A
D. vitamin D deficiency
E. vitamin E deficiency   (11:34)

11. An infant usually triples its weight by

A. 3 months
B. 6 months
C. 12 months
D. 18 months
E. 24 months   (11:3)

12. Most infants (75%) can sit alone by the age of

A. 1 month
B. 6 months
C. 12 months
D. 15 months
E. 24 months   (11:14)

13. The following mineral requirements for a child are all correct *except*

A. sodium: 3 g/day
B. potassium: 0.25 mg/kg/day
C. calcium: 50-70 mg/kg/day
D. magnesium: 13 mg/kg/day
E. phosphorus: 1.5 g/day   (12:137)

14. A school-age boy suffered from upper respiratory infection three weeks ago. Now he complains of fever, fatigue, and pain in both knee joints. The involved joints are tender, swollen, and hot. Tachycardia is also noted. The most likely diagnosis is

A. sickle cell anemia
B. acute glomerulonephritis
C. rheumatoid arthritis
D. rheumatic fever
E. acute pericarditis   (12:590)

14. The earliest sign of heart involvement in rheumatic fever is usually detected by

A. auricular fibrillation
B. apical systolic murmur
C. apical late diastolic rumbling
D. gallop rhythm
E. bradycardia   (12:591)

15. In nephrotic syndrome, diuresis is most reliably initiated by

A. thiazide diuretics
B. deliberate exposure to German measles
C. restriction of sodium intake
D. corticosteroids
E. intravenous infusion of normal saline   (12:1322)

16. All of the following statements concerning acute glomerulonephritis are true *except*

A. an increase of both systolic and diastolic blood pressure is frequently seen
B. it may follow impetigo
C. serum complement activity is elevated
D. there is periorbital edema in morning
E. there are hematuria and proteinuria   (11:305-308)

17. Which of the following statements concerning enuresis is *not* true?

A. organic disease can be an etiological factor

B. premature toilet training can be an etiological factor

C. enuresis is frequently found to occur in more than one member of a family

D. enuresis is urinary incontinence past seven years of age

E. diurnal enuresis is more indicative of organic causation than is nocturnal enuresis   *(11:54)*

18. A 13-year-old girl who is in the third percentile for height and has no evidence of sexual maturation most likely

A. is a pituitary dwarf

B. has gonadal dysgenesis

C. is a primordial dwarf

D. has hypothyroidism

E. has no endocrine disturbance   *(11:17-18)*

19. A male infant who weighed five pounds, four ounces at term developed jitteriness, cyanosis, apathy, apnea, a weak and high pitched cry, limpness, and eye rolling at 29 hours of age. The pregnancy had been complicated by albuminuria, excessive weight gain, and hypertension. However, the delivery was atraumatic and was not accompanied by any recognized trauma or anoxia. Despite his birthweight, the infant appeared quite mature. He was alert and was thought to have been normal at birth and for the first 24 hours of life. The most likely diagnosis is

A. hypoglycemia

B. congenital heart disease

C. intracranial bleeding

D. neonatal tetany

E. adrenal hemorrhage   *(12:397)*

Pediatrics/183

20. A four-year-old boy suddenly developed a high fever, chilliness, and vomiting. On examination he was found to have nuchal rigidity and positive Kernig's sign. Petechial lesions have been noted on both extremities and over the abdomen. The most likely diagnosis is

A. pneumococcal meningitis

B. encephalitis

C. brain tumor

D. meningococcal meningitis

E. aseptic meningitis   *(11:218-219)*

21. Meningitis in children is most frequently caused by which of the following microorganisms?

A. *Staphylococcus*

B. *Hemophilus influenzae*

C. *E. coli*

D. *Pneumococcus*

E. *Meningococcus*   *(49:867-868)*

22. The following statements about febrile convulsions are all true *except* that

A. they occur in about 6-8% of all children

B. they frequently occur between 6 and 48 months

C. a family history of febrile convulsions is rarely obtained

D. seizures are symmetrical and usually last less than 15 minutes

E. the child is neurologically normal before and after the convulsion   *(11:336)*

23. Petit mal (absence seizure) usually begins in childhood. It may be characterized by all of the following *except*

A. impairment of consciousness with mild clonic movements

B. either increased or decreased postural tone

C. 5/second spike on EEG

D. automatic movements

E. autonomic phenomena   *(13:1843-1844)*

24. Your sweet two-year-old daughter is put to bed and she begins to cry. You will

A. let her cry and ignore her

B. pick her up and kiss her

C. change her diaper

D. give her antihistamines

E. feed her with baby food   *(24:171)*

25. Evaluation of the emotional aspects of the child's life

A. is outside of the competence of the family physician

B. should only be done by pediatricians

C. should only be done by psychiatrists

D. is within the area of responsibility of the family physician

E. should only be done by child psychologists   *(12:10)*

26. The parental disciplinary behavior most conducive to delinquency is

A. excessive corporal punishment
B. avoidance of all corporal punishment
C. marked laxness
D. marked inconsistency
E. marked strictness   (3:689)

27. If a child screams when he becomes angry, it is mostly likely due to

A. normal reaction
B. childhood schizophrenia
C. hyperkinesis
D. childhood neurosis
E. separation anxiety   (5:533-534)

28. Institutionalized children are usually

A. overstimulated
B. overindulged
C. oversocialized
D. understimulated
E. overfed   (1:906)

29. Harry is a two-year-old boy who was toilet trained at age 12 months, but lost bladder and bowel control after his younger brother was born. Harry's adjustive pattern is an example of

A. repression
B. suppression
C. projection
D. regression
E. rationalization   (4:39-40)

30. Defiance, rebellion, antisocial feelings, and demands for independence in an adolescent boy

A. can usually be controlled by stricter rules and punishment
B. should be turned over to the courts for disposition
C. can be seen as the expected behavior during this stage of development
D. are usually accompanied by inner feelings of security, confidence, and masculinity
E. are psychotic behaviors   (5:575)

31. A 10-year-old boy has been bitten by a skunk. To rule out rabies, which is the rapid, reliable test?

A. antibody titer of the rabies
B. stain of the brain tissue of the skunk to find the Negri bodies
C. virus culture from the skunk's brain tissue

D. examination of the skunk's brain tissue by the fluorescent antibody test
E. immune fluorescent antibody titer of the boy   (12:805)

32. The administration of gamma-globulin (0.25 ml/kg of body weight) to a child susceptible to mumps between the second and fifth day after exposure to the disease will probably

A. prevent the development of mumps in almost all patients
B. sensitize the patient to gamma-globulin
C. prolong the incubation period
D. be followed in four to six weeks by infectious hepatitis
E. have little beneficial effect on the complications of mumps   (12:772)

33. In treating the asthmatic attack, which of the following is helpful?

A. epinephrine
B. aminophylline
C. large volumes of fluids IV
D. aerosol inhalation
E. all of the above   (11:459)

34. Successful therapy of hyaline membrane disease entails

A. reducing the metabolic rate
B. administering high levels of oxygen
C. correcting alkalosis
D. monitoring the infant's arterial pH and O_2
E. antibiotics   (12:325)

35. A 10-month-old infant is hospitalized because of dyspnea, cough, stridor, and high fever. The present illness began with irritability and slight fever 36 hours before admission. Breathing soon became audible and raspy. A high-pitched barking cough developed, and the temperature rose rapidly. When his respirations became labored, he was brought to the hospital. His past medical history is negative and he has received two of his three diphtheria-pertussis-tetanus immunizations. The most likely diagnosis is

A. parainfluenza laryngotracheitis
B. diphtheritic laryngotracheitis
C. spasmodic croup (acute allergic subglottic edema)
D. H. influenzae Type B laryngotracheitis
E. foreign body obstruction in trachea
                                    (11:240-241)

36. A roentgenogram of the chest of a 9-month-old infant reveals pleural fluid and pneumatoceles. These findings are probably caused by

A. *Klebsiella pneumoniae*
B. Group A beta-hemolytic *Streptococcus*
C. *Streptococcus pneumoniae*
D. *H. influenzae,* Type B
E. *S. aureus*   (12:1250)

37. Recurrent abdominal pain in a child is most likely

A. psychological
B. caused by worm infestation
C. caused by peptic ulcer
D. caused by abdominal epilepsy
E. an indication for an IVP study   (11:281)

38. An 11-month-old girl has developed diarrhea that is watery in nature. No other symptoms are noted and no abnormalities are found in the physical examination. You would now

A. prescribe oral ampicillin
B. advise that solid foods be discontinued
C. start oral tetracyclines
D. institute paregoric syrup
E. offer skim milk fortified with vitamin D
                                   (12:291-293)

39. Cromolyn sodium is useful in

A. status asthmaticus treatment
B. hay fever treatment
C. the maintenance therapy of asthma
D. the prophylaxis of asthma
E. the treatment of bronchiectasis   (12:535)

40. Measles vaccine is

A. recommended for newborns
B. recommended for infants at 12 months of age
C. recommended for routine immunization at the age of 15 months with live attenuated vaccine
D. recommended for routine immunization at age of 15 months with inactivated virus vaccine
E. not effective if given with mumps vaccines
                                   (12:192)

41. At 15 months of age, a male infant is noted to have an open anterior fontanel during a routine visit to your office. You would

A. order a skull x-ray

B. order T3 and T4
C. administer MMR
D. administer corticosteroids
E. order a chromosomal study   (12:192)

42. A two-week-old white boy is seen because of vomiting for one day. He has had four stools and wet 12 diapers within the last 24 hours. His weight is 300 g (10 oz) less than at birth, his fontanelle is depressed, and his peripheral pulse is barely palpable. Electrolyte determination in his serum indicates Na^+ 120 mEq/liter, K^+ 7.6 mEq/liter, Cl^- 82 mEq/liter, CO_2 16 mEq/liter, and glucose 40 mg%. The most likely diagnosis is

A. pyloric stenosis
B. pneumococcal meningitis
C. adrenogenital syndrome
D. bilateral hydronephrosis due to urethral valves
E. diabetes mellitus   (12:1482-1488)

43. A five-year-old girl has had abdominal pain and vomiting for one day. She was lethargic but her appetite was good. Compared to 8 months ago, she has lost 6.5 lb (3 kg). You would now

A. order urinalysis
B. order SGPT and SGOT
C. order a plain film of the abdomen
D. order intravenous urography
E. order a skull CT scan   (12:1406-1407)

44. A full-time working mother brings her four-week-old baby for the first office visit. Her birth was 7 lb 4 oz and the weight in the office 8 lb 8 oz. She is bottle feeding the baby and is worried about adequate nutrition and weight gain. You would

A. reassure her
B. order CBC for the baby
C. order CBC for the mother
D. advise breast feeding
E. advise the use of soybean milk   (12:18)

45. A newborn baby presents with jaundice, hepatomegaly, and seizure. The eye ground reveals retinal hemorrhages, and skull x-rays show multiple punctate calcifications. The most likely diagnosis is

A. cystocercosis
B. cytomegalic inclusion disease
C. toxoplasmosis
D. Wilson's disease

E. biliary obstruction   (26:271)

46. A 50-year-old woman has Huntington's disease. The risk of her 30-year-old daughter developing the condition is

   A. 100%
   B. 50%
   C. 25%
   D. 5%
   E. 0%   (76:2121)

47. A 28-year-old school teacher has brought her three-year-old boy to your office. She states that her father-in-law stayed with them for three weeks last month and she has just learned that he has had active tuberculosis. The boy is asymptomatic and the physical examinations are essentially normal. The tuberculin test is negative. Now you would

   A. start isoniazid and rifampin combination therapy for 18 months
   B. reassure the mother that no medications are necessary at this point
   C. give the booster of rubeola vaccine
   D. start isoniazid for three months and reevaluate the situation
   E. give influenza immunization for preventive protection   (12:722)

48. Methylmalonic acidemia of the fetus can be treated by the mother's ingestion of

   A. thiamine
   B. vitamin B2
   C. alcohol
   D. vitamine B12
   E. steroids   (12:426)

Directions: For each of the incomplete statements below, ONE or MORE of the numbered completions is correct. In each case select:

   A. if only 1, 2, and 3 are correct
   B. if only 1 and 3 are correct
   C. if only 2 and 4 are correct
   D. if only 4 is correct
   E. if all are correct

49. The causes of increased IgM concentrations in infants in the first week of life include

   1. chronic intrauterine infection
   2. normalcy

   3. perinatal infection
   4. maternal narcotic addiction   (12:507)

50. The breasts of a five-day-old male infant are found to be engorged. You would

   1. perform incision and drainage
   2. institute a hormonal therapy
   3. admit the patient and order a chromosome study
   4. leave him alone and reassure the parents   (11:200)

51. Causes of jaundice during the first week of life include

   1. enclosed hemorrhage
   2. rubella syndrome
   3. transient familial neonatal hyperbilirubinemia
   4. Crigler-Najjar's syndrome   (12:356)

52. Juvenile rheumatoid arthritis is characterized by

   1. stiffness following inactivity
   2. nephritis
   3. fever and rash
   4. rheumatic carditis   (11:364-366)

53. The signs and symptoms of hypervitaminosis D include

   1. polyuria
   2. pallor
   3. hypercalcemia
   4. decreased serum phosphorus level   (11:35)

54. Delayed dentition may be due to

   1. cretinism
   2. malnutrition
   3. familial tendency
   4. fluoridation of drinking water   (12:22)

55. At eight weeks of age, the infant

   1. no longer displays tonic neck attitude
   2. follows a moving object 180° with its eyes
   3. has sagging of the head on ventral suspension
   4. smiles on social contact, listens to voices and coos   (12:23)

56. At 40 weeks of age, the infant

   1. sits erect for sustained periods
   2. pulls himself to a standing position

3. grasps objects with his thumb and forefinger
4. responds to his name, waves bye-bye
(12:25)

57. Which of the following is true of subacute bacterial endocarditis?

1. frequently shows Osler's nodes
2. gallop rhythm may be present
3. EKG may show prolongation of the P-R interval
4. *Streptococcus faecalis* is involved in the majority of cases   (11:274-276)

58. Features associated with sickle cell anemia are

1. autosplenectomy
2. bone infarcts
3. *Salmonella* infection
4. pain crisis   (12:1223-1225)

59. Acute renal failure is characterized by

1. hyperkalemia
2. acidosis
3. high serum creatinine
4. low serum concentration of urea   (12:1357)

60. Severe reactions to stings of *Hymenoptera* (bees, wasps, hornets, etc.)

1. may be local in nature
2. may be anaphylactic in nature
3. may recur if the patient is bitten again by an insect of the same species
4. require desensitization therapy   (11:462)

61. Tick paralysis

1. is produced by the saliva of the tick
2. usually begins in the arms
3. is marked by a rapid and complete recovery if the tick is removed quickly
4. is a flaccid descending motor paralysis   (12:871)

62. Following adequate therapy for influenzal meningitis, the focal neurological signs and fever persist and the spinal fluid does not become sterile. You will give a(n)

1. pleural tap
2. urinary catheterization
3. abdominal tap
4. subdural tap   (11:219)

63. Which of the following features is characteristic of influenzal meningitis?

1. often preceded by an upper respiratory infection
2. often accompanied by otitis media
3. smear and culture on chocolate agar of spinal fluid reveals Gram-negative pleomorphic coccobacillis
4. purpuric lesions are the most frequent presenting signs   (12:656)

64. The causes of neonatal convulsions include

1. anoxia
2. addicted mother
3. maple syrup urine disease
4. severe infections   (12:1531)

65. In order to teach a new task to a child, it is wise to

1. reinforce immediately after the act
2. allow a delay between the response and reinforcement
3. gradually shift to unpredictable intermittent reinforcement
4. insist on perfect performance on the first try   (24:35)

66. In children, a good way to modify behavior is to

1. specify signals to the children so that they understand what is expected of them
2. ignore disruptive behaviors
3. praise children for improvement in behavior
4. award privileges to those showing good behavior   (24:13)

67. Effective punishment includes

1. preventing avoidance of and escape from the punisher
2. reducing the need for subsequent punishment
3. not providing a model of aggressive behavior
4. avoidance of producing in the child a hateful attitude towards the punisher   (24:124)

68. In order to change inappropriate behavior in children, it is best to

1. immediately reinforce favorable behaviors

by attention, praise, and physical contact
2. punish inappropriate behaviors to weaken the responses
3. punish disruptive behaviors by withholding all forms of reinforcement
4. repeatedly attend undesirable behaviors
(24:15)

69. A six-year-old boy is admitted for elective surgery. There are many signs that he is fearful of body damage. In order to minimize lasting emotional trauma, the doctor should

1. explain to the child before the operation what he will experience and what he will likely feel
2. after the operation, be available to him to elicit his reactions
3. encourage the mother to remain with the child during most of the day and, if possible, overnight
4. guarantee the child that the procedure will not hurt
(1:605)

70. An infant who does not have a mother or a mother substitute and who is raised under conditions where little attention is given to his psychological needs may show signs of

1. marasmus
2. adequate ego development
3. delayed development
4. manic behavior
(1:974)

71. Factors known to be strongly associated with battered children are

1. young parents
2. age less than three years
3. drug-addicted parents
4. adoptive parents
(1:976-977)

72. Clinical features that should arouse suspicion of the battered-child syndrome are a

1. five-month-old with a fractured femur caused by getting his leg caught in the crib sides
2. 10-month-old with height and weight less than the third percentile who is unable to crawl or sit and lies in bed motionless with an intense gaze
3. five-month-old with a burn of the perineum who was placed in a bathtub of water that was too hot
4. six-month-old with an acute subdural

hematoma found on investigation for repeated vomiting without any history of head trauma
(12:109)

73. Correct statements about cat-scratch disease include which of the following?

1. local lymph nodes are enlarged
2. there is conjunctival involvement
3. granulomatous lesions are typical
4. meningoencephalitis is a complication
(12:949-950)

74. Smallpox vaccination

1. should be given routinely to American children
2. should be given to children in the endemic area
3. improves eczema
4. may produce postvaccinal encephalomyelitis (allergic encephalitis) as a complication
(12:761-763)

75. Therapeutic administration of oxygen to a premature infant may cause

1. retrolental fibroplasia
2. Wilson-Mikity's syndrome
3. bronchopulmonary dysplasia
4. cerebral hemorrhage
(12:347)

76. *Mycoplasma pneumoniae* (Eaton agent) infections may be manifested by

1. cervical adenitis
2. lung infiltrates on roentgenogram of the chest
3. clinical responsiveness to erythromycin therapy
4. increased cold agglutinin titer
(12:742)

77. Bronchiolitis

1. is the same as asthma
2. may be caused by the respiratory syncytial and influenzal viruses
3. is most commonly seen in children over nine years of age
4. is usually preceded by upper respiratory infection
(11:242)

78. The common causes of vomiting in children include

1. URI
2. gastroenteritis

3. GU infection
4. intestinal obstructions   *(12:888)*

79. A child who is more than 10% dehydrated should be

1. kept on a regular diet
2. treated by diuretics
3. kept on fluid-restriction diet
4. corrected by immediate intravenous feeding   *(12:235)*

80. Goodpasture's syndrome is a combination of

1. pulmonary alveolar hemorrhage
2. lupus
3. glomerulonephritis
4. erythema nodosum   *(12:585)*

81. All American children should receive immunization during the first year of life against

1. diphtheria and pertussis
2. poliomyelitis
3. tetanus
4. smallpox   *(12:187)*

82. A baby in the nursery has developed diarrhea. You would now

1. culture the stool
2. discharge all the infants from the nursery
3. enforce handwashing by the nursery personnel
4. initiate erythromycin therapy   *(12:408)*

83. The following statements are true for the comparison of human milk and cow's milk:

1. the water content of human milk is much higher than that of cow's milk
2. human milk provides more calories per ounce than cow's milk
3. cow's milk contains a higher proportion of fat than human milk
4. cow's milk contains a higher proportion of protein than human milk   *(12:150)*

84. A nine-year-old girl has recovered from acute rheumatic fever. You would now

1. reassure her that she has acquired an immunity toward rheumatic fever
2. prescribe oral penicillin (200,000 units daily) for 10 days
3. prescribe tetracyclines (2 g daily) for 2 weeks

4. continue administration of benzathine penicillin G (1,200,000 units IM) every four weeks   *(12:594)*

85. A six-month-old black infant is seen in the office for the first time after birth. His birth weight was 4 lb (1.8 kg) and he weighs 13 lb (6 kg) now. He was breast-fed without any supplements. On physical examination, he appears to be alert and well developed but pale. The remaining examination is unremarkable. His hemoglobin is 9.0 g%. You would now

1. order a bilirubin level test
2. perform bone marrow aspiration
3. order a serum ion level test
4. examine a blood smear   *(12:1214-1216)*

86. A 10-month-old girl is brought to your office by her mother for diarrhea and vomiting for the past 24 hours. She has had 16 to 18 watery stools which are hard to distinguish from urine. She is pale, cyanotic, lethargic, and irritable, with doughy skin and parcheal tongue. You would now

1. order blood gasses
2. order serum electrolytes
3. order a barium enema
4. measure body weight   *(12:233)*

87. A differential diagnosis of wheezing in children may include

1. cystic fibrosis
2. asthma
3. foreign body aspiration
4. atelectasis   *(12:1076)*

88. A two-year-old girl has been found to be loosing weight during the past three monthly visits. You would now

1. order brain scans
2. perform detailed physical examinations
3. order intravenous urography
4. take a detailed psychosocial history   *(12:253-254)*

89. A seven-year-old boy is brought to your office by his mother for his first medical care since birth. Physical examinations are essentially normal. However, he has never received any immunizations before. You would now

1. agree with the mother that regular well child care is useless
2. administer Salk vaccine
3. give pertussis vaccine
4. perform a tuberculin test   (104:902)

Directions: Each group of numbered words or phrases is followed by a list of lettered statements. MATCH the lettered statement most closely associated with the numbered word or phrase.

Questions 90 to 93

90. Congenital porphyria
91. Blue-diaper syndrome
92. Abeta-lipoproteinemia
93. Homogentisic acid

A. Acanthocytes
B. Dark-brown-stained diaper
C. Hypercalcemia, nephrocalcinosis, and indicanuria
D. Burgundy-red urine   (11:103-110)

Questions 94 and 95

94. 45 chromosome XO
95. Trisomy 21

A. Turner's syndrome
B. Down's syndrome   (1:5417)

Questions 96 to 99

96. Mental retardation; dry, baggy skin; scanty, coarse hair; thick tongue; umbilical hernia; coarse, harsh voice; short, pudgy extremities; delayed dentition
97. Mental retardation; congenital heart disease; speckling of the iris; traverse fissure of the palm; high palatal arch; incurving little finger
98. Mental retardation; thick lips and tongue; enlargement of the liver and spleen with a protruding belly; large head; membranous corneal veil
99. Viral infection in the mother during the early months of pregnancy

A. Down's syndrome
B. Gargoylism
C. Cretinism
D. None of the above   (73:131-145)

Questions 100 to 104

100. Sustained muscular contraction on the attempted use of a muscle after rest
101. Abnormal fatigability of skeletal muscles
102. Pseudohypertrophy of muscles
103. Reversible paralysis of striated muscle
104. Fine fasciculations of the tongue, often with atrophy

A. Infantile muscular atrophy (Werdnig-Hoffmann's disease)
B. Myotonia congenita
C. Progressive muscular dystrophy
D. Myasthenia gravis
E. Familial periodic paralysis   (12:1610)

Questions 105 to 108

105. Age 18 months
106. Age 10 months
107. Age 12 months
108. Age 3 years

A. Rides a tricycle, counts from one to three
B. Says two or three words
C. Stands without support
D. Builds a tower of three or four blocks   (12:23-25)

Questions 109 to 112

109. Atrial septal defect (ASD)
110. Patent ductus arteriosus (PDA)
111. Aortic insufficiency
112. Mitral insufficiency

A. Holosystolic murmur
B. Continuous murmur
C. High-pitched decrescendo diastolic murmur
D. Constant splitting of pulmonary second sound (P_2)   (12:1103-1104)

Questions 113 to 117

113. Boot-shaped heart on roentgenogram
114. Left-axis deviation on electrocardiogram
115. Palliative therapy by balloon septostomy
116. May be caused by rubella virus
117. Peripheral pulses of poor quality

A. Peripheral pulmonary arterial stenosis
B. Hypoplastic left ventricle
C. Tetralogy of Fallot

D. Transposition of the great vessels
E. Tricuspid atresia   (12:1123-1167)

Questions 118 to 121
118. Atypical lymphocytes
119. Conversion to leukemia
120. Viral etiology
121. Intestinal obstruction

   A. Infectious mononucleosis
   B. Lymphosarcoma
   C. Both
   D. Neither   (12:766,947)

Questions 122 to 125
122. Positive tourniquet test
123. Prolonged PTT
124. CNS hemorrhage
125. Hemarthrosis

   A. Idiopathic thrombocytopenic purpura (ITP)
   B. Classic hemophilia
   C. Both
   D. Neither   (12:1244,1251)

Questions 126 to 129

For each numbered disease below, select the lettered characteristic that would be present in a 13-month-old infant with that disease.

126. Acute lymphocytic leukemia
127. Hereditary spherocytosis
128. Folic acid deficiency
129. Iron deficiency anemia   (12:1214-1263)

   A. Microcytosis
   B. Autosomal recessive inheritance
   C. Hypersegmented neutrophils
   D. Thrombocytopenia
   E. Increased osmotic fragility

Questions 130 to 132
130. Pyloric stenosis
131. Infantile diarrhea
132. Salicylate intoxication

   A. Increase in pH
   B. Decrease in pH
   C. No change in pH   (11:79-80)

Questions 133 to 137
133. CSF cell 120; L:N = 95:5; sugar 70
134. CSF cell 1200; L:N = 5:95; sugar 20
135. CSF cell 120; L:N = 60:40; sugar 20; chloride 400 mg/100 ml
136. CSF protein 150; albuminocytologic dissociation
137. CSF cell 30, mostly lymphocytes; protein 30; sugar 60; pressure 250 mmH$_2$O

   A. Meningococcal meningitis
   B. Tuberculous meningitis
   C. Guillain-Barré's syndrome
   D. Brain tumor
   E. Aseptic meningitis   (11:216-222)

Questions 138 to 141
138. The lungs are the most frequent site for metastases
139. When the tumor is treated in the first year of life, the cure rate is greater than 20%
140. Ranks among the four most common malignant diseases in children less than 16 years of age
141. Can sometimes be found by bone marrow aspiration

   A. Neuroblastoma
   B. Wilm's tumor
   C. Both
   D. Neither   (11:419-420)

Questions 142 and 143
142. Kayser-Fleischer ring
143. Optic glioma

   A. Wilson's disease
   B. Von Recklinghausen's disease   (11:108,448)

Questions 144 to 147
144. Korsakoff's syndrome
145. Infantile autism
146. Lead poisoning
147. Encopresis

   A. Fecal soiling
   B. Pica
   C. Twirling
   D. Confabulation   (1:248-253)

Questions 148 to 151
148. Ethosuximide (Zarontin)   (3:258-259; 296)
149. EDTA

150. Imipramine (Tofranil)   *(3:557-559)*
151. Penicillamine   *(3:285-287)*

A. Enuresis
B. Petit mal
C. Hepatolenticular degeneration
D. Chronic lead poisoning

Questions 152 to 154
152. IQ 68-85
153. IQ < 20
154. IQ 36-51

A. Profound mental retardation
B. Severe mental retardation
C. Moderate mental retardation
D. Mild mental retardation
E. Borderline mental retardation   *(1:851)*

Questions 155 to 161
155. Positive culture from vesicles
156. Eruptions appear in various stages
157. Skin lesions primarily involve the trunk
158. Skin lesions primarily involve extremities
159. Active immunization with live attenuated virus after exposure can prevent the disease
160. Kaposi's varicelliform eruptions
161. Eruptions appear in the same stage

A. Smallpox
B. Chicken pox
C. Both
D. Neither   *(11:189)*

Questions 162 to 166
162. Scarlet fever
163. Diphtheria
164. Poliomyelitis
165. Measles
166. Chicken pox

A. Incubation period: 1 to 5 days
B. Incubation period: 7 to 10 days
C. Incubation period: 10 to 20 days
     (11:190-205)

Questions 167 and 168
167. Uroporphyrinogen-1 synthetase
168. C₁-esterase inhibitor

A. Hereditary spherocytosis
B. G6PD deficiency
C. Pseudocholinesterase deficiency
D. Acute intermittent porphyria
E. Hereditary angioedema   *(78:452)*

Questions 169 and 170
169. Basophilic stippling
170. Ovalocytes

A. folic acid deficiency
B. Elliptocytosis
C. lead poisoning
D. pernicious anemia
E. iron deficiency anemia   *(73:893-900)*

Directions: The following clinical set problem consists of clinical information presented in the format of questions or incomplete statements followed by a group of the numbered options. Indicate "T" if the option is true; indicate "F" if the option is false.

A four-year-old boy was brought to a Family Practice Center located at the underserved inner city by his mother. Both the mother and the boy are recent immigrants from Mexico and speak only a little English. The boy's aunt presented his complaints as sore throat and loss of appetite. The aunt also indicated that the boy has been treated for anemia back home and requested that you give him strong iron and vitamin shots. The physical examination revealed injected pharynx and enlarged red tonsils. The remaining examinations were unremarkable. You would now:

171. Prescribe vitamin E 100 IU 1 tablet t.i.d. for 1 month
172. Give him a shot of 0.5 ml (0.5 mg) vitamin B 12 (cyanocobalamin)
173. Administer 0.5 ml (25 mg) of ferrous gluconate injection
174. Administer I.M. pencillin G 1 million units
175. Take a throat culture
176. Prescribe erythromycin 250 mg b.i.d. for 5 days
177. Order hemoglobin, hematocrit and RBC count
178. Prescribe ampicillin 250 mg q.i.d. for 10 days
179. Prescribe ampicillin 250 mg in 5 ml syrup q.i.d for 10 days

One week later the boy returned to the Family Practice Center with his aunt. The aunt reported that sore throat has been resolved but the boy has had vague epigastric discomfort for almost a year without improvement. Physical examinations were essentially normal. You would now:
180. Order upper GI series
181. Order gastroendoscopy
182. Order stool examination for parasitic ova
183. Order gastric juice analysis

184. Prescribe cimetidine (Tagamet) 200 mg t.i.d. for 1 week

Ascariasis is suspected to be the diagnosis. Which of the following statements aid in identification of its eggs?

185. Yellowish oval shape with plug-like ends; measuring 50 × 23 μ

186. Asymmetric, flattened on one side; measuring 30 × 60 μ

187. Outer mamillated coverings, measuring 40 × 60 μ

Which of the following medications are effective for Ascariasis?

188. Piperazine (Antepar)

189. Pyrantel Pamoate (Antiminth)

190. Chlorquine (Aralen)   (*12:855*)

Answers and Explanations

1. **(A)** Because of a deficiency of pancreatic enzyme, pebble-like hard masses of tenacious meconium block the terminal ileum; the bowel proximal to this area is greatly dilated and filled with pasty meconium. Volvulus and gangrene of the dilated loops may occur with perforation. Sweat-electrolyte levels are elevated and a chloride level above 60 mEq/liter is significant. The gamma-globulin is also elevated.

2. **(A)** The cause is unknown, but a deficiency of surfactin and hypoperfusion may be associated. This condition is the major cause of death in the newborn period, with high incidence among premature babies.

3. **(E)** The routine administration to each infant in the nursery of full therapeutic doses of an antibiotic effective against the staphylococcal strain from the day of admission through the day of discharge is not a preferable aspect of management. Erythromycin is usually the drug of choice; kanamycin is too toxic.

4. **(D)** Niemann-Pick's disease is characterized in the tissues by vacuolated foam cells whose most striking chemical feature is the cytoplasmic accumulation of sphingomyelin (a phospholipid).

5. **(B)** Where normal parents have a child with harelip (with or without cleft palate), the average risk that another child will have a

similar malformation is about 5%. If the parents have had two affected children, the risk of having still another is about 10%. If one parent has the anomaly, the average risk for a child is 5%.

6. **(D)** Synthesis of red cell G6PD is determined by genes borne on the X chromosome. Thus G6PD deficiency is an X-linked recessive disease like hemophilia. Since the father's X chromosome carries the pathological trait of G6PD deficiency, all the daughters will become carriers of G6PD deficiency (each daughter has one X chromosome from the father; another X from the mother) and none of the sons will have G6PD deficiency traits (the Y of each son comes from the father and the X of each son comes from the mother). Since the sister of the mother has hemophilia, the sister's two Xs are both affected; one of the affected Xs is derived from the grandfather and another is derived from the grandmother. The grandfather is a hemophiliac, but the mother is not affected. She carries one affected X for hemophilia (received from the grandfather) and one normal X (received from the grandmother). The father carries normal XY for hemophilia. Thus half of the daughters will be carriers for hemophilia (one affected X from mother and one normal X from father), half of the daughters will be normal (one normal X from mother and one normal X from father), half of the sons will be normal (one normal X from mother and one Y from father) and

half of the sons will be carriers of hemophilia (one affected X from the mother and one Y from the father).

7. **(A)** Cholesterol is deposited in the reticulum cells in the disease. The classic triad consists of punched-out lesions in the skull, bilateral exophthalmos, and diabetes insipidus. There is a variety of skin lesions, including a diffuse papular eruption of vesicular nature in the young patient, a scaly and petechial dermatitis, and a moist, denuded involvement in intertriginous areas.

8. **(D)** Evaporated milk provides 40 cal/oz; thus it provides 40 cal/oz $\times$ 6 oz = 240 cal. Sugar provides 120 cal/oz; thus it provides 120 cal/oz $\times$ 3/4 oz = 90 cal.

Total calories: 240 cal + 90 cal = 330 cal

$$\text{Total fluid: } 6 \text{ oz} + 14 \text{ oz} + 3/4 \text{ oz} = 20.75 \text{ oz}$$
$$\text{cal/oz} = 330 \text{ cal}/20.75 \text{ oz}$$
$$= 16 \text{ cal}$$

9. **(C)** Symptoms of hypervitaminosis A can occur after a period of several weeks of 10 times the prophylactic dosage (1500-5000 IU). Bone pain, loss of hair, cheilosis, and benign intracranial hypertension (pseudotumor cerebri) may be noted as well.

10. **(C)** At birth, 7½ lb is the average weight; the weight is usually doubled by the fifth month and tripled by 12 months (22 lb). The birth weight is quadrupled (30 lb) at 2½ years of age. At 10 years of age the weight is 10 times that at birth (75 lb).

11. **(B)** The infant will be able to sit steadily by the age of 28 weeks.

12. **(B)** The daily requirement of potassium is 1-2 g or 1.5 mEq/kg.

13. **(D)** The symptoms of rheumatic fever usually do not develop until some time after the manifestations of the preceding streptococcal infection have disappeared. This latent period lasts from one to five weeks, and in chorea this may be two to six months. The presenting manifestation of acute rheumatic fever is commonly arthritis or choreiform movements in school-age children and carditis in very young children.

14. **(B)** Carditis occurs in 40% of patients during the first attack of rheumatic fever and may be the only major manifestation in infants and young children. Tachycardia and apical systolic murmur (sometimes with apical middiastolic murmur) are usually present.

15. **(A)** Excessive edema should be reduced by thiazides to improve the overall condition before instituting prednisolone therapy. Sodium intake is also to be restricted.

16. **(C)** Acute glomerulonephritis is probably due to hypersensitivity to an extrarenal infection with certain types of beta-hemolytic streptococci—e.g., Group A, Type 12. The antistreptolysin-O titer is elevated but the serum complement is diminished during the acute phase.

17. **(D)** Enuresis is urinary incontinence, usually nocturnal, past three years of age. Children develop bladder control at different ages. Many normal children may not develop bladder control until four years of age. Organic causes of enuresis include pyelitis, congenital malformation of the urinary tract, irritation of the genitalia, and spina bifida. Most commonly, enuresis is due to psychological maladjustment.

18. **(E)** Although girls are usually two years ahead of boys in growth, the changes can begin as early as six to eight years of age or as late as 15 to 17 years of age. Usually the "tincture of time" (the old remedy of the family doctor) will result in a satisfactory outcome. A healthy girl will usually reveal the appearance of pubic hair (which appears earlier than axillary hair), breast enlargement, sudden gain in height, and acne vulgaris as early signs of puberty.

19. **(A)** Four pathophysiological groups of neonatal infants are at high risk of developing hypoglycemia: (1) infants of diabetic mothers and infants with severe erythroblastosis fetalis; (2) low-birthweight infants (particularly infants of toxemic mothers); (3) very immature or severely ill infants; (4) infants with galactosemia, glycogen storage disease, maple syrup urine disease, leucine sensitivity, insulinomas, or Beckwith's syndrome. Onset is from a few hours to a week after birth. Symptoms include jitteriness or trem-

ors, cyanosis, apathy, convulsions, tachypnea, weak or high-pitched cry, limpness, difficulty in feeding, eye rolling, sudden pallor, sweating, and hypothermia. If the symptoms persist with the administration of sufficient glucose, other causes must be considered (including infections such as meningitis).

20. **(D)** The meningitic form presents symptoms and signs of meningitis plus those of septicemia (purpura). Endotoxic shock with disseminated intravascular coagulation (DIC) leading to adrenal hemorrhage and circulatory collapse (Waterhouse-Friderichsen's syndrome) occurs frequently with meningococcemia (hypotension, widespread purpura, rapid thready pulse, and coma). The treatment of shock includes hydrocortisone, isoproterenol, antibiotics, and adequate blood-volume replacement.

21. **(B)** In the newborn period, meningitis may occur secondary to *E. coli* infection. In later infancy, influenzal meningitis is most frequent, especially between the ages of six and 12 months. *Pneumococcus, Meningococcus,* and tuberculosis are also frequently encountered.

22. **(C)** There is frequently a family history of febrile convulsions. A normal electroencephalogram is obtained about one week after the seizure and prognosis is good. Convulsions usually disappear by the age of three years.

23. **(C)** Petit mal is characterized by episodes of abrupt, momentary loss of consciousness accompanied by cessation of voluntary activities. While having a petit mal attack, some children may perform semipurposeful motor acts, such as snapping of fingers, patting movements, or walking around in circles (petit mal automatism). When attacks occur in close succession for a prolonged period of time, mental function is continually impaired and the child remains dazed and confused. Myoclonic jerks may also present, known as petit mal status. The EEG abnormality consists of bursts of generalized bilaterally synchronous 3/second spikes, and wave complexes appear, usually against a background of normal activity. Bursts lasting longer than five seconds are often associated with clinical attacks.

24. **(A)** Bedtime crying is easily cured from the start by following a consistent bedtime routine, putting your child to bed, and leaving her. If she cries on being left, it should be ignored. The young child will quickly learn not to cry at bedtime.

25. **(D)** Pediatricians and family physicians have the responsibility of the total health needs of children, including the quality of the child's life in providing comprehensive and continuous care.

26. **(D)** The parents of delinquent children usually communicate their permissiveness to the children, though mostly through unconsciously driven behavior. Approval of the delinquent behavior of the children is often expressed in nonverbal forms, and parental disciplinary behavior usually lacks consistency.

27. **(A)** Screaming is a normal reaction for a child who becomes angry, usually because of frustration at failing to gain his desires, antagonism between himself and his parents, or jealousy between siblings. The behavioral syndrome that includes screaming, breath holding, kicking, and throwing himself on the floor is called a temper tantrum. Most preschool children have tantrums; they are considered pathological only when frequent and severe.

28. **(D)** Institutionalized children are frequently deprived of maternal care (or receive multimothering). The prolonged residence in poor environments often will lead to intellectual and personality deficiencies and also failure to develop normal patterns of social responsiveness due to understimulation. The child thus often becomes withdrawn and apathetic.

29. **(D)** This is a typical example of regression. A toilet-trained, first-born child may temporarily lose bladder and bowel control in response to the arrival of a second child in the family. Regression is the return to an earlier level of emotional adjustment (e.g., not toilet-trained) at which gratification was assured.

30. **(C)** Normal adolescence is characterized by a multitude of personality changes. The turmoil involves the adolescent's attempts to

establish himself as an independent individual. His efforts are often of a rebellious and radical nature. The adolescent boy may show rebellion, defiance, and antisocial feelings.

31. **(D)** The pathognomonic sign of rabies is to find the neuronal cytoplasm of the Negri body (inclusion body) in the skunk's brain or salivary gland. Examination of these tissues by the fluorescent antibody test is a rapid, reliable means of diagnosis. However, it's sometimes difficult to obtain the biting skunk for observations and examinations.

32. **(E)** The treatment of mumps is entirely by general measures. The use of hyperimmune mumps gamma-globulin not only does not significantly reduce complications, in some instances it actually increases their incidence. A live attenuated vaccine is available for prophylaxis.

33. **(E)** The acute asthmatic attack is usually treated with epinephrine, hydration, sedation, antibiotics, corticosteroids, and aminophylline. Hospitalization is often needed.

34. **(D)** Successful therapy may consist of the use of oxygen, sodium bicarbonate to correct acidosis, and adequate warm temperature. Monitoring of arterial pH and O_2 is indicated. Too high a level of oxgen administration may cause retrolental fibroplasia.

35. **(D)** Spasmodic croup is called midnight croup and is characterized by barking cough that improves with fresh air and IPPB. Bacterial (vast majority—*H. influenzae* Type B) croup occurs day or night with high fever and inflamed epiglottis. Treatment is by tracheostomy (in a third of cases), ampicillin, cool humidity, adequate fluids, and sometimes corticosteroids.

36. **(E)** Most commonly, the patient with staphylococcal pneumonia is an infant less than a year of age, often with a history of staphylococcal skin lesions and upper respiratory infection for several days to a week. Abrupt onset of fever, cough, and respiratory distress (grunting respirations, subcostal retractions, cyanosis), radiographic evidence of bronchopneumonia (mostly in the right lung), pleural effusion, empyema, pneumothorax, and pneumatoceles develop. Methi-

cillin is used before the sensitivity test. Surgical drainage of collections of pus may also be indicated.

37. **(A)** Recurrent abdominal pain in a child is usually caused by emotional stress. Abdominal epilepsy is a rare condition. The incidence of positive organic disorders in recurrent abdominal pain in children is about 7%. Although an IVP study is not required immediately, a urinalysis should be performed to rule out disease in the urinary tract. The family and personal history, together with the clinical examination and minimal investigation, will provide important evidence that there is no demonstrable organic disease and that there is an emotional disorder to account for the symptoms. These patients are usually tense, fussy, timid, anxious, and overconscientious. These children may also show emotional disturbance such as fears, sleep disorders, and school difficulties.

38. **(B)** Simple diarrhea in the child is best treated by supportive measures. Formula and solid foods are temporarily withheld to reduce the solute load reaching the diseased bowel and to diminish fecal water loss. Oral fluids, including warm dilute sugar solution, soft drinks exhausted of carbonation, and solutions of flavored gelatin mixes, are given frequently. More advanced cases may require intravenous fluid replacement.

39. **(D)** Cromolyn sodium (Intal, Aarane) is used for chemoprophylaxis of asthma and is not effective for acute asthmatic attack. It prevents antigen-induced release of chemical mediators. It is useful in the treatment of extrinsic or allergic asthma (such as exercise-induced asthma). The drug is used in children with intrinsic asthma who do not respond to theophylline and adrenergic agents.

40. **(C)** The live attenuated measles vaccine is recommended for primary immunization at age 15 months. Some infants less than 15 months of age fail to produce antibody for the vaccine due to persistent maternal antibody. Killed virus vaccine is not recommended; individuals receiving killed virus vaccine may develop a severe atypical form of measles when they are exposed to natural

measles later. Measles vaccine is also effective if given just after exposure.

41. **(C)** In a normal infant, the anterior fontanel closes between 9 and 18 months of age, and an open anterior fontanel occurring at 15 months of age is within the limits of the normal developmental stage; no work-ups are necessary at this time. MMR (measles, mumps, and rubella) primary immunization is recommended at 15 months of age. Persistent open fontanel may be caused by chromosomal abnormalities (Down's syndrome, trisomy 13 or 18), hypothyroidism, malnutrition, rubella syndrome, and skeletal disorders.

42. **(C)** The weight loss and physical examination of the infant suggest severe dehydration and impending shock. Twelve wet diapers in 24 hours suggest that the dehydration was caused by polyuria rather than by vomiting for one day. The chemical determinations reveal very low concentrations of Na and Cl and an elevated level of K. Glucose is low, ruling out diabetes mellitus. The large amount of urine and the four stools are incompatible with a diagnosis of pyloric stenosis; also, pyloric stenosis does not cause severe dehydration in one day of vomiting and usually presents with metabolic alkalosis and a low K level. Hydronephrosis would not cause the weight loss and severe shock-like picture at the age of two weeks. The hyperkalemia would be very unusual with pneumococcal meningitis, although the other signs could be present. With any form of meningitis, the fontanel would be bulging, whereas with dehydration it is usually depressed. The diagnosis of salt-losing adrenogenital syndrome is suggested by the chemical data, especially the high K concentration. In female infants, adrenogenital syndrome is associated with various forms of masculinization of the genitalia, which may be noticed at the time of birth. In males, the physical examination gives no clue, and the disease usually presents at any time between one and 10 weeks of age with vomiting and the clinical features described above. Saline infusion, or even oral saline administration, has a dramatic and life-saving effect and may even mask the clinical and chemical signs. Although cortisone is the rational therapy for the essential defect (inability of

the adrenal cortex to make cortisol), it does not work rapidly enough.

43. **(A)** A five-year-old child is expected to gain at least 3 lb during an eight-month period. Weight loss of 6.5 lb usually indicates a serious illness which has probably existed for longer than one day. Serum transaminase level (SGPT and SGOT) is useful in the diagnosis of hepatitis, which usually causes anorexia. An acute abdominal problem (acute appendicitis) usually does not cause weight loss and lethargy. Intravenous urography is useful in identifying renal diseases, which usually do not cause lethargy after one day of vomiting. Hyperthyroidism and diabetes mellitus may cause weight loss with a good appetite. Abdominal pain, vomiting, and lethargy are suspicious of diabetic ketoacidosis, and a thorough history (family history), physicals, and work-ups are mandatory.

44. **(A)**

$$7 \text{ lb } 4 \text{ oz} = 7.25 \text{ lb}$$
$$= 3.3 \text{ kg } (1 \text{ lb} = 0.45 \text{ kg})$$
$$8 \text{ lb } 8 \text{oz} = 3.8 \text{ kg}$$
$$3.8 \text{ kg} - 3.3 \text{ kg} = 0.5 \text{ kg} = 500 \text{ g}$$
$$4 \text{ weeks} = 28 \text{ days } (1 \text{ week} = 7 \text{ days})$$

The baby is presumed to regain her prior weight at 10 days of age; so that during the past 18 days (28 days − 10 days = 18 days) the baby has gained 28 g/day (500 g/ 18 days = 28 g/day). The average baby gains 25 g/day over this period, and anything over 20 g/day is normal. Although the mother's desire for breast feeding should be encouraged, it may not be practical for a full-time working mother to breastfeed her baby during working hours.

45. **(B)** Cytomegalic inclusion disease usually presents with jaundice, hepatosplenomegaly, prematurity, microcephaly, chorditis, necrotizing retinitis, retinal hemorrhages, microphthalmia, cataract, optic atrophy, and optic disk malformation. Interferon inducers (poly I:C) and arabinoside (Vidarabine) may be useful.

46. **(B)** Huntington's disease is characterized by choreiform movement, mental deterioration (dementia), and rigidity. It is transmitted by an autosomal dominant trait, with late onset

at 30 to 50 years. Thus the chance for children of an affected individual of eventually developing the disease is one in two.

47. **(D)** Isoniazid single-drug therapy should be instituted for the close contacts (such as household contacts) of patients with an active case of tuberculosis, even though the contacts' tuberculin skin tests are negative; early treatment prior to the hematogenous dissemination will promptly eradicate the tubercle bacilli before hypersensitivity develops. Isoniazid should continue for three months if the tuberculin test remains negative and no evidence of disease is present. If there is positive conversion of the tuberculin test, isoniazid (10-20 mg/kg) should be continued for a total of 12 months of chemoprophylaxis. In a tuberculin-positive child who receives rubeola vaccine or who has had rubeola, pertussis, or influenza, one month of isoniazid chemoprophylaxis is required. The initial therapy for tuberculosis is isoniazid and rifampin (10 mg/kg) for 12 months.

48. **(D)** Methylmalonic acidemia is associated with mental retardation and metabolic acidosis. In vitamin B12 responsive variant, prenatal diagnosis can be done and the mother can be treated with large doses of vitamin B12 during her last trimester.

49. **(B)** The IgM concentrations in infants during the first week of life will be increased beyond the level of 17 mg/100 ml in patients with chronic intrauterine infections or perinatal infection.

50. **(D)** Engorgement of the infant's breasts due to maternal (placental and ovarian) estrogen stimulation may occur a few days after birth in either sex. The maternal hormone prolactin, from the anterior pituitary, may produce oozing of milk ("witch's milk"). These signs subside spontaneously and no treatment is indicated.

51. **(E)** The causes of jaundice during the first week of life include physiological jaundice, cretinism. Crigler-Najjar's syndrome, transient familial hyperbilirubinemia, novobiocin, vitamin K, sepsis, hepatitis, toxoplasmosis, cytomegalic inclusion disease, rubella, and galactosemia.

52. **(B)** Only a small percentage of children with rheumatoid arthritis will be found positive for the tests for rheumatic factors (e.g., latex). C-reactive protein is frequently positive, sedimentation rate is usually increased, and antistreptolysin-O titer is usually elevated. Gamma-globulin is usually elevated and LE cells may be observed in up to 5% of patients.

53. **(A)** Hypervitaminosis D results in increased serum phosphorus and calcium crystals and casts in the urine, with eventual renal damage and nitrogen retention. Hypertension may develop.

54. **(A)** Delay in eruption of deciduous teeth occurs in hypothyroidism (cretinism) and in other nutritional and growth disturbances (e.g., prolonged illness in infancy). In some families, the children have conspicuously early or late dentition without other signs of retardation or acceleration of growth. Thus the delay in dentition is not a good index of growth disorder.

55. **(C)** At eight weeks, the head is sustained in the plane of the body on ventral suspension; tonic neck posture predominates.

56. **(E)** At 40 weeks, in addition, an infant will be able to creep or crawl.

57. **(A)** Osler's nodes are pathognomonic erythematous painful nodules in the fingertips. *Streptococcus viridans* is involved in the majority of cases. Murmurs of changing character are heard.

58. **(E)** Sickle cell anemia is a severe, chronic, hemolytic anemia occurring mainly in Blacks with the homozygous sickle gene (hemoglobin S 75-98%; fetal hemoglobin 2-25%). The clinical course is marked by episodes of pain (crisis) due to occlusion of small blood vessels by spontaneously sickled red cells. Patients with sickle cell anemia frequently also suffer from gallstones, nephrotic syndrome (renal concentrating defect), pneumococcal meningitis, autosplenectomy, *Salmonella* osteomyelitis, infarctions, and delayed puberty.

59. **(A)** Acute renal failure is due to markedly

disturbed tubular function resulting from mechanical (calculi), chemical (sulfa drugs), or hypoxic (dehydration, shock, burns) damage which impairs the ability to conserve water. Oliguria or anuria is characteristic, with low blood pressure and shock. Hyperkalemia; hyponatremia; metabolic acidosis; elevation of serum concentrations of urea, phosphate, uric acid and creatinine; hypocalcemia; and anemia are often present.

60. **(E)** Stinging insect allergy is best managed by desensitization therapy. The reactions after subsequent stingings have been markedly reduced in 90% of hyposensitized individuals. Local reaction includes swelling, itching, and burning; the systemic reaction includes generalized urticaria, anaphylactic shock (hypotension, cyanosis, unconsciousness), wheezing, dyspnea, laryngeal edema with hoarseness, abdominal pain, vomiting, and angioedema.

61. **(B)** Tick paralysis can be produced by the Rocky Mountain wood tick and is characterized by a flaccid ascending motor paralysis that begins in the legs.

62. **(D)** Subdural collections of fluid may be associated with meningitis, particularly *H. influenzae* meningitis. If subdural taps produce fluid, it should be removed by repeated aspirations.

63. **(A)** Purpuric lesions are suggestive of meningococcal meningitis.

64. **(E)** Neonatal convulsions usually point to a disorder of the central nervous system and suggest anoxic brain damage, intracranial hemorrhage, cerebral anomaly, subdural effusion, meningitis, tetany, or, rarely, pyridoxine deficiency, hypoglycemia, hyponatremia, or hypernatremia.

65. **(B)** There are three useful rules concerning the proper method of reinforcement. They are:
1. In teaching new tasks, reinforce immediately rather than permitting a delay between the response and reinforcement.
2. In the early stages of learning a task, reinforce every correct response. As the behavior becomes stronger, require more and more responses before reinforcing

(shift gradually to unpredictable intermittent reinforcement).
3. Reinforce improvement or steps in the right direction. Do not insist on perfect performance on the first try.

66. **(E)** The following three procedures are useful in changing children's behavior:
1. Give clear signals. Make the rules clear so that the children know what is expected of them. Repeat the rules as necessary.
2. Ignore disruptive behaviors. Do not attend to the behaviors you wish to weaken. Get involved with other children showing behaviors you wish to strengthen. Praise a child showing behavior incompatible with disruptive behaviors.
3. Praise the children for improvement in behavior. Notice the children who are being good, rather than bad. Tell them what it is they're doing that you like. Award privileges to those showing good behavior.

67. **(E)** Effective punishment must do at least four things:
1. Prevent avoidance of and escape from the punisher
2. Reduce the need for subsequent punishment
3. Not provide a model of aggressive behavior
4. Avoid teaching the child a hateful attitude towards the punisher

68. **(A)** To change the inappropriate behavior of children, the following rules are very useful:
1. Follow responses you wish to strengthen with reinforcing events (e.g., attention, praise, physical contact).
2. Follow reponses you wish to weaken with punishing events.
3. Withhold all forms of reinforcement for specified time periods.
4. Responses can be weakened by not reinforcing (e.g., ignoring) them.

69. **(A)** To minimize the child's emotional reaction and to prevent long-term psychological difficulties, he should be prepared to cope with the stress of either elective or emergency surgery. The realistic situation should be explained to him in terms he can understand. Parents should possess cheerful attitudes; the mother should stay if at all

possible. The anesthesiologist should familiarize the child preoperatively with a light sleep premedication. Following the operation, the family physician should be available to support the child.

70. **(B)** An infant without adequate mothering will frequently develop intellectual and language retardation and at times severe debility (marasmus). The infant will tend to become withdrawn and apathetic.

71. **(A)** The child abuse (battered child) syndrome is frequently associated with young, addicted, unhappily married parents. The parents committing the abuse frequently were themselves abused as children. Child abuse occurs less often in children older than three years and less often involves adoptive parents. The children abused are frequently children with low birthweight.

72. **(E)** Battered child syndrome is frequently diagnosed by a high index of suspicion. Subdural hematoma with absence of diagnostic evidence of hemorrhagic diathesis or accidental trauma is frequently caused by violent shaking. Stories of babies under six months old trying to get out of the crib and fracturing the femur are usually fabrications. The child with failure to thrive due to caloric deprivation usually has a weight and height less than the third percentile. Hot water burns on the perineum are usually done by parents for the punishment of enuresis or resistance to toilet training.

73. **(E)** The cat-scratch disease is thought to be due to a large virus and is possibly due to contact with a domestic cat. Clinical manifestations include cervical adenitis, transient pulmonary infiltration, conjunctivitis, and enlargement of preauricular and cervical lymph nodes. Erythema multiforme and nodosum, and meningoencephalitis have also been observed.

74. **(C)** If all American children were to receive smallpox vaccinations, the risk of vaccination complications would be considerably higher than the present risks of smallpox.

75. **(E)** Oxygen tension in the arterial blood is kept in the range of 50-80 mmHg when assisted ventilation is being used. The princi-

ple of using as little oxygen as possible for the shortest possible time must be rigidly adhered to in the therapy of infants. Premature infants receiving 30-40% oxygen may develop retrolental fibroplasia.

76. **(E)** A few patients have no abnormal physical findings, although some have maculopapular or urticarial rash, which usually disappears within 48 hours. Chest x-ray usually shows evidence of pneumonia before physical signs are apparent.

77. **(C)** Bronchiolitis can be a severe infection and is rarely seen in patients over two years old. It may be caused by virus (ECHO 11, adenovirus, influenza A, parainfluenza, and respiratory syncytial) or bacteria (*H. influenzae*).

78. **(E)** Children react by vomiting to most insults, especially infections. Not infrequently, vomiting will precede fever.

79. **(D)** Losses of body weight in excess of 1% per day represent loss of body water. A 5-10% loss represents moderate dehydration; a 10-15% loss is severe and is frequently associated with or indicates approaching peripheral circulatory failure.

80. **(B)** Goodpasture's syndrome, a combination of pulmonary alveolar hemorrhage and glomerulonephritis, overlaps with polyarteritis nodosa and idiopathic pulmonary hemosiderosis. Antibiotics reactive with glomerular and alveolar basement membranes are involved in pathogenesis. The clinical syndrome includes hemoptysis, anemia, and nephritis. Corticosteroids may be helpful.

81. **(A)** The smallpox vaccination is not recommended for American children except those traveling to endemic areas.

82. **(B)** Epidemic diarrhea of the newborn may be caused by pathogenic *E. coli, Salmonella,* echovirus, and adenovirus. Stool culture and antibiotic sensitivity should be performed to initiate effective therapy, when indicated. The afflicted infants should be monitored for fluid and electrolyte balance. The handwashing technique should be enforced for all nursery personnel to control the spread of the disease. If the disease is under control, there

is no need to discharge all infants from the nursery. Follow-up stool cultures for recovered infants are necessary.

83. (D)

Constituents	Human milk (%)	Cow's milk (%)
Water	88	88
Protein	1.1	3.3
Fat	3.8	3.8
Sugar	7.0	4.8

The energy values of human milk and cow's milk are essentially the same: 20 kcal/oz or 0.67 kcal/ml.

84. (D) Continuous administration of chemoprophylaxis will prevent streptococcal infections and recurrences of acute rheumatic fever. Regimens of oral penicillin have met with poor compliance by patients and should only be reserved for patients who are reliable, who have had minimal heart disease, and who have suffered from initial attacks of rheumatic fever. Chemoprophylaxis should be continued through childhood. During adulthood, patients who are at high risk of exposure to streptococcal infections (such as school teachers or people in the military services) should continue the chemoprophylaxis.

85. (D) Breast milk contains only trace amounts of iron and of vitamin D, both of which are required in higher than average amounts in an infant who has more than tripled his birth weight in 6 months. Iron deficiency anemia is the most likely diagnosis and a blood smear would characteristically show microcytosis, anisocytosis, poikilocytosis, and hypochromia. Microcytosis and hypochromia can also be shown by the erythrocyte indices. However, sickle cell anemia is a possibility and blood smear examination yields more information than the measurement of erythrocyte indices.

86. (C) The large number of watery stools and vomiting are responsible for severe dehydra-

tion. Lethargy, irritability, and "doughy" skin are characteristic of hypertonic dehydration, which requires rapid intravenous infusion of saline (half isotonic and contains glucose) to restore the circulating blood volume and glomerular filtration.

87. (E) Wheezing is a musical, high-pitched, continuous, expiratory (and sometimes inspiratory) sound, usually associated with a prolonged expiratory phase. It is caused by partial obstruction of the central and medium-sized airway. Wheezing is a common complaint in children, and the list of differential diagnoses includes asthma, cystic fibrosis, bronchiectasis, bronchiolitis, pneumonias, atelectasis, pulmonary tuberculosis, alpha-1-antitrypsin deficiency, foreign body aspiration, hypersensitivity pneumonitis, and chronic aspiration.

88. (C) Failure to thrive (inadequate weight gain) may be caused by many problems, including malignancies (especially of the kidney, adrenal, and brain) and endocrine disorders (hypothyroidism), but is most commonly due to emotional deprivation, environmental disruptions, inadequate food intake, child abuse, or maternal neglect. A detailed history (including dietary and psychosocial histories) and physicals should first be obtained to identify the causes.

89. (D) Primary immunization for children not immunized in infancy is as follows.

Schedule	Under 6 years	Over 6 years
First visit	DPT$_1$, TOPV$_1$, TT	Td$_1$, TOPV$_1$, TT
1 month	MMR (over 15 months)	MMR
2 months	DPT$_2$, TOPV$_2$	Td$_2$, TOPV$_2$
4 months	DPT$_3$	
10-16 months	DPT$_4$, TOPV$_3$	Td$_3$, TOPV$_3$
14-16 years	Td (every 10 years)	Td (every 10 years)

DPT: diphtheria, pertussis, tetanus.
Td: tetanus, diphtheria (no pertussis).
TOPV: trivalent oral polio, TOPV primary immu-

nizations require only two doses (TOPV$_1$, and TOPV$_2$); the third dose (at 6 months) is only required in endemic areas; Salk vaccine is not commonly used.

MMR: measles, mumps, rubella (German measles), given when the child is over 15 months of age.

90. (D)

91. (C)

92. (A)

93. (B) Congenital porphyria is characterized by the excretion of urine that is burgundy-red as passed or becomes so upon exposure to light; this begins at birth or shortly thereafter. Blue-diaper syndrome is a familial disorder of Hartnup's disease characterized by hypercalcemia, nephrocalcinosis, and indicanuria. Abeta-lipoproteinemia is an autosomal recessive disease characterized by steatorrhea, ataxia, acanthocytosis, and retinitis pigmentosa. Alkaptonuria is due to the absence in the liver of the enzyme homogentisic acid oxidase. The accumulation of homogentisic acid causes the dark brown staining of urine-moistened diapers.

94. (A)

95. (B) Turner's syndrome (female gonadal dysgenesis) is manifested by females with 45 chromosome XO. Patients are short and stocky, with webbing of the neck and lack of secondary sexual characteristics at puberty. Down's syndrome (mongolism) is associated with trisomy at the twenty-first autosomal chromosome.

96. (C)

97. (A)

98. (B)

99. (D) Congenital rubella, associated with rubella infection of the mother in the first trimester, causes mental retardation, deafness, cataract, and cardiac anomalies.

100. (B)

101. (D)

102. (C)

103. (E)

104. (A) Myotonia congenita (Thomsen's disease) is transmitted by dominant inheritance. Slow swallowing and gagging in infancy and inability to release a firm hand grip in childhood may arouse attention. The muscles are still upon the first attempt to carry out a motion; the stiffness subsides when the movement is repeated a few times. Myasthenia gravis is frequently associated with thymoma and lupus erythematosus. Ptosis, double vision, and muscle weakness without muscular atrophy are usually present. Muscle strength will be increased by administration of Tensilon or neostigmine. Progressive muscular dystrophy (the childhood or Duchenne type) is characterized by pseudohypertrophy of calf, deltoid, brachioradialis, and tongue muscle. Familial periodic paralysis is transmitted in a dominant manner. Paralysis of striated muscle is reversible and frequently follows large carbohydrate meals or rest after strong exercise. Serum potassium is low during paralysis. Werdnig-Hoffman's disease is transmitted by a recessive trait with atrophy of anterior horn cells in the spinal cord and of motor nuclei in the brainstem. The legs tend to lie in a frog-leg position, with hips abducted and knees flexed. Fibrillations usually are visible in the tongue.

105. (D)

106. (C)

107. (B)

108. (A) The child smiles (on social contact) by two months of age; can stand without support by 10 months of age; can say two or three words (e.g., Mama, Dada) communicatively by one year of age; and can ride a tricycle at three years.

109. (D)

110. (B)

111. (C)

112. (A) Early, high-pitched diastolic murmurs are usually due to incompetence of the aortic or pulmonary valves. Pansystolic (regurgitation) murmurs are from mitral or tricuspid insufficiency and VSD. Wide splitting of second sound is seen in ASD. The continuous "machinery" murmur is classic for PDA.

113. (C)

114. (E)

115. (D)

116. (A)

117. (B) Tetralogy of Fallot includes pulmonary stenosis, ventricular septal defect, hypertrophic right ventricle, and dextroposition of the aorta. Roentgenogram reveals a normal-sized, boot-shaped heart with decrease of pulmonary markings. Tricuspid atresia causes cyanosis, polycythemia, exertional dyspnea, and anoxic hypercyanotic attacks early in life. EKG shows left axis deviation, left ventricular hypertrophy, and peaked P-wave. Transposition of the great vessels causes intense cyanosis and dyspnea observed within the first week of life with possible cardiac failure. After the diagnosis has been confirmed in the catheterization laboratory on an emergency basis, a large interatrial communication is created by the balloon atrial septostomy to rupture the foramen ovale until surgical correction is undertaken. Single or multiple constrictions may occur anywhere along the major branches of the pulmonary artery. Peripheral pulmonary stenosis may be caused by congenital rubella syndrome and has a familial tendency. Hypoplastic left ventricle causes weak peripheral pulses; heart failure often appears in the first week of life.

118. (C)

119. (B)

120. (A)

121. (B) Lymphosarcoma is the most common malignant neoplasm of the gastrointestinal tract in early life. Presenting complaints include abdominal pain and palpable mass, which may be the neoplasm or an intussusception. Some cases are difficult to distinguish from acute lymphatic leukemia.

Infectious mononucleosis is caused by Epstein and Barr's (EB) virus and is characterized by fever, cervical adenopathy, sore throat, maculopapular rash, and splenomegaly. Atypical lymphocytes (at least 10%) and heterophil agglutination are helpful for diagnosis.

122. (A)

123. (B)

124. (C)

125. (B) ITP is characterized by generalized petechiae. Intracranial hemorrhage is the most serious complication; platelet count is usually below 20,000, resulting in positive tourniquet test. Bleeding time and clot retraction time are prolonged. Classic hemophilia is an X-linked disease due to deficiency of factor Vlll in the plasma. The hallmark is hemarthrosis; the partial prothrombin time (PTT) is greatly prolonged.

126. (D)

127. (E)

128. (C)

129. (A) About 80% of childhood leukemias are of the acute lymphoblastic type, causing anemia, neutropenia, thrombocytopenia, and diffuse infiltration of organs and tissues. Folic acid deficiency, possibly due to feeding of goat's milk, usually causes megaloblastic anemia to develop at four to seven months of age, with hypersegmented neutrophils. Hereditary spherocytosis is transmitted by dominant inheritance and causes familial hemolytic anemia and acholuric jaundice with splenomegaly. The spherocytic red cell is smaller than the normal erythrocyte and lacks the central pallor of the biconcave disk; the osmotic fragility is increased. Iron deficiency anemia is frequently seen in infants nine to 24 months of age who consume large amounts of milk and carbohydrates without iron supplements. The erythrocytes are microcytic, hypochromic, and poikilocytotic.

130. (A)

131. (B)

132. **(A)** Pyloric stenosis causes metabolic alkalosis (later changing to metabolic acidosis), infantile diarrhea causes metabolic acidosis, and salicylate intoxication causes respiratory alkalosis. Acidosis causes pH to decrease and alkalosis causes pH to increase.

133. **(E)**

134. **(A)**

135. **(B)**

136. **(C)**

137. **(D)** Bacterial meningitis is most frequently confused with aseptic meningitis due to a variety of viruses. Differentiation by spinal fluid findings is at times difficult, but usually possible. When the patient presents with ambiguous CSF findings, they usually should be treated as if they had bacterial meningitis with suboptimal antibiotic therapy.

138. **(B)**

139. **(C)**

140. **(C)**

141. **(A)** Wilm's tumor (embryonal adenomyosarcoma of the kidney) metastasizes to the lung, very rarely to the bone, while neuroblastoma metastasizes early (70% of patients at time of initial diagnosis) in orbital involvement. The prognosis of both tumors is grave and the better result is for patients whose tumors are discovered during the first year of life. Bone marrow metastases have occurred in some patients with neuroblastoma; bone marrow aspiration smears occasionally reveal the characteristic pseudorosette of tumor cells. Catecholamine secretions may be increased in patients with neuroblastoma.

142. **(A)**

143. **(B)** Wilson's disease (hepatolenticular degeneration) is characterized by Kayser-Fleischer ring, a greenish-yellow ring near the margin of the iris; liver cirrhosis; and mental retardation.

144. **(D)**

145. **(C)**

146. **(B)**

147. **(A)** Korsakoff's syndrome is a chronic brain syndrome characterized by confabulation, disorientation, amnesia, and peripheral neuropathy. It is associated with chronic alcoholism and results from thiamine and niacin deficiencies. Infantile autism is characterized by lack of communicative skills, interpersonal sensitivities, and obsessive need for sameness, as well as twirling. Pica is the compulsive eating of nonfood substances; it is a characteristic feature of lead poisoning. Encopresis is the syndrome of psychogenic fecal soiling.

148. **(B)**

149. **(D)**

150. **(A)**

151. **(C)** Imipramine is the drug of choice for enuresis; calcium disodium versenate (EDTA) is frequently used for chronic lead poisoning; ethosuximide is effective in treating children with petit mal; penicillamine has been used for Wilson's disease (hepatolenticular degeneration).

152. **(E)**

153. **(A)**

154. **(C)** The levels of mental retardation are classified as follows: borderline (IQ 68-85); mild (IQ 52-67); moderate (IQ 36-51); severe (IQ 20-35); and profound (IQ < 20).

155. **(C)**

156. **(B)**

157. **(B)**

158. **(A)**

159. **(A)**

160. **(D)**

161. **(A)** Kaposi's varicelliform eruptions are caused by herpes simplex. The distribution

of eruptions in smallpox is centrifugal with the same stage of eruptions, while the distribution of eruptions in chicken pox is centripetal, with different stages (macules, papules, vesicles, and crusts) all simultaneously present.

162. (A)

163. (A)

164. (C)

165. (B)

166. (C)

Incubation period (days)	Illness
10-21	Chicken pox
7-14	Measles
7-14	Poliomyelitis
2-6	Diphtheria
2-5	Scarlet fever

167. (D)

168. (E) Acute intermittent porphyria is characterized by intermittent abdominal pain and neuropathies (paresthesia, wrist drop, foot drop, psychosis, convulsion). It is an autosomal dominant disease with defect of uroporphyrinogen-1 synthetase. Hereditary spherocytosis is due to the increased osmotic fragility of the erythrocyte. Pseudocholinesterase deficiency is an autosomal recessive disease which is sensitive to succinylcholine. G6PD deficiency is an X-linked recessive disease which may cause hemolysis by ingestion of certain drugs (sulfonamide). Hereditary angioedema is an autosomal dominant disease with defect on C_1-esterase inhibitor. It is treated with the androgen derivative, danazol.

169. (C)

170. (B) In folic acid deficiency, oval macrocytes and hypersegmented neutrophils are seen. Elliptocytosis (ovalocytosis) is inherited with autosomal dominance. Ovalocytes are increased, with increased erythrocyte osmotic fragility. Lead poisoning may cause basophilic stippling of erythrocytes and hypochromia. Iron deficiency anemia is characterized by hypochromia and microcytosis.

171-F, 172-F, 173-F, 174-F, 175-T, 176-F, 177-T, 178-F, 179-F; 180-F, 181-F, 182-T, 183-F, 184-F; 185-F, 186-F, 187-T; 188-T, 189-T, 190-F

Most common cause of pharyngotonsillitis is viral in orgin and the treatment is symptomatic. Streptococcal sore throat requires a 10-day course of pencillin treatment. The identification of beta *Streptococcus* often needs positive throat culture in addition to clinical findings. This patient's laboratory results fail to confirm the suspicion of anemia and the initiation of therapy can be delayed at this time. The eggs of *Ascaria lumbricoides* are characterized by bile-strained mamillated outer shells. A single dose of pyrantel pamoate (11 mg/kg) is effective; a 2-day-course of piperazine (75 mg/l kg) is also commonly administered.

References

Below is a numbered list of reference books pertaining to the material in the book.

On the last line of each test item at the right hand side, there appears a number combination that identifies the reference source and the page or pages where the information relating to the question and the correct answer may be found. The first number refers to the textbook or journal in the list and the second number refers to the page of that textbook or journal.

For example: (3:200) is a reference to the third book in the list, page 200 of Kolb's *Modern Clinical Psychiatry*.

1. Kaplan, H.I. *Modern Synopsis of Comprehensive Textbook of Psychiatry,* 3rd edition. Baltimore: Williams & Wilkins Co., 1981.

2. Shaw, C. *The Psychiatric Disorders of Childhood,* 2nd edition. New York: Appleton-Century-Crofts, 1970.

3. Kolb, L. *Modern Clinical Psychiatry,* 10th edition. Philadelphia: W.B. Saunders Co., 1982.

4. Rowe, C. *An Outline of Psychiatry,* 7th edition. Dubuque, Iowa: Wm. C. Brown Co., 1980.

5. Solomon, P. *Handbook of Psychiatry,* 3rd edition. Los Altos, Calif.: Lange Medical, 1974.

6. Jone, H.W. *Novak's Textbook of Gynecology,* 10th edition. Baltimore: Williams & Wilkins Co., 1981.

7. Kistner, R.W. *Gynecology: Principles and Practice,* 3rd edition. Chicago: Year Book Medical, 1979.

8. Green, T.H. *Gynecology: Essentials of Clinical Practice,* 3rd edition. Boston: Little, Brown & Co., 1977.

9. Disaia, P.J. *Synopsis of Gynecologic Oncology.* New York: John Wiley & Sons, 1975.

10. Niswander, K.R. *Obstetric and Gynecologic Disorders: A Practitioner's Guide.* Flushing, N.Y.: Medical Examination, 1975.

11. Wasserman, E. *Survey of Clinical Pediatrics,* 7th edition. New York: McGraw-Hill, 1981.

12. Behrman, R.E. *Nelson Textbook of Pediatrics,* 12th edition. Philadelphia: W.B. Saunders Co., 1983.

13. Barnett, H.L. *Pediatrics,* 16th edition. New York: Appleton-Century-Crofts, 1977

14. Aladjem, S. *Clinical Perinatology,* 2nd edition. St. Louis: C.V. Mosby Co., 1980.

15. Burrow, G.N. *Medical Complications During Pregnancy.* 2nd edition. Philadelphia: W.B. Saunders Co., 1982.

16. Benson, R.C. *Handbook of Obstetrics and Gynecology,* 7th edition. Los Altos, Calif.: Lange Medical, 1980.

17. Willson, J.R. *Obstetrics and Gynecololgy,* 7th edition. St. Louis: C.V. Mosby Co., 1983.

18. Pritchard, J.A. *Williams Obstetrics,* 16th edition. New York: Appleton-Century-Crofts, 1980.

19. Page, E.W. *Human Reproduction: Essentials of Reproductive and Perinatal Medicine.* 3rd edition. Philadelphia: W.B. Saunders Co., 1981.

20. Danforth, D. *Textbook of Obstetrics and Gynecology,* 4th edition. New York: Harper & Row, 1982.

21. Garrey, M.M. *Obstetrics Illustrated,* 3rd edition. Edinburgh and London: Churchill Livingston, 1980.

22. McLennan, C.E. *Synopsis of Obstetrics,* 9th edition. St. Louis: C.V. Mosby Co., 1974.

23. Sheps, M.C. *Public Health and Population Change: Current Research Issues.* Pittsburgh: University of Pittsburgh Press, 1965.

24. Becker, W. C. *Parents Are Teachers: A Child Management Program.* Champaign, Ill.: Research Press Co., 1971.

25. Stewart, W.D. *Dermatology Diagnosis and Treatment of Cutaneous Disorders,* 4th edition. St. Louis: C.V. Mosby Co., 1978.

26. Vaughan, D. *General Ophthalmology,* 10th edition. Los Altos, Calif.: Lange Medical, 1983.

27. Scott, P.R. *An Aid to Clinical Surgery,* 9th edition. London: Churchill Livingston, 1971.

28. Illingworth, C.A. *Short Textbook of Surgery,* 9th edition. London: Churchill Livingstone, 1972.

29. Lowenfels, A.B. *Companion Guide to Surgical Diagnosis.* Baltimore: Williams & Wilkins Co., 1975.

30. Schwartz, S.I. *Principles of Surgery,* 4th edition. New York: McGraw-Hill, 1984.

31. Way, L.W. *Current Surgical Diagnosis and Treatment.* Los Altos, Calif.: Lange Medical, 1983.

32. Egdahl, R.H. *Core Textbook of Surgery.* New York: Grune & Stratton, 1972.

33. Long, R.H. *The Physician and the Law,* 3rd edition. New York: Appleton-Century-Crofts, 1968.

34. DeWeese, D.D. *Textbook of Otolaryngology,* 5th edition. St. Louis: C.V. Mosby Co., 1977.

35. Ausband, J.R. *Ear, Nose and Throat Disorders: A Practitioner's Guide.* Flushing, N.Y.: Medical Examination, 1974.

36. Foxen, E.M. *Lecture Notes on Diseases of the Ear, Nose and Throat,* 3rd edition. Oxford: Blackwell Scientific, 1972.

37. Gordon, R.A. *Anesthesia and Resuscitation: A Manual for Medical Students,* 2nd edition. Toronto: University of Toronto Press, 1973.

38. Smith, D.R. *General Urology,* 10t edition. Los Altos, Calif.: Lange Medical, 1981.

39. Krupp, M.A. *Curren Medical Diagnosis and Treatment.* Los Altos, Calif.: Lange Medical, 1984.

40. Mausner, J.S. *Epidemiology: An Introductory Text.* W.B. Saunders Co., 1974.

41. Last J.M. *Maxcy-Rosenau Public Health and Preventive Medicine,* 12th edition. New York: Appleton-Century-Crofts, 1986.

42. MacMahon, B. *Epidemiology: Principles and Methods.* Boston: Little, Brown & Co., 1970.

43. Clark, D.W. *Preventive Medicine.* Boston: Little, Brown & Co., 1967.

44. Grant, M. *Handbook of Community Health,* 2nd edition. Philadelphia: Lea & Febiger, 1975.

45. Bjorn, J.C. *The Problem-oriented Private Practice of Medicine: A System for Comprehensive Health Care.* Chicago: Modern Hospital Press, 1970.

46. Shindell, S. *A Coursebook in Health Care Delivery.* New York: Appleton-Century-Crofts, 1976.

47. Bahn, A.K. *Basic Medical Statistics.* New York: Grune & Stratton, 1972.

48. Hall, E.J. *Radiobiology for the Radiologist.* Hagerstown, Md.: Harper & Row, 1973.

49. Frolich, E.D. *Rypins' Medical Licensure Examinations: Topical Summaries and Questions,* 13th edition. Philadelphia: J.B. Lippincott Co., 1981.

50. Rakel, R.E. *Family Practice,* 3rd edition. Philadelphia: W.B. Saunders Co., 1984.

51. *Med. Clin of North Am* 57 (6): 1973.

52. Thomas, A. *Temperament and Behavior Disorders in Children.* New York: New York University Press, 1969.

53. *JAMA* (Suppl) 227 (7): 1974.

54. Kagan, B.M. *Antimicrobial Therapy,* 3rd edition. Philadelphia: W.B. Saunders Co., 1980.

55. Robbins, S.L. *Pathologic Basis of Disease,* 2nd edition. Philadelphia: W.B. Saunders Co., 1979.

56. Pratt, P.C. "A Modern Concept of the Emphysemas Based on Correlations of Structure and Function." *Hum Pathol* 1:443-463, 1970.

57. Kueppers, F. "Alpha-antitrypsin and its Deficiency: State of the Art." *Am Rev Respir Dis* 110:176-94, 1974.

58. Gennaro, A.R. "Pathogenesis of Diverticulosis of the Colon." *Dis Colon Rectum* 17:64-73, 1974.

59. Morson, B.C. "The Technique and Interpretation of Rectal Biopsies in Inflammatory Bowel Disease." In Sommers, S.C. (ed.), *Pathology Annual 1974.* New York: Appleton-Century-Crofts, 1975.

60. McCluskey, R.T. "Immunologically Mediated Glomerular, Tubular and Interstitial Renal Disease." *N Engl J Med* 288:564-570, 1973.

61. Thompson, T.T. *Primer of Clinical Radiology.* Boston: Little, Brown & Co., 1973.

62. Hamby, R.L. "Clinical Hemodynamic Aspects of Single Vessel Coronary Artery Disease." *Am Heart J* 85:458-66, 1973.

63. Hamby, R.L.; *et al.* "Coronary Artery Calcification: Clinical Implications and Angio-

graphic Correlates." *Am Heart J* 87:565-70, 1974.

64. Berman, P.M. "Diverticular Disease of the Colon: The Possible Role of 'Roughage' in Both Food and Life." *Am J Dig Dis* 18:506-507, 1973.

65. Baylis, T.M. "Lactose and Milk Intolerance: Clinical Implications." *N Engl J Med* 292:1156-59, 1975.

66. *AFP* 24(6): 160-163, 1981.

67. *AFP* 29(1): 147-153, 1984.

68. *Postgraduate Medicine* 72(5): 281-288, 1982.

69. *JFP* 20(6): 551-557, 1985.

70. Williams, W.J. *Hematotogy,* 3rd edition. New York: McGraw-Hill, 1983.

71. Baum, G.L. *Textbook of Pulmonary Diseases,* 2nd edition. Boston: Little, Brown & Co., 1974.

72. Goldberger, E. *A Primer of Water, Electrotyte and Acid-Base Syndromes,* 5th edition. Philadelphia: Lea & Febiger, 1975.

73. Wyngarden, J.B. *Textbook of Medicine,* 17th edition. Philadelphia: W.B. Saunders Co., 1985.

74. Williams, R.H. *Textbook of Endocrinology,* 6th edition. Philadelphia: W.B. Saunders Co., 1981.

75. Cumming, G. *Disorders of the Respiratory System.* Oxford: Blackwell Scientific, 1973.

76. Petersdorf, R.G. *Harrison's Principles of Internal Medicine,* 10th edition. New York: McGraw-Hill, 1983.

77. Aegerter, E. *Orthopedic Diseases.: Physiology, Pathology, Radiology,* 4th edition, Philadelphia: W.B. Saunders Co., 1975.

78. Harvey, A.M. *The Principles and Practice of Medicine,* 21st edition. New York, Appleton-Century-Crofts, 1984.

79. Latner, A.L. *Cantarow and Trumper Clinical Biochemistry,* 7th edition, Philadelphia: W.B. Saunders Co., 1975.

80. Weiner, H.L. *Neurology for the House Officer,* New York: MEDCOM, 1974.

81. DePalma, A.F. *The Management of Fractures and Dislocations.: An Atlas,* 2nd edition. Philadelphia: W.B. Saunders Co., 1970.

82. McCarty, D.J. *Arthritis and Allied Conditions.: A Textbook of Rheumatology,* 10th edition. Philadelphia: Lea & Febiger, 1985.

83. Wintrobe, M.M. *Clinical Hematology,* 8th edition. Philadelphia: Lea & Febiger, 1981.

84. Merritt, H.H. *A Textbook of Neurology,* 6th edition. Philadelphia: Lea & Febiger, 1979.

85. Hoeprich, P.D. *Infectious Diseases: A Guide to the Understanding and Management of Infectious Processes.* New York: Harper & Row, 1972.

86. Sleisenger, M.H. *Gastrointestinal Disease: Pathophysiology, Diagnosis, Management,* 2nd edition. Philadelphia: W.B. Saunders Co., 1978.

87. Ezrin, C. *Systematic Endocrinology,* 2nd edition. New York: Harper & Row, 1979.

88. Carter, S. *Neurology of Infancy and Childhood.* New York: Appleton-Century-Crofts, 1974.

89. Stollerman, G.H. *Advances in Internal Medicine.* Chicago: Year Book Medical, 1976, vol. 21.

90. James, A.E., Jr. *Exercises in Diagnostic Radiology, 6.: Nuclear Radiology.* Philadelphia: W.B. Saunders Co., 1973.

91. Sell, S. *Immunology, Immunopathology and Immunity,* 3rd edition. New York: Harper & Row, 1980.

92. Dubin, D. *Rapid Interpretation of EKG's.: A Programmed Course,* 2nd edition. Tampa, Fla.: Cover, 1972.

93. New, P.F.J. "Computerized Axial Tomography with the EMI Scanner." *Radiology* 110: 109-123, 1974.

94. Potchen, E.J. *Principles of Diagnostic Radiology.: Companion Volume to Internal Medicine.* New York: McGraw-Hill, 1971.

95. Teplick, J.G. *Roentgenologic Diagnosis: A Complement in Radiology to the Beeson and McDermott Textbook of Medicine,* 3rd edition. Philadelphia: W.B. Saunders Co., 1976.

96. Shneidman, E.S. *Clues to Suicide.* New York: McGraw-Hill, 1957.

97. Josselyn, I.M. *The Adolescent and His World.* New York: Family Service Association of America, 1952.

98. *First International Conference on the Mental Health Aspects of Sickle-cell Anemia.* NIMH Center for Studies of Child and Family Mental Health. Nashville, Tenn.: Community Mental Health Center, Meharry Medical College.

99. Noland, R.L. *Counselling Parents of the Emotionally Disturbed Child.* Springfield, Ill.: Charles C. Thomas, 1972.

100. Sager, C.J. *Progress in Group and Family Therapy.* New York: Brunner/ Mazel, 1972.

101. Smith, J.R. *Beyond Monogamy: Recent Studies of Sexual Alternatives in Marriage.* Baltimore: Johns Hopkins University Press, 1974.

102. Schumacher, S.S. "The Reproductive Biology Research Foundation Treatment Ap-

224

proach to Sexual Inadequacy." *Professional Psychology,* Fall 1971, pp. 363-65.

103. Mazzaferri, E.L. *Endocrinology: A Review of Clinical Endocrinology.* Flushing, N.Y.: Medical Examination, 1974.

104. Taylor, R.B. *Family Medicine: Principles and Practice.* New York: Springer-Verlag, 1978.

105. Fitzpatrick, T.B. *Dermatology in General Medicine,* 2nd edition. McGraw-Hill, New York, 1979.

106. *Am Fam Physician* 23 (1): 1981.

107. *Am Fam Physician* 24 (2): 1981.

108. Ryan, G.M. *Ambulatory Care in Obstetrics and Gynecology.* New York: Grune & Stratton, 1980.

109. Kaplan, H.F., *Comprehensive Textbook of Psychiatry, IV,* 4th edition. Baltimore: Williams & Wilkins, 1985.

110. Usdin, G. *Psychiatry in General Medical Practice.* New York: McGraw-Hill, 1979.

111. Freeman, A.M. *Psychiatry for the Primary Care Physician.* Baltimore: Williams & Wilkins, 1979.

112. Rakel, R.E. *Principles of Family Medicine.* Philadelphia: W.B. Saunders Co., 1977.

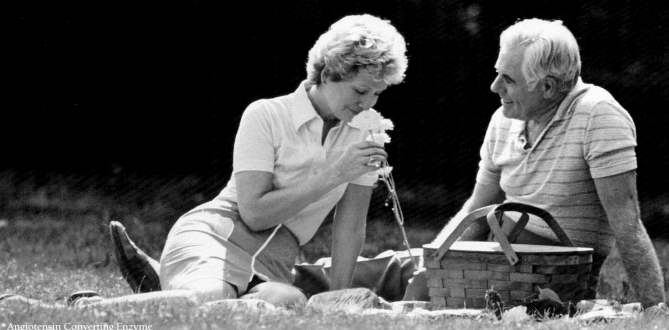

CAPOTEN® TABLETS
Captopril Tablets

DESCRIPTION

CAPOTEN (captopril) is the first of a new class of antihypertensive agents, a specific competitive inhibitor of angiotensin I-converting enzyme (ACE), the enzyme responsible for the conversion of angiotensin I to angiotensin II. Captopril is also effective in the management of heart failure.

CAPOTEN (captopril) is designated chemically as 1-[(2S)-3-mercapto-2-methylpropionyl]-L-proline [MW 217.29].

Captopril is a white to off-white crystalline powder that may have a slight sulfurous odor; it is soluble in water (approx. 160 mg/mL), methanol, and ethanol and sparingly soluble in chloroform and ethyl acetate.

CAPOTEN (captopril) is available in potencies of 12.5 mg, 25 mg, 50 mg, and 100 mg as scored tablets for oral administration. Inactive ingredients: cellulose, corn starch, lactose, and stearic acid.

CLINICAL PHARMACOLOGY

Mechanism of Action

The mechanism of action of CAPOTEN (captopril) has not yet been fully elucidated. Its beneficial effects in hypertension and heart failure appear to result primarily from suppression of the renin-angiotensin-aldosterone system. However, there is no consistent correlation between renin levels and response to the drug. Renin, an enzyme synthesized by the kidneys, is released into the circulation where it acts on a plasma globulin substrate to produce angiotensin I, a relatively inactive decapeptide. Angiotensin I is then converted by angiotensin converting enzyme (ACE) to angiotensin II, a potent endogenous vasoconstrictor substance. Angiotensin II also stimulates aldosterone secretion from the adrenal cortex, thereby contributing to sodium and fluid retention.

CAPOTEN (captopril) prevents the conversion of angiotensin I to angiotensin II by inhibition of ACE, a peptidyldipeptide carboxy hydrolase. This inhibition has been demonstrated in both healthy human subjects and in animals by showing that the elevation of blood pressure caused by exogenously administered angiotensin I was attenuated or abolished by captopril. In animal studies, captopril did not alter the pressor responses to a number of other agents, including angiotensin II and norepinephrine, indicating specificity of action.

ACE is identical to "bradykininase," and CAPOTEN (captopril) may also interfere with the degradation of the vasodepressor peptide, bradykinin. Increased concentrations of bradykinin or prostaglandin E_2 may also have a role in the therapeutic effect of CAPOTEN.

Inhibition of ACE results in decreased plasma angiotensin II and increased plasma renin activity (PRA), the latter resulting from loss of negative feedback on renin release caused by reduction in angiotensin II. The reduction of angiotensin II leads to decreased aldosterone secretion, and, as a result, small increases in serum potassium may occur along with sodium and fluid loss.

The antihypertensive effects persist for a longer period of time than does demonstrable inhibition of circulating ACE. It is not known whether the ACE present in vascular endothelium is inhibited longer than the ACE in circulating blood.

Pharmacokinetics

After oral administration of therapeutic doses of CAPOTEN (captopril), rapid absorption occurs with peak blood levels at about one hour. The presence of food in the gastrointestinal tract reduces absorption by about 30 to 40 percent; captopril therefore should be given one hour before meals. Based on carbon-14 labeling, average minimal absorption is approximately 75 percent. In a 24-hour period, over 95 percent of the absorbed dose is eliminated in the urine; 40 to 50 percent is unchanged drug; most of the remainder is the disulfide dimer of captopril and captopril-cysteine disulfide.

Approximately 25 to 30 percent of the circulating drug is bound to plasma proteins. The apparent elimination half-life for total radioactivity in blood is probably less than 3 hours. An accurate determination of half-life of unchanged captopril is not, at present, possible, but it is probably less than 2 hours. In patients with renal impairment, however, retention of captopril occurs (see DOSAGE AND ADMINISTRATION).

Pharmacodynamics

Administration of CAPOTEN (captopril) results in a reduction of peripheral arterial resistance in hypertensive patients with either no change, or an increase, in cardiac output. There is an increase in renal blood flow following administration of CAPOTEN (captopril) and glomerular filtration rate is usually unchanged.

Reductions of blood pressure are usually maximal 60 to 90 minutes after oral administration of an individual dose of CAPOTEN (captopril). The duration of effect is dose related. The reduction in blood pressure may be progressive, so to achieve maximal therapeutic effects, several weeks of therapy may be required. The blood pressure lowering effects of captopril and thiazide-type diuretics are additive. In contrast, captopril and beta-blockers have a less than additive effect.

Blood pressure is lowered to about the same extent in both standing and supine positions. Orthostatic effects and tachycardia are infrequent but may occur in volume-depleted patients. Abrupt withdrawal of CAPOTEN has not been associated with a rapid increase in blood pressure.

In patients with heart failure, significantly decreased peripheral (systemic vascular) resistance and blood pressure (afterload), reduced pulmonary capillary wedge pressure (preload) and pulmonary vascular resistance, increased cardiac output, and increased exercise tolerance time (ETT) have been demonstrated. These hemodynamic and clinical effects occur after the first dose and appear to persist for the duration of therapy. Placebo controlled studies of 12 weeks duration show no tolerance to beneficial effects on ETT; open studies, with exposure up to 18 months in some cases, also indicate that ETT benefit is maintained. Clinical improvement has been observed in some patients where acute hemodynamic effects were minimal.

Studies in rats and cats indicate that CAPOTEN (captopril) does not cross the blood-brain barrier to any significant extent.

INDICATIONS AND USAGE

Hypertension: CAPOTEN (captopril) is indicated for the treatment of hypertension.

In using CAPOTEN, consideration should be given to the risk of neutropenia/agranulocytosis (see WARNINGS).

CAPOTEN may be used as initial therapy for patients with normal renal function, in whom the risk is relatively low. In patients with impaired renal function, particularly those with collagen vascular disease, captopril should be reserved for hypertensives who have either developed unacceptable side effects on other drugs, or have failed to respond satisfactorily to drug combinations.

CAPOTEN is effective alone and in combination with other antihypertensive agents, especially thiazide-type diuretics. The blood pressure lowering effects of captopril and thiazides are approximately additive.

Heart Failure: CAPOTEN (captopril) is indicated in patients with heart failure who have not responded adequately to or cannot be controlled by conventional diuretic and digitalis therapy. CAPOTEN is to be used with diuretics and digitalis.

WARNINGS

Neutropenia/Agranulocytosis

Neutropenia ($<1000/mm^3$) with myeloid hypoplasia has resulted from use of captopril. About half of the neutropenic patients developed systemic or oral cavity infections or other features of the syndrome of agranulocytosis.

The risk of neutropenia is dependent on the clinical status of the patient:

In clinical trials in patients with hypertension who have normal renal function (serum creatinine less than 1.6 mg/dL and no collagen vascular disease), neutropenia has been seen in one patient out of over 8,600 exposed.

In patients with some degree of renal failure (serum creatinine at least 1.6 mg/dL) but no collagen vascular disease, the risk of neutropenia in clinical trials was about 1 per 500, a frequency over 15 times that for uncomplicated hypertension. Daily doses of captopril were relatively high in these patients, particularly in view of their diminished renal function. In foreign marketing experience in patients with renal failure, use of allopurinol concomitantly with captopril has been associated with neutropenia but this association has not appeared in U.S. reports.

In patients with collagen vascular diseases (e.g., systemic lupus erythematosus, scleroderma) and impaired renal function, neutropenia occurred in 3.7 percent of patients in clinical trials.

While none of the over 750 patients in formal clinical trials of heart failure developed neutropenia, it has occurred during the subsequent clinical experience. About half of the reported cases had serum creatinine ≥ 1.6 mg/dL and more than 75 percent were in patients also receiving procainamide. In heart failure, it appears that the same risk factors for neutropenia are present.

The neutropenia has usually been detected within three months after captopril was started. Bone marrow examinations in patients with neutropenia consistently showed myeloid hypoplasia, frequently accompanied by erythroid hypoplasia and decreased numbers of megakaryocytes (e.g., hypoplastic bone marrow and pancytopenia); anemia and thrombocytopenia were sometimes seen.

In general, neutrophils returned to normal in about two weeks after captopril was discontinued and serious infections were limited to clinically complex patients. About 13 percent of the cases of neutropenia have ended fatally, but almost all fatalities were in patients with serious illness, having collagen vascular disease, renal failure, heart failure or immunosuppressant therapy, or a combination of these complicating factors.

Evaluation of the hypertensive or heart failure patient should always include assessment of renal function.

If captopril is used in patients with impaired renal function, white blood cell and differential counts should be evaluated prior to starting treatment and at approximately two-week intervals for about three months, then periodically.

In patients with collagen vascular disease or who are exposed to other drugs known to affect the white cells or immune response, particularly when there is impaired renal function, captopril should be used only after an assessment of benefit and risk, and then with caution.

All patients treated with captopril should be told to report any signs of infection (e.g., sore throat, fever). If infection is suspected, white cell counts should be performed without delay.

Since discontinuation of captopril and other drugs has generally led to prompt return of the white count to normal, upon confirmation of neutropenia (neutrophil count $<1000/mm^3$) the physician should withdraw captopril and closely follow the patient's course.

Proteinuria

Total urinary proteins greater than 1 g per day were seen in about 0.7 percent of patients receiving captopril. About 90 percent of affected patients had evidence of prior renal disease or received relatively high doses of captopril (in excess of 150 mg/day), or both. The nephrotic syndrome occurred in about one-fifth of proteinuric patients. In most cases, proteinuria subsided or cleared within six months whether or not captopril was continued. Parameters of renal function, such as BUN and creatinine, were seldom altered in the patients with proteinuria.

Since most cases of proteinuria occurred by the eighth month of therapy with captopril, patients with prior renal disease or those receiving captopril at doses greater than 150 mg per day, should have urinary protein estimations (dip-stick on first morning urine) prior to treatment, and periodically thereafter.

Hypotension

Excessive hypotension was rarely seen in hypertensive patients but is a possible consequence of captopril use in severely salt/volume depleted persons such as those treated vigorously with diuretics, for example, patients with severe congestive heart failure (see PRECAUTIONS [Drug Interactions]).

In heart failure, where the blood pressure was either normal or low, transient decreases in mean blood pressure greater than 20 percent were recorded in about half of the patients. This transient hypotension may occur after any of the first several doses and is usually well tolerated, producing either no symptoms or brief mild lightheadedness, although in rare instances it has been associated with arrhythmia or conduction defects. Hypotension was the reason for discontinuation of drug in 3.6 percent of patients with heart failure.

BECAUSE OF THE POTENTIAL FALL IN BLOOD PRESSURE IN THESE PATIENTS, THERAPY SHOULD BE STARTED UNDER VERY CLOSE MEDICAL SUPERVISION. A starting dose of 6.25 or 12.5 mg tid may minimize the hypotensive effect. Patients should be followed closely for the first two weeks of treatment and whenever the dose of captopril and/or diuretic is increased.

Hypotension is not per se a reason to discontinue captopril. Some decrease of systemic blood pressure is a common and desirable observation upon initiation of CAPOTEN (captopril) treatment in heart failure. The magnitude of the decrease is greatest early in the course of treatment; this effect stabilizes within a week or two, and generally returns to pretreatment levels, without a decrease in therapeutic efficacy, within two months.

PRECAUTIONS

General

Impaired Renal Function

Hypertension—Some patients with renal disease, particularly those with severe renal artery stenosis, have developed increases in BUN and serum creatinine after reduction of blood pressure with captopril. Captopril dosage reduction and/or discontinuation of diuretic may be required. For some of these patients, it may not be possible to normalize blood pressure and maintain adequate renal perfusion.

Heart Failure—About 20 percent of patients develop stable elevations of BUN and serum creatinine greater than 20 percent above normal or baseline upon long-term treatment with captopril. Less than 5 percent of patients, generally those with severe preexisting renal disease, require discontinuation of treatment due to progressively increasing creatinine; subsequent improvement probably depends upon the severity of the underlying renal disease.

See CLINICAL PHARMACOLOGY, DOSAGE AND ADMINISTRATION, ADVERSE REACTIONS [Altered Laboratory Findings].

Valvular Stenosis: There is concern, on theoretical grounds, that patients with aortic stenosis might be at particular risk of decreased coronary perfusion when treated with vasodilators because they do not develop as much afterload reduction as others.

Surgery/Anesthesia: In patients undergoing major surgery or during anesthesia with agents that produce hypotension, captopril will block angiotensin II formation secondary to compensatory renin release. If hypotension occurs and is considered to be due to this mechanism, it can be corrected by volume expansion.

Information for Patients

Patients should be told to report promptly any indication of infection (e.g., sore throat, fever), which may be a sign of neutropenia, or of progressive edema which might be related to proteinuria and nephrotic syndrome.

All patients should be cautioned that excessive perspiration and dehydration may lead to an excessive fall in blood pressure because of reduction in fluid volume. Other causes of volume depletion such as vomiting or diarrhea may also lead to a fall in blood pressure; patients should be advised to consult with the physician.

Patients should be warned against interruption or discontinuation of medication unless instructed by the physician.

Heart failure patients on captopril therapy should be cautioned against rapid increases in physical activity.

Patients should be informed that CAPOTEN (captopril) should be taken one hour before meals (see DOSAGE AND ADMINISTRATION).

g Interactions

otension—Patients on Diuretic Therapy: Patients on diuretics and especially those in whom ·etic therapy was recently instituted, as well as those on severe dietary salt restriction or dialysis, / occasionally experience a precipitous reduction of blood pressure usually within the first hour r receiving the initial dose of captopril.

he possibility of hypotensive effects with captopril can be minimized by either discontinuing the ·etic or increasing the salt intake approximately one week prior to initiation of treatment with ?OTEN (captopril) or initiating therapy with small doses (6.25 or 12.5 mg). Alternatively, provide dical supervision for at least one hour after the initial dose. If hypotension occurs, the patient uld be placed in a supine position and, if necessary, receive an intravenous infusion of normal ne. This transient hypotensive response is not a contraindication to further doses which can be n without difficulty once the blood pressure has increased after volume expansion.

gents Having Vasodilator Activity: Data on the effect of concomitant use of other vasodilators in ents receiving CAPOTEN (captopril) for heart failure are not available; therefore, nitroglycerin or er nitrates (as used for management of angina) or other drugs having vasodilator activity should, ossible, be discontinued before starting CAPOTEN. If resumed during CAPOTEN therapy, such nts should be administered cautiously, and perhaps at lower dosage.

gents Causing Renin Release: Captopril's effect will be augmented by antihypertensive agents cause renin release. For example, diuretics (e.g., thiazides) may activate the renin-angiotensin-osterone system.

gents Affecting Sympathetic Activity: The sympathetic nervous system may be especially impor- in supporting blood pressure in patients receiving captopril alone or with diuretics. Therefore, nts affecting sympathetic activity (e.g., ganglionic blocking agents or adrenergic neuron block- agents) should be used with caution. Beta-adrenergic blocking drugs add some further hypertensive effect to captopril, but the overall response is less than additive.

gents Increasing Serum Potassium: Since captopril decreases aldosterone production, eleva- of serum potassium may occur. Potassium-sparing diuretics such as spironolactone, triamterene, miloride, or potassium supplements should be given only for documented hypokalemia, and 1 with caution, since they may lead to a significant increase of serum potassium. Salt substitutes taining potassium should also be used with caution.

hibitors Of Endogenous Prostaglandin Synthesis: It has been reported that indomethacin may uce the antihypertensive effect of captopril, especially in cases of low renin hypertension. Other steroidal anti-inflammatory agents (e.g., aspirin) may also have this effect.

g/Laboratory Test Interaction

otopril may cause a false-positive urine test for acetone.

cinogenesis, Mutagenesis and Impairment of Fertility

-year studies with doses of 50 to 1350 mg/kg/day in mice and rats failed to show any evidence of cinogenic potential.

tudies in rats have revealed no impairment of fertility.

mal Toxicology

onic oral toxicity studies were conducted in rats (2 years), dogs (47 weeks; 1 year), mice (2 rs), and monkeys (1 year). Significant drug related toxicity included effects on hematopoiesis, al toxicity, erosion/ulceration of the stomach, and variation of retinal blood vessels.

eductions in hemoglobin and/or hematocrit values were seen in mice, rats, and monkeys at es 50 to 150 times the maximum recommended human dose (MRHD). Anemia, leukopenia, mbocytopenia, and bone marrow suppression occurred in dogs at doses 8 to 30 times MRHD. reductions in hemoglobin and hematocrit values in rats and mice were only significant at 1 year returned to normal with continued dosing by the end of the study. Marked anemia was seen at dose levels (8 to 30 times MRHD) in dogs, whereas moderate to marked leukopenia was noted / at 15 and 30 times MRHD and thrombocytopenia at 30 times MRHD. The anemia could be ersed upon discontinuation of dosing. Bone marrow suppression occurred to a varying degree, ng associated only with dogs that died or were sacrificed in a moribund condition in the 1 year dy. However, in the 47-week study at a dose 30 times MRHD, bone marrow suppression was nd to be reversible upon continued drug administration.

aptopril caused hyperplasia of the juxtaglomerular apparatus of the kidneys at doses 7 to 200 es the MRHD in rats and mice, at 20 to 60 times MRHD in monkeys, and at 30 times the MRHD logs.

astric erosions/ulcerations were increased in incidence at 20 and 200 times MRHD in male rats l at 30 and 65 times MRHD in dogs and monkeys, respectively. Rabbits developed gastric and stinal ulcers when given oral doses approximately 30 times MRHD for only 5 to 7 days.

1 the two-year rat study, irreversible and progressive variations in the caliber of retinal vessels al sacculations and constrictions) occurred at all dose levels (7 to 200 times MRHD) in a se-related fashion. The effect was first observed in the 88th week of dosing, with a progressively eased incidence thereafter, even after cessation of dosing.

gnancy: Category C

otopril was embryocidal in rabbits when given in doses about 2 to 70 times (on a mg/kg basis) the ximum recommended human dose, and low incidences of craniofacial malformations were n. These effects in rabbits were most probably due to the particularly marked decrease in blood ssure caused by the drug in this species.

aptopril given to pregnant rats at 400 times the recommended human dose continuously during tation and lactation caused a reduction in neonatal survival.

lo teratogenic effects (malformations) have been observed after large doses of captopril in nsters and rats.

aptopril crosses the human placenta.

here are no adequate and well-controlled studies in pregnant women. Captopril should be used ing pregnancy or for patients likely to become pregnant, only if the potential benefit justifies a ential risk to the fetus.

sing Mothers

ncentrations of captopril in human milk are approximately one percent of those in maternal od. The effect of low levels of captopril on the nursing infant has not been determined. Caution uld be exercised when captopril is administered to a nursing woman, and, in general, nursing uld be interrupted.

liatric Use

ety and effectiveness in children have not been established although there is limited experience 1 the use of captopril in children from 2 months to 15 years of age with secondary hypertension l varying degrees of renal insufficiency. Dosage, on a weight basis, was comparable to that used adults. CAPOTEN (captopril) should be used in children only if other measures for controlling od pressure have not been effective.

VERSE REACTIONS

oorted incidences are based on clinical trials involving approximately 7000 patients.

Renal—About one of 100 patients developed proteinuria (see WARNINGS).

ach of the following has been reported in approximately 1 to 2 of 1000 patients and are of ertain relationship to drug use: renal insufficiency, renal failure, polyuria, oliguria, and urinary quency.

Hematologic—Neutropenia/agranulocytosis has occurred (see WARNINGS). Cases of anemia, mbocytopenia, and pancytopenia have been reported.

Dermatologic—Rash, often with pruritus, and sometimes with fever, arthralgia, and eosinophilia, curred in about 4 to 7 (depending on renal status and dose) of 100 patients, usually during the four weeks of therapy. It is usually maculopapular, and rarely urticarial. The rash is usually mild l disappears within a few days of dosage reduction, short-term treatment with an antihistaminic ent, and/or discontinuing therapy; remission may occur even if captopril is continued. Pruritus, nout rash, occurs in about 2 of 100 patients. Between 7 and 10 percent of patients with skin rash have shown an eosinophilia and/or positive ANA titers. A reversible associated pemphigoid-like lesion, and photosensitivity, have also been reported.

Angioedema of the face, mucous membranes of the mouth, or of the extremities has been observed in approximately 1 of 1000 patients and is reversible on discontinuance of captopril therapy. One case of laryngeal edema has been reported.

Flushing or pallor has been reported in 2 to 5 of 1000 patients.

Cardiovascular—Hypotension may occur; see WARNINGS and PRECAUTIONS [Drug Interactions] for discussion of hypotension on initiation of captopril therapy.

Tachycardia, chest pain, and palpitations have each been observed in approximately 1 of 100 patients.

Angina pectoris, myocardial infarction, Raynaud's syndrome, and congestive heart failure have each occurred in 2 to 3 of 1000 patients.

Dysgeusia—Approximately 2 to 4 (depending on renal status and dose) of 100 patients developed a diminution or loss of taste perception. Taste impairment is reversible and usually self-limited (2 to 3 months) even with continued drug administration. Weight loss may be associated with the loss of taste.

The following have been reported in about 0.5 to 2 percent of patients but did not appear at increased frequency compared to placebo or other treatments used in controlled trials: gastric irritation, abdominal pain, nausea, vomiting, diarrhea, anorexia, constipation, aphthous ulcers, peptic ulcer, dizziness, headache, malaise, fatigue, insomnia, dry mouth, dyspnea, cough, alopecia, paresthesias.

Altered Laboratory Findings

Elevations of liver enzymes have been noted in a few patients but no causal relationship to captopril use has been established. Rare cases of cholestatic jaundice, and of hepatocellular injury with or without secondary cholestasis, have been reported in association with captopril administration.

A transient elevation of BUN and serum creatinine may occur, especially in patients who are volume-depleted or who have renovascular hypertension. In instances of rapid reduction of long-standing or severely elevated blood pressure, the glomerular filtration rate may decrease transiently, also resulting in transient rises in serum creatinine and BUN.

Small increases in the serum potassium concentration frequently occur, especially in patients with renal impairment (see PRECAUTIONS).

OVERDOSAGE

Correction of hypotension would be of primary concern. Volume expansion with an intravenous infusion of normal saline is the treatment of choice for restoration of blood pressure.

Captopril may be removed from the general circulation by hemodialysis.

DOSAGE AND ADMINISTRATION

CAPOTEN (captopril) should be taken one hour before meals. Dosage must be individualized.

Hypertension—Initiation of therapy requires consideration of recent antihypertensive drug treatment, the extent of blood pressure elevation, salt restriction, and other clinical circumstances. If possible, discontinue the patient's previous antihypertensive drug regimen for one week before starting CAPOTEN.

The initial dose of CAPOTEN (captopril) is 25 mg bid or tid. If satisfactory reduction of blood pressure has not been achieved after one or two weeks, the dose may be increased to 50 mg bid or tid. Concomitant sodium restriction may be beneficial when CAPOTEN is used alone.

The dose of CAPOTEN in hypertension usually does not exceed 50 mg tid. Therefore, if the blood pressure has not been satisfactorily controlled after one to two weeks at this dose (and the patient is not already receiving a diuretic), a modest dose of a thiazide-type diuretic (e.g., hydrochlorothiazide, 25 mg daily), should be added. The diuretic dose may be increased at one- to two-week intervals until its highest usual antihypertensive dose is reached.

If CAPOTEN (captopril) is being started in a patient already receiving a diuretic, CAPOTEN therapy should be initiated under close medical supervision (see WARNINGS and PRECAUTIONS [Drug Interactions] regarding hypotension), with dosage and titration of CAPOTEN as noted above.

If further blood pressure reduction is required, the dose of CAPOTEN may be increased to 100 mg bid or tid and then, if necessary, to 150 mg bid or tid (while continuing the diuretic). The usual dose range is 25 to 150 mg bid or tid. A maximum daily dose of 450 mg CAPOTEN should not be exceeded.

For patients with severe hypertension (e.g., accelerated or malignant hypertension), when temporary discontinuation of current antihypertensive therapy is not practical or desirable, or when prompt titration to more normotensive blood pressure levels is indicated, diuretic should be continued but other current antihypertensive medication stopped and CAPOTEN dosage promptly initiated at 25 mg bid or tid, under close medical supervision.

When necessitated by the patient's clinical condition, the daily dose of CAPOTEN may be increased every 24 hours or less under continuous medical supervision until a satisfactory blood pressure response is obtained or the maximum dose of CAPOTEN (captopril) is reached. In this regimen, addition of a more potent diuretic, e.g., furosemide, may also be indicated.

Beta-blockers may also be used in conjunction with CAPOTEN therapy (see PRECAUTIONS [Drug Interactions]), but the effects of the two drugs are less than additive.

Heart Failure—Initiation of therapy requires consideration of recent diuretic therapy and the possibility of severe salt/volume depletion. In patients with either normal or low blood pressure, who have been vigorously treated with diuretics and who may be hyponatremic and/or hypovolemic, a starting dose of 6.25 or 12.5 mg tid may minimize the magnitude or duration of the hypotensive effect (see WARNINGS, [Hypotension]); for these patients, titration to the usual daily dosage can then occur within the next several days.

For most patients the usual initial daily dosage is 25 mg tid. After a dose of 50 mg tid is reached, further increases in dosage should be delayed, where possible, for at least two weeks to determine if a satisfactory response occurs. Most patients studied have had a satisfactory clinical improvement at 50 or 100 mg tid. A maximum daily dose of 450 mg of CAPOTEN (captopril) should not be exceeded.

CAPOTEN is to be used in conjunction with a diuretic and digitalis. CAPOTEN therapy must be initiated under very close medical supervision.

Dosage Adjustment in Renal Impairment—Because CAPOTEN (captopril) is excreted primarily by the kidneys, excretion rates are reduced in patients with impaired renal function. These patients will take longer to reach steady-state captopril levels and will reach higher steady-state levels for a given daily dose than patients with normal renal function. Therefore, these patients may respond to smaller or less frequent doses.

Accordingly, for patients with significant renal impairment, initial daily dosage of CAPOTEN (captopril) should be reduced, and smaller increments utilized for titration, which should be quite slow (one- to two-week intervals). After the desired therapeutic effect has been achieved, the dose should be slowly back-titrated to determine the minimal effective dose. When concomitant diuretic therapy is required, a loop diuretic (e.g., furosemide), rather than a thiazide diuretic, is preferred in patients with severe renal impairment.

HOW SUPPLIED

12.5 mg tablets in bottles of 100, **25 mg tablets** in bottles of 100 and 1000, **50 mg tablets** in bottles of 100, and **100 mg tablets** in bottles of 100. Bottles contain a desiccant-charcoal canister.

Unimatic® unit-dose packs containing 100 tablets are also available for each potency: **12.5 mg, 25 mg, 50 mg.** and **100 mg.**

The **12.5 mg tablet** is a flat oval with a partial bisect bar; the **25 mg tablet** is a biconvex rounded square with a quadrisect bar; the **50 and 100 mg tablets** are biconvex ovals with a bisect bar.

All captopril tablets are white and may exhibit a slight sulfurous odor. Tablet identification numbers: 12.5 mg, **450**; 25 mg, **452**; 50 mg, **482**; and 100 mg, **485**.

Storage

Do not store above 86° F. Keep bottles tightly closed (protect from moisture). (J3-658D)

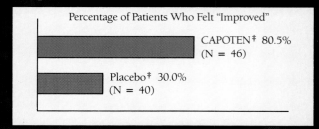